Role
Development
in Professional Nursing Practice

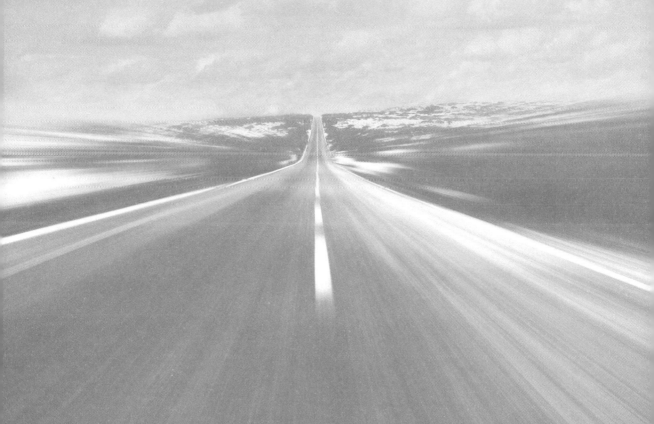

Welcome to *Role Development in Professional Nursing Practice, Second Edition!*

Along with useful tables and figures, each chapter includes:

KEY TERMS

Found in a list at the beginning of each chapter, these terms will create an expanded vocabulary in role development. Visit **http://nursing.jbpub.com/ roledevelopment** to see these terms in an interactive glossary and use word puzzles to nail the definitions!

CLASSROOM LEARNING OBJECTIVES

Found at the beginning of each chapter, these objectives provide instructors and students with a snapshot of the key information they will encounter in each chapter. They can serve as a checklist to help guide and focus study.

Framework for Professional Nursing Practice

Kathleen Masters

LEARNING OBJECTIVES

After completing this chapter, the student should be able to:
1. Identify the four metaparadigm concepts of nursing.
2. Identify and describe several theoretical works in nursing.
3. Begin the process of identifying theoretical frameworks of nursing that are consistent with a personal belief system.

Key Terms and Concepts
- Concept
- Conceptual model
- Propositions
- Assumptions
- Theory
- Metaparadigm
- Person
- Environment
- Health
- Nursing
- Philosophies

Although the beginning of nursing theory development can be traced to Florence Nightingale, it was not until the second half of the 1900s that nursing theory caught the attention of nursing as a discipline. During the decades of the 1960s and 1970s, theory development was a major topic of discussion and publication. During the 1970s, much of the discussion was related to the development of one global theory for nursing. However, in the 1980s, attention turned from the development of a global theory for nursing as scholars began to recognize multiple approaches to theory development in nursing.

Because of the plurality in nursing theory, this information must be organized in order to be meaningful for practice, research, and further knowledge development. The goal of this chapter is to present an organized and practical overview of the major concepts, models, philosophies, and theories that are essential in professional nursing practice.

45

CRITICAL THINKING QUESTIONS

An integral part of the learning process, critical thinking scenarios and questions are presented by the authors to spark thought and provide insight into the situations you may face in practice. Thought-provoking questions appear throughout each chapter.

CONVENIENT MARGIN NOTES

Located throughout the entire book, margin notes reiterate the most important messages and main ideas for students to take from their reading.

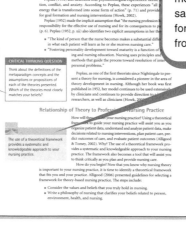

62 CHAPTER 2: Framework for Professional Nursing Practice

Peplau (1952) also described six nursing roles that emerge during the phases of the nurse–patient relationship: the role of the stranger, the role of the resource person, the teaching role, the leadership role, the surrogate role, and the counseling role. Peplau (1952) also described four psychobiological experiences: needs, frustration, conflict, and anxiety. According to Peplau, these experiences "all provide energy that is transformed into some form of action" (p. 71) and provide a basis for goal formation and nursing interventions (Howk, 2002).

Peplau (1952) made the implicit assumption that "the nursing profession has legal responsibility for the effective use of nursing and for its consequences to patients" (p. 6). Peplau (1952, p. xii) also identifies two explicit assumptions in her theory:

- "The kind of person that the nurse becomes makes a substantial difference in what each patient will learn as he or she receives nursing care."
- "Fostering personality development toward maturity is a function of nursing and nursing education. Nursing uses principles and methods that guide the process toward resolution of interpersonal problems."

Peplau, as one of the first theorists since Nightingale to present a theory for nursing, is considered a pioneer in the area of theory development in nursing. Although her book was first published in 1952, her model continues to be used extensively by clinicians and continues to provide direction to nurse researchers, as well as clinicians (Howk, 2002).

CRITICAL THINKING QUESTION

Think about the definitions of the metaparadigm concepts and the assumptions or propositions of each of the theories presented. Which of the theories most closely matches your beliefs?

Relationship of Theory to Professional Nursing Practice

How will theory affect your nursing practice? Using a theoretical framework to guide your nursing practice will assist you as you organize patient data, understand and analyze patient data, make decisions related to nursing interventions, plan patient care, predict outcomes of care, and evaluate patient outcomes (Alligood & Tomey, 2002). Why? The use of a theoretical framework provides a systematic and knowledgeable approach to your nursing practice. The framework also becomes a tool that will assist you to think critically as you plan and provide nursing care.

The use of a theoretical framework provides a systematic and knowledgeable approach to your nursing practice.

How do you begin? Now that you know why nursing theory is important to your nursing practice, it is time to identify a theoretical framework that fits you and your practice. Alligood (2006) presented guidelines for selecting a framework for theory-based practice. The steps include:

- Consider the values and beliefs you truly hold in nursing.
- Write a philosophy of nursing that clarifies your beliefs related to person, environment, health, and nursing.

CASE STUDIES

Found in select chapters, these vignettes illustrate research questions and studies in actual clinical settings.

patient's case. In Table 4–1, each box includes principles appropriate for each of the four topics. The additional principles of fairness and loyalty are included in the contextual features section.

Intense emotional conflicts between healthcare professionals and the patient and family may occur and hurt feelings can result. Nurses need to be sensitive and open to the needs of patients and families, particularly during these times. As information is passed back and forth between healthcare professionals and patients and families, an attitude of respect is indispensable in keeping the lines of communication open. Nurses play an essential role in the decision-making process in bioethical cases because of their traditional roles as patient advocate, caregiver, and educator. Nurses must attempt to maximize the values and needs of patients

CASE STUDY MS. CRANFORD

You are a student nurse who is caring for Ms. Cranford. She is an 87-year-old mentally competent woman who has lived alone since her husband died 10 years ago. She was admitted to the hospital with chest pain, feeling faint, and a pulse of 48, and a blood pressure of 98/56. The physician and nurses stabilized Ms. Cranford with medications and intravenous fluids but later informed Ms. Cranford and her only son that she would need a heart pacemaker to regulate her heartbeat. After the physician explained the procedure and risks involved, Ms. Cranford pondered the situation for a long while before discussing it with her son and the physician. Her medical history includes long-term adult-onset diabetes, chronic renal failure, and arterial insufficiency. She feels very tired. She decides that she does not want a pacemaker. Once Ms. Cranford tells her son her wishes, he is quite upset, and, thus, he meets with the physician to discuss the options. The physician and Ms. Cranford's son revisited this issue with her in an attempt to persuade her to change her mind, but she continues to refuse the recommended treatment. She and her son argue. The physician tries to explain to Ms. Cranford that the pacemaker is for her benefit, in her "best inter-

est," and involves very minimal risks to her. She feels as if they are "ganging up" on her. Once the registered nurse becomes aware of the problem, you and the nurse visit with Ms. Cranford and her son to assess and evaluate the ethical issues involved with her case.

CASE STUDY QUESTIONS:

Imagine that you are a nurse on the ethics committee consulted about Ms. Cranford's case. Answer the following questions:

1. What are the central ethical issues and questions in this case?
2. What principles are in conflict in this case?
3. What did the physician mean by "best interest" for Ms. Cranford?
4. Use the Four Topics Method to discuss issues, to identify additional information that may be needed, and to analyze this case. What are your recommendations on behalf of the ethics committee?
5. What is the role of the nurses caring for Ms. Cranford in resolving this situation with the ethics team, her other healthcare providers, Ms. Cranford, and her son?

CLASSROOM ACTIVITIES

From informal presentations to small group case evaluations, classroom learning activities bring this resource to life. Learn how the information in this text applies to the everyday practice of the professional nurse! Classroom activities can be found at the end of most chapters.

- Survey definitions of person, environment, health, and nursing in nursing models
- Select two or three frameworks that best fit with your beliefs related to the concepts of person, environment, health, and nursing.
- Review the assumptions of the frameworks that you have selected.
- Make applications of those frameworks in a selected area of nursing practice.
- Compare the frameworks on client focus, nursing action, and client outcome.
- Review the nursing literature written by persons who have used the frameworks.
- Select a framework and develop its use in your nursing practice.

Conclusion

As demonstrated by the descriptions of the philosophies, conceptual models, and theories presented in this chapter, there is a wide variety of perspectives and frameworks from which to practice nursing. There is no one right or wrong answer. Begin with whichever one seems to "fit," and then practice using it as you provide nursing care. "The full realization of nursing theory-guided practice is perhaps the greatest challenge that nursing as a scholarly discipline has ever faced" (Cody, 2006). So, be patient; developing your nursing practice guided by nursing theory will take time and practice. All nursing theories require in-depth study over time to master fully (this chapter has provided only a brief introduction), but the incorporation of theory into your practice will transform your nursing practice. The end result of this process will be seen in the excellent nursing care that you are able to provide to patients over the course of your professional nursing career.

CLASSROOM ACTIVITY 1

Divide into small groups and give each group a copy of the same case study. Assign a different nursing theory to each group, and ask the groups to develop a plan of care with the assigned nursing theory as the basis for practice. Each group should share the plan of care with the class. Discuss the differences and similarities in the foci of care based upon each of the selected theories.

CLASSROOM ACTIVITY 2

Think about the metaparadigm concepts of nursing. Draw each of the concepts in relation to the other concepts to show your ideas of how each of the concepts interface with one another. Present your "conceptual model" to the class, and discuss your ideas about each of the concepts represented. This activity works best if colored pencils, crayons, or markers and a large piece of paper are provided for students. Actual student examples are presented in Figure 2–1 and Figure 2–2.

What's New to the Second Edition of *Role Development in Professional Nursing Practice!*

New! Now Divided into Two Units!
- **Unit I** focuses on the foundational concepts that are essential to the development of the individual professional nurse
- **Unit II** addresses the issues related to professional nursing practice and the management of patient care

New Chapters!
- **Chapter 10** on evidence-based practice
- **Chapter 15** on the future direction of nursing
- **Chapters 8 & 9** geared toward beginning nursing students

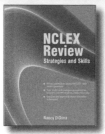
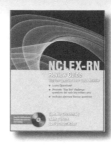
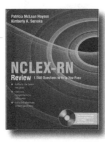
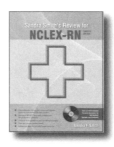
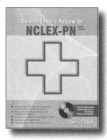
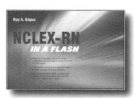

Role
Development

SECOND EDITION

in Professional Nursing Practice

Edited by

Kathleen Masters, DNS, RN

Associate Professor
Associate Director for Undergraduate Programs
School of Nursing
University of Southern Mississippi
Hattiesburg, Mississippi

JONES AND BARTLETT PUBLISHERS

Sudbury, Massachusetts

BOSTON   TORONTO   LONDON   SINGAPORE

World Headquarters

Jones and Bartlett Publishers	Jones and Bartlett Publishers Canada	Jones and Bartlett Publishers International
40 Tall Pine Drive	6339 Ormindale Way	Barb House, Barb Mews
Sudbury, MA 01776	Mississauga, Ontario L5V 1J2	London W6 7PA
978-443-5000	Canada	United Kingdom
info@jbpub.com		
www.jbpub.com		

Jones and Bartlett's books and products are available through most bookstores and online booksellers. To contact Jones and Bartlett Publishers directly, call 800-832-0034, fax 978-443-8000, or visit our website www.jbpub.com.

Substantial discounts on bulk quantities of Jones and Bartlett's publications are available to corporations, professional associations, and other qualified organizations. For details and specific discount information, contact the special sales department at Jones and Bartlett via the above contact information or send an email to specialsales@jbpub.com.

The authors, editor, and publisher have made every effort to provide accurate information. However, they are not responsible for errors, omissions, or for any outcomes related to the use of the contents of this book and take no responsibility for the use of the products and procedures described. Treatments and side effects described in this book may not be applicable to all people; likewise, some people may require a dose or experience a side effect that is not described herein. Drugs and medical devices are discussed that may have limited availability controlled by the Food and Drug Administration (FDA) for use only in a research study or clinical trial. Research, clinical practice, and government regulations often change the accepted standard in this field. When consideration is being given to use of any drug in the clinical setting, the health care provider or reader is responsible for determining FDA status of the drug, reading the package insert, and reviewing prescribing information for the most up-to-date recommendations on dose, precautions, and contraindications, and determining the appropriate usage for the product. This is especially important in the case of drugs that are new or seldom used.

Production Credits
Publisher: Kevin Sullivan
Acquisitions Editor: Emily Ekle
Acquisitions Editor: Amy Sibley
Associate Editor: Patricia Donnelly
Editorial Assistant: Rachel Shuster
Production Editor: Carolyn F. Rogers
Associate Marketing Manager: Ilana Goddess
Manufacturing and Inventory Control Supervisor: Amy Bacus
Composition: Circle Graphics
Cover Design: Kristin E. Ohlin
Cover, Section Opener, and Key Term Box Image: © Mikhail/ShutterStock, Inc.
Printing and Binding: Malloy, Inc.
Cover Printing: Malloy, Inc.

Library of Congress Cataloging-in-Publication Data

Role development in professional nursing practice / [edited by] Kathleen Masters.—2nd ed.
    p. ; cm.
 Includes bibliographical references and index.
 ISBN 978-0-7637-5603-1 (pbk.)
 1. Nursing. 2. Nursing—Standards. 3. Nursing—Practice—United States. I. Masters, Kathleen.
 [DNLM: 1. Nursing—standards. 2. Nursing—trends. 3. Nurse's Role. 4. Philosophy, Nursing. 5. Professional Practice. WY 16 R745 2009]
 RT82.R587 2009
 610.73—dc22

                        2008024795

6048

Printed in the United States of America
13 12 11 10 09   10 9 8 7 6 5 4 3 2

Dedication

This book is dedicated to my Heavenly Father and to my loving family: my husband, Eddie, and my two daughters, Rebecca and Rachel. Words cannot express my appreciation for their ongoing encouragement and support throughout my career.

Contents

Preface

Although the process of professional development is a lifelong journey, it is a journey that begins in earnest during the time of academic preparation. The goal of this book is to provide nursing students with a roadmap to help guide them along their journey as a professional nurse.

This book is organized into two units. The chapters in the first unit focus on the foundational concepts that are essential to the development of the individual professional nurse. The chapters in Unit II address issues related to professional nursing practice and the management of patient care.

The chapters included in Unit I will provide the student nurse with a basic foundation in areas such as nursing history, theory, philosophy, ethics, socialization into the nursing role, and the social context of nursing. Also included in Unit I is content related to the care of the professional self and career development in nursing.

The chapters in Unit II are more directly related to patient care issues. Included are topics such as patient education, ethical issues in nursing practice, the law as it relates to patient care and nursing, clinical judgment, informatics and technology, as well as a new chapter on evidence-based nursing practice. Unit II concludes with a chapter addressing future directions in professional nursing practice.

Although the topics included in this textbook are not inclusive of all that could potentially be discussed in relationship to the broad topic of role development in professional nursing practice, it is my prayer that the topics included will make a contribution to the profession of nursing by providing the student with a solid foundation and a desire to grow as a professional nurse throughout the journey that we call a professional nursing career. Let the journey begin.

Kathleen Masters

Contributors

Janie B. Butts, DSN, RN
University of Southern Mississippi
School of Nursing
Hattiesburg, Mississippi

Kay Coltharp Cater, MN, RN
William Carey University
School of Nursing
Hattiesburg, Mississippi

Luann M. Daggett, DSN, RN
William Carey University
School of Nursing
Hattiesburg, Mississippi

Kathleen Driscoll, JD, MS, RN
Professor
University of Cincinnati
College of Nursing
Cincinnati, Ohio

Patricia Becker Hentz, EdD, RN, PMH-NP
Associate Professor
University of Southern Maine
Portland, Maine

Melanie Gilmore, PhD, RN
University of Southern Mississippi
School of Nursing
Meridian, Mississippi

Karen Saucier Lundy, PhD, RN, FAAN
Professor
University of Southern Mississippi
School of Nursing
Hattiesburg, Mississippi

Evadna Lyons, PhD, RN
University of Southern Mississippi
School of Nursing
Meridian, Mississippi

Katherine Nugent, PhD, RN
Director
University of Southern Mississippi
School of Nursing
Hattiesburg, Mississippi

Karen Rich, MN, PhD, RN
University of Southern Mississippi
School of Nursing
Long Beach, Mississippi

Jill Rushing, MSN, RN
University of Southern Mississippi
School of Nursing
Hattiesburg, Mississippi

Mary W. Stewart, PhD, RN
Dean and Professor
William Carey University
School of Nursing
Hattiesburg, Mississippi

Sharon Vincent, MSN, RN, CNOR
Nurse Instructor
University of Southern Mississippi
School of Nursing
Hattiesburg, Mississippi

Unit I

Foundations of Professional Nursing Practice

chapter 1

A History of Health Care and Nursing

Karen Saucier Lundy

LEARNING OBJECTIVES

After completing this chapter, the student should be able to:

1. Identify social, political, and economic influences on the development of professional nursing practice.
2. Identify important leaders and events that have significantly affected the development of professional nursing practice.

Although no specialized nurse role per se developed in early civilizations, human cultures recognized the need for nursing care. The truly sick person was weak and helpless and could not fulfill the duties that were normally expected of a member of the community. In such cases, someone had to watch over the patient, nurse him or her, and provide care. In most societies, this nurse role was filled by a family member, usually female. As in most cultures, the childbearing woman had special needs that often resulted in a specialized role for the caregiver. Every society since the dawn of time had someone to nurse and take care of the mother and infant around the childbearing events. In whatever form the nurse took, the role was associated with compassion, health promotion, and kindness (Bullough & Bullough, 1978).

Note: This chapter is adapted from Lundy, K. S., & Bender, K. W. (2009). History of community health and public health nursing, in K. S. Lundy and S. Janes (Eds.), *Community health nursing: Caring for the public's health* (2nd ed.). Sudbury, MA: Jones and Bartlett.

Key Terms and Concepts

- Greek era
- Roman era
- Deaconesses
- Black Death
- Edward Jenner
- Louis Pasteur
- Joseph Lister
- Robert Koch
- Edwin Klebs
- Saint Vincent de Paul
- Reformation
- Chadwick Report
- Shattuck Report
- John Snow
- Florence Nightingale
- William Rathbone
- Goldmark Report
- Brown Report
- Isabel Hampton Robb
- American Nurses Association
- Lavinia Lloyd Dock
- *American Journal of Nursing (AJN)*
- Margaret Sanger
- Jane A. Delano
- Annie Goodrich
- Lillian Wald
- Mary Brewster
- Henry Street Settlement
- Elizabeth Tyler
- Jessie Sleet Scales
- Dorothea Linde Dix
- Clara Barton
- Frontier Nursing Service
- Mary Breckenridge
- Mary D. Osborne
- Cadet Nurse Corps
- Frances Payne Bolton
- *Nursing's Agenda for Health Care Reform*
- Managed care

3

Classical Era

More than 4000 years ago, Egyptian physicians and nurses used an abundant pharmacological repertoire to cure the ill and injured. The Ebers Papyrus lists more than 700 remedies for ailments ranging from snake bites to puerperal fever. The Kahun Papyrus (circa 1850 BC) identified suppositories (e.g., crocodile feces) that could be used for contraception (Kalisch & Kalisch, 1986). Healing appeared in the Egyptian culture as the successful result of a contest between invisible beings of good and evil (Shryock, 1959). The physician was not a shaman; instead there was specialization and separation of function, with physicians, priests, and sorcerers all practicing separately and independently. Some clients would consult the physician, some the shaman, and others sought healing from magical formulas. Many tried all three approaches. The Egyptians, quite notably, did not accept illness and death as inevitable but believed that life could be indefinitely prolonged. Because Egyptians blended medicine and magic, the concoctions believed to be the most effective were often bizarre and repulsive by today's standards. For example, lizard's blood, swine's ears and teeth, putrid meat and fat, tortoise brains, the milk of a lactating woman, the urine of a chaste woman, and excreta of donkeys and lions were frequently used ingredients. At least some explanation for these odd ingredients can be found in the following: "These pharmacological mixtures were intended to sicken and drive out the intruding demon which was thought to cause the disease. Drugs containing fecal matter were in fact used until the end of the 1700s in Europe as common practice" (Kalisch & Kalisch, 1986).

As early as 3000 to 1400 BC, the Minoans created ways to flush water and construct drainage systems. Around 1000 BC, the Egyptians constructed elaborate drainage systems, developed pharmaceutical herbs and preparations, and embalmed the dead. The Hebrews formulated an elaborate hygiene code that dealt with laws governing both personal and community hygiene, such as contagion, disinfection, and sanitation through the preparation of food and water. Hebrews, although few in number, exercised great influence in the development of religious and health doctrine. According to Bullough and Bullough (1978), most of their genius was religious, giving birth to both Christianity and Islam. The Jewish contribution to public health is greater in sanitation than in their concept of disease. Garbage and excreta were disposed of outside the city or camp, infectious diseases were quarantined, spitting was outlawed as unhygienic, and bodily cleanliness became a prerequisite for moral purity. Although many of the Hebrew ideas about hygiene were Egyptian in origin, Moses and the Hebrews were the first to codify them and link them with spiritual godliness. Their notion of disease was rooted in the "disease as God's punishment for sin" idea.

The civilization that grew up between the Tigris and Euphrates Rivers is known geographically as Mesopotamia (modern Iraq) and includes the Sumerians. Disease and disability in the Mesopotamian area, at least in the earlier period, were considered a great curse, a divine punishment for grievous acts against the gods. Having such a curse of illness resulting from sin did not exactly put the sick person in a valued status in the society. Experiencing illness as punishment for a sin linked the sick person to anything even remotely deviant; such things as murder, perjury, adultery, or drunkenness could be the identified sins. Not only was the person suffering from the illness, he or she was branded by all of society as having deserved it. The illness made the sin apparent to all; the sick person was isolated and disgraced. Those who obeyed God's law lived in health and happiness. Those who transgressed the law were punished, with illness and suffering thought to be consequences. The sick person then had to make atonement for the sins, enlist a priest or other spiritual healer to lift the spell or curse, or live with the illness to its ultimate outcome. In simple terms, the person had to get right with the gods or live with the consequences (Bullough & Bullough, 1978). Nursing care by a family member or relative would be needed in any case, regardless of the outcome of the sin, curse, disease-atonement-recovery or death cycle. This logic became the basis for explanation of why some people "get sick and some don't" for many centuries and still persists to some degree in most cultures today.

The Greeks and Health

In Greek mythology, the god of medicine, Asclepias, cured disease. One of his daughters, Hygeia, from whom we derive the word *hygiene,* was the goddess of preventive health and protected humans from disease. Panacea, Asclepias' other daughter, was known as the all-healing "universal remedy," and today is used to describe any ultimate cure-all in medicine. She was known as the "light" of the day, and her name was invoked and shrines built to her during times of epidemics (Brooke, 1997).

During the **Greek era**, Hippocrates of Cos emphasized the rational treatment of sickness as a natural rather than god-inflicted phenomenon. Hippocrates (460–370 BC) is considered the father of medicine because of his arrangements of the oral and written remedies and diseases, which had long been secrets held by priests and religious healers, into a textbook of medicine that was used for centuries (Bullough & Bullough, 1978). Hippocrates' contribution to the science of public health was his recognition that making accurate observations of and drawing general conclusions from actual phenomena formed the basis of sound medical reasoning (Shryock, 1959).

In Greek society, health was considered to result from a balance between mind and body. Hippocrates wrote a most important book, *Air, Water and Places,* which detailed the relationship between humans and the environment. This is considered a milestone in the eventual development of the science of epidemiology as the first such treatise on the connectedness of the web of life. This topic of the relationship between humans and their environment did not reoccur until the development of bacteriology in the late 1800s (Rosen, 1958).

Hippocrates wrote a most important book, *Air, Water and Places,* which detailed the relationship between humans and the environment. This is considered a milestone in the eventual development of the science of epidemiology as the first such treatise on the connectedness of the web of life.

Perhaps the idea that most damaged the practice and scientific theory of medicine and health for centuries was the doctrine of the four humors, first spoken of by Empedodes of Acragas (493–433 BC). Empedodes was a philosopher and a physician, and as a result, he synthesized his cosmological ideas with his medical theory. He believed that the same four elements (or "roots of things") that made up the universe were found in humans and in all animate beings (Bullough & Bullough, 1978). Empedodes believed that man was a microcosm, a small world within the macrocosm, or external environment. The four humors of the body (blood, bile, phlegm, and black bile) corresponded to the four elements of the larger world (fire, air, water, and earth) (Kalisch & Kalisch, 1986). Depending on the prevailing humor, a person was sanguine, choleric, phlegmatic, or melancholic. Because of this strongly held and persistent belief in the connection between the balance of the four humors and health status, treatment was aimed at restoring the appropriate balance of the four humors through the control of their corresponding elements. By manipulating the two sets of opposite qualities—hot and cold, wet and dry—balance was the goal of the intervention. Fire was hot and dry, air was hot and wet, water was cold and wet, and earth was cold and dry. For example, if a person had a fever, cold compresses would be prescribed for a chill and the person would be warmed. Such doctrine gave rise to faulty and ineffective treatment of disease that influenced medical education for many years (Taylor, 1922).

Plato, in *The Republic,* detailed the importance of recreation, a balanced mind and body, nutrition, and exercise. There was a distinction made among gender, class, and health as early as the Greek era; only males of the aristocracy could afford the luxury of maintaining a healthful lifestyle (Rosen, 1958).

In *The Iliad,* a poem about the attempts to capture Troy and rescue Helen from her lover Paris, 140 different wounds are described. The mortality rate averaged 77.6%, the highest as a result of sword and spear thrusts and the lowest from superficial arrow wounds. There was considerable need for nursing care, and Achilles, Patroclus, and other princes often acted as nurses to the injured. The early stages of Greek medicine reflected the influences of Egyptian, Babylonian, and Hebrew medicine. Therefore, good medical and nursing techniques were used to treat these war wounds: The arrow was drawn or cut out, the wound washed, soothing herbs applied, and the wound bandaged. However, in sickness in which no wound occurred, an evil spirit was considered the cause. For example, the cause of the plague was unknown, so the question became how and why affected soldiers had angered the gods. According to *The Iliad,* the true healer of the plague was the prophet who prayed for Apollo to stop shooting the "plague arrows." The Greeks applied rational causes and cures to external injuries, while internal ailments continued to be linked to spiritual maladies (Bullough & Bullough, 1978).

Roman Era

During the rise and the fall of the **Roman era** (31 BC–AD 476), Greek culture continued to be a strong influence. The Romans easily adopted Greek culture and expanded the Greeks' accomplishments, especially in the fields of engineering, law, and government. The development of policy, law, and protection of the public's health was an important precursor to our modern public health systems. For Romans, the government had an obligation to protect its citizens, not only from outside aggression such as warring neighbors, but from inside the civilization, in the form of health laws. According to Bullough and Bullough (1978, p. 20), Rome was essentially a "Greek cultural colony."

During the third century BC, Rome began to dominate the Mediterranean, Egypt, the Tigris-Euphrates Valley, the Hebrews, and the Greeks (Boorstin, 1985). Greek science and Roman engineering then spread throughout the ancient world, providing a synthesized Greco-Roman foundation for eventual public health policies (Bullough & Bullough, 1978).

Galen of Pergamum (AD 129–199), often known as the greatest Greek physician after Hippocrates, left for Rome after studying medicine in Greece and Egypt and gained great fame as a medical practitioner, lecturer, and experimenter. In his lifetime, medicine evolved into a science; he submitted traditional healing practices to experimentation and was possibly the greatest medical researcher before the 1600s (Bullough & Bullough, 1978). He was considered the last of the great physicians of antiquity (Kalisch & Kalisch, 1978).

The Greek physicians and healers certainly made the most contributions to medicine, but the Romans surpassed the Greeks in promoting the evolution of nursing. Roman armies developed the notion of a mobile war nursing unit as their battles took them far from home where they could be cared for by their wives and family. This portable hospital was a series of tents arranged in corridors; as battles wore on, these tents gave way to buildings that became permanent convalescent camps along the battle sites (Rosen, 1958). Many of these early military hospitals have been excavated by archaeologists along the banks of the Rhine and Danube Rivers. They had wards, recreation areas, baths, pharmacies, and even rooms for officers who needed a "rest cure" (Bullough & Bullough, 1978). Coexisting were the Greek dispensary forms of temples, or the *iatreia,* which started out as a type of physician waiting room. These eventually developed into a primitive type of hospital, places for surgical clients to stay until they could be taken home by their families. Although nurses during the Roman era were usually family members, servants, or slaves, nursing had strengthened its position in medical care and emerged during the Roman era as a separate and distinct specialty.

The Greek physicians and healers certainly made the most contributions to medicine, but the Romans surpassed the Greeks in promoting the evolution of nursing.

The Romans developed massive aqueducts, bathhouses, and sewer systems during this era. At the height of the Roman Empire, Rome provided 40 gallons of water per person per day to its 1 million inhabitants, which is comparable to our rates of consumption today (Rosen, 1958). Even though these engineering feats were remarkable at the time, poorer and less fortunate residents often did not benefit from the same level of public health amenities, such as sewer systems and latrines (Bullough & Bullough, 1978). However, the Romans did provide many of their citizens with what we would consider public health services.

Middle Ages

Many of the advancements of the Greco-Roman era were reversed during the Middle Ages after the decline of the Roman Empire (AD 476–1453). The Middle Ages, or the medieval era, served as a transition between ancient and modern civilizations. Once again, myth, magic, and religion were explanations and cures for illness and health problems. The medieval world was the result of a fusion of three streams of thought, actions, and ways of life—Greco-Roman, Germanic, and Christian—into one (Donahue, 1985). Nursing was most influenced by Christianity with the beginning of **deaconesses**, or female servants, doing the work of God by ministering to the needs of others. Deacons in the early Christian churches were apparently available only to care for men, while deaconesses cared for the needs of the women. This role of the deaconess in the church was considered a forward step in the development of nursing, and in the 1800s would strongly influence the young Florence Nightingale. During this era, Roman military hospitals were replaced by civilian ones. In early Christianity, the Jiakonia, a kind of combination outpatient and welfare office, was managed by deacons and deaconesses and served as the equivalent of a hospital. Jesus served as the example of charity and compassion for the poor and marginal of society.

Communicable diseases were rampant during the Middle Ages, primarily because of the walled cities that emerged in response to the paranoia and isolation of the populations. Infection was next to impossible to control. Physicians had little to offer, deferring to the church for management of disease. Nursing roles were carried out primarily by religious orders. The oldest hospital (other than military hospitals in the Roman era) in Europe was most likely the Hôtel-Dieu in Lyons, France, founded about 542 by Childebert I, king of France. The Hôtel-Dieu in Paris was founded around 652 by Saint Landry, bishop of Paris. During the Middle Ages, charitable institutions, hospitals, and medical schools increased in number, with the religious leaders as caregivers. The word *hospital*, which is derived from the Latin word *hospitalis*, meaning service of guests, was most likely more of a shelter for travelers and other pilgrims as well as the occasional person who needed extra care (Kalisch & Kalisch, 1986). Early European hospitals were more like hospices or homes for the aged, sick pilgrims, or orphans. Nurses in these early hospitals were religious deaconesses who chose to care for others in a life of servitude and spiritual sacrifice.

Black Death

During the Middle Ages, a series of horrible epidemics, including the **Black Death** or bubonic plague, ravaged the civilized world (Diamond, 1997). In the 1300s, Europe, Asia, and Africa saw nearly half their populations lost to the bubonic plague. According to Bullough and Bullough (1978), an interesting account of the arrival of the bubonic plague in 1347 claims that the disease had started in the Genoese colony of Kaffa in the Crimea. The story passed down through the ages was that the city was being besieged by a Mongol khan. When the disease broke out among the khan's men, he catapulted the bodies of its victims into Kaffa to infect and weaken his enemies. The soldiers and colonists of Kaffa carried the disease back to Genoa. Worldwide, more than 60 million deaths were eventually attributed to this horrible plague. In some parts of Europe, only one-fourth of the population survived, with some places having too few people to bury the dead. Families abandoned sick children, and the sick were often left to die alone (Cartwright, 1972).

Nurses and physicians were powerless to avert the disease. Black spots and tumors on the skin appeared and petechiae and hemorrhages gave the skin a darkened appearance. There was also acute inflammation of the lungs, burning sensations, unquenchable thirst, and inflammation of the entire body. Hardly anyone afflicted survived the third day of the attack. So great was the fear of contagion that ships were set to sail with bodies of infected persons without a crew, drifting through the North, Black, and Mediterranean Seas from port to port with their dead passengers (Cohen, 1989). Bubonic plague is caused by the bacillus *Pasteurella pestis,* which is usually transmitted by the bite of a flea carried by an animal vector, typically a rat. After the initial flea bite, the infection spreads through the lymph nodes and the nodes swell to enormous size; the inflamed nodes are called bubos, from which the bubonic plague derives its name. Medieval people knew that this disease was in some way communicable, but they were unsure of the mode of transmission (Diamond, 1997), hence the avoidance of victims and a reliance on isolation techniques. The practice of quarantine in city ports was developed as a preventive measure and is still used today (Bullough & Bullough, 1978; Kalisch & Kalisch, 1986).

The Renaissance

During the rebirth of Europe, great political, social, and economic advances occurred along with a tremendous revival of learning. Donahue (1985, p. 188) contends that the Renaissance has been "viewed as both a blessing and a curse." There was a renewed interest in the arts and sciences, which helped advance medical science (Boorstin, 1985; Bullough & Bullough, 1978). Columbus and other explorers discovered new worlds, and belief in a sun-centered rather than earth-centered universe was promoted by Copernicus (1473–1543); Sir Isaac Newton's (1642–1727) theory of gravity changed the world forever. Gunpowder was introduced, and social and religious upheavals resulted in the American and French Revolutions at the end of the 1700s. In the arts and sciences, Leonardo da Vinci, known as one of "the greatest geniuses of all time," made a number of anatomical drawings based on dissection experiences. These drawings have become classics in the progression of knowledge about the human anatomy. Many artists of this time left an indelible mark and continue to exert influence today, including Michelangelo, Raphael, and Titian (Donahue, 1985).

The Advancement of Science and Health of the Public

It took the first 50 years of the 1700s for the new knowledge from the Enlightenment to be organized and digested.

It took the first 50 years of the 1700s for the new knowledge from the Enlightenment to be organized and digested, according to Donahue (1985). In Britain, **Edward Jenner** discovered an effective method of vaccination against the dreaded smallpox virus in 1798. Psychiatry developed as a separate branch of medicine, and instruments that measured and allowed for assessment of the body such as the pulse watch and the stethoscope were invented.

One of the greatest scientists of this period was **Louis Pasteur** (1822–1895). A French chemist, Pasteur first became interested in pathogenic organisms through his studies of the diseases of wine. He discovered if wine was heated to a temperature of 55°C to 60°C, the process killed the microorganisms that spoiled wine. This discovery was critical to the wine industry's success in France. This process of pasteurization led Pasteur to investigate many fields and save many lives from contaminated milk and food.

Joseph Lister (1827–1912) was a physician who set out to decrease the mortality resulting from infection after surgery. He used Pasteur's research to eventually arrive at a chemical antiseptic solution of carbolic acid for use in surgery. Widely regarded as the father of modern surgery, he practiced his antiseptic surgery with great results, and the Listerian principles of asepsis changed the way physicians and nurses practice to this day (Dietz & Lehozky, 1963). **Robert Koch** (1843–1910), a physician known for his research in anthrax, is regarded as the father of microbiology. By identifying the organism that caused cholera, *Vibrio cholerae,* he also demonstrated its transmission by water, food, and clothing. **Edwin Klebs** (1834–1913) proved the germ theory, that is, that germs are the causes of infectious diseases. This discovery of the bacterial origin of diseases may be considered the greatest achievement of the 1800s. Although the microscope had been around for two centuries, it remained for Lister, Pasteur, and Koch—and ultimately Klebs—to provide the missing link (Dietz & Lehozky, 1963; Rosen, 1958).

The Emergence of Home Visiting

In 1633, **Saint Vincent de Paul** founded the Sisters of Charity in France, an order of nuns who traveled from home to home visiting the sick. As the services of the sisters grew, St. Vincent appointed Mademoiselle Le Gras as supervisor of these visitors. These nurses functioned as the first organized visiting nurse service, making home visits and caring for the sick in their homes. De Paul believed that for family members to go to the hospital was disruptive to family life and that taking nursing services to the home enabled health to be restored more effectively and more efficiently.

The Reformation

Religious changes during the Renaissance were to influence nursing perhaps more than any other aspect of society. Particularly important was the rise of Protestantism as a result of the reform movements of Martin Luther (1483–1546) in Germany and John Calvin (1509–1564) in France and Geneva. Although the various sects were numerous in the Protestant movement, the agreement among the leaders was almost unanimous on the abolition of the monastic or cloistered career. The effects

> Religious changes during the Renaissance were to influence nursing perhaps more than any other aspect of society.

on nursing were drastic: monastic-affiliated institutions, including hospitals and schools, were closed, and orders of nuns, including nurses, were dissolved. Even in countries where Catholicism flourished, seizures of monasteries by royal leaders occurred frequently.

Religious leaders, such as Martin Luther in Germany who led the **Reformation** in 1517, were well aware of the lack of adequate nursing care as a result of these sweeping changes. Luther advocated that each town establish something akin to a "community chest" to raise funds for hospitals and nurse visitors for the poor (Dietz & Lehozky, 1963). For example, in England, where there had been at least 450 charitable foundations before the Reformation, only a few survived the reign of Henry VIII, who closed most of the monastic hospitals (Donahue, 1985). Eventually, Henry VIII's son, Edward VI, who reigned from 1547 to 1553, was convinced and did endow some hospitals, namely St. Bartholomew's Hospital and St. Thomas' Hospital, which would eventually house the Nightingale School of Nursing later in the 1800s (Bullough & Bullough, 1978).

The Dark Period of Nursing

The last half of the period between 1500 and 1860 is widely regarded as the "dark period of nursing" because nursing conditions were at their worst (Donahue, 1985). Education for girls, which had been provided by the nuns in religious schools, was lost. Because of the elimination of hospitals and schools, there was no one to pass on knowledge about caring for the sick. As a result, the hospitals were managed and staffed by municipal authorities; women entering nursing service often came from illiterate classes, and even then there were too few to serve (Dietz & Lehozky, 1963). The lay attendants who filled the nursing role were illiterate, rough, inconsiderate, and often immoral and alcoholic. Intelligent women and men could not be persuaded to accept such a degraded and low-status position in the offensive municipal hospitals of London. Nursing slipped back into a role of servitude as menial, low-status work. According to Donahue (1985), when a woman could no longer make it as a gambler, prostitute, or thief, she might become a nurse. Eventually, women serving jail sentences for crimes such as prostitution and stealing were ordered to care for the sick in the hospitals instead of serving their sentences in the city jail (Dietz & Lehozky, 1963). The nurses of this era took bribes from clients, became inappropriately involved with them, and survived the best way they could, often at the expense of their assigned clients.

Nursing had, during this era, virtually no social standing or organization. Even Catholic sisters of the religious orders throughout Europe "came to a complete standstill" professionally because of the intolerance of society (Donahue, 1985, p. 231). Charles Dickens, in *Martin Chuzzlewit* (1910), created the immortal characters of Sairey Gamp and Betsy Prig. Sairey Gamp was a visiting nurse based on an actual hired attendant whom Dickens had met in a friend's home. Sairey Gamp was hired to care for sick family members but was instead cruel to her clients, stole from them, and ate their rations; she was an alcoholic and has been immortalized forever as a reminder of the world in which Florence Nightingale came of age (Donahue, 1985).

> She was a fat old woman, this Mrs. Gamp, with a husky voice and a moist eye, which she had a remarkable power of turning up and showing the white of it. Having very little neck, it cost her some trouble to look over herself, if one may say so, to those to whom she talked. She wore a very rusty black gown, rather the worse for snuff, and a shawl and bonnet to correspond. . . . The face of Mrs. Gamp—the nose in particular—was somewhat red and swollen, and it was difficult to enjoy her society without becoming conscious of the smell of spirits. Like most persons who have attained to great eminence in their profession, she took to hers very kindly; insomuch, that setting aside her natural predilections as a woman, she went to a lying-in [birth] or a laying-out [death] with equal zest and relish.
>
> *Charles Dickens,* 1844

Early Organized Health Care in the Americas: A Brave New World

In the New World, the first hospital in the Americas, the Hospital de la Purisima Concepcion, was founded some time before 1524 by Hernando Cortez, the conqueror of Mexico. The first hospital in the continental United States was erected in Manhattan in 1658 for the care of sick soldiers and slaves. In 1717, a hospital for infectious diseases was built in Boston; the first hospital established by a private gift was the Charity Hospital in New Orleans. A sailor, Jean Louis, donated the endowment for the hospital's founding (Bullough & Bullough, 1978).

During the 1600s and 1700s, colonial hospitals were often used to house the poor and downtrodden with little resemblance to modern hospitals. Hospitals called "pesthouses" were created to care for clients with contagious diseases; their primary purpose was to protect the public at large, rather than to treat and care for the clients. Contagious diseases were rampant during the early years of the American colonies, often being spread by the large number of immigrants who brought these diseases with them on their long journeys to America. Medicine was not as developed as in Europe, and nursing remained in the hands of the uneducated. Average life expectancy at birth was only around 35 years by 1720. Plagues were a constant nightmare, with outbreaks of smallpox and yellow fever. In 1751, the first true hospital in the new colonies, Pennsylvania Hospital, was erected in Philadelphia on the recommendation of Benjamin Franklin (Kalisch & Kalisch, 1986).

By today's standards, hospitals in the 1800s were disgraceful, dirty, unventilated, and contaminated by infections; to be a client in a hospital actually increased one's risk of dying. As in England, nursing was considered an inferior occupation. After the sweeping changes of the Reformation, educated religious health workers were replaced with lay people who were "down and outers," in prison, or had no option left but to work with the sick (Kalisch & Kalisch, 1986).

The Chadwick Report and the Shattuck Report

Edwin Chadwick became a major figure in the development of the field of public health in Great Britain by drawing attention to the cost of the unsanitary conditions that shortened the life span of the laboring class and the threats to the wealth of Britain. Although the first sanitation legislation, which established a National Vaccination Board, was passed in 1837, Chadwick found in his classic study, *Report on an Inquiry into the Sanitary Conditions of the Laboring Population of Great Britain,* that death rates were high in large industrial cities such as Liverpool. A more startling finding, from what is often referred to simply as the **Chadwick Report**, was that more than half the children of labor-class workers died by age 5, indicating poor living conditions that affected the health of the most vulnerable. Laborers lived only half as long as the upper classes.

One consequence of the report was the establishment of the first board of health, the General Board of Health for England, in 1848 (Richardson, 1887). More legislation followed that initiated social reform in the areas of child welfare, elder care, the sick, the mentally ill, factory health, and education. Soon sewers and fire plugs, based on an available water supply, appeared as indicators that the public health linkages from the Chadwick Report had an impact.

In the United States during the 1800s, waves of epidemics of yellow fever, smallpox, cholera, typhoid fever, and typhus continued to plague the population as in

England and the rest of the world. As cities continued to grow in the industrialized young nation, poor workers crowded into larger cities and suffered from illnesses caused by the unsanitary living conditions (Hanlon & Pickett, 1984). Similar to Chadwick's classic study in England, Lemuel Shattuck, a Boston bookseller and publisher who had an interest in public health, organized the American Statistical Society in 1839 and issued a census of Boston in 1845. Shattuck's census revealed high infant mortality rates and high overall population mortality rates. In his *Report of the Massachusetts Sanitary Commission in 1850,* Shattuck not only outlined his findings on the unsanitary conditions but made recommendations for public health reform that included the bookkeeping of population statistics and development of a monitoring system that would provide information to the public about environmental, food, and drug safety and infectious disease control (Rosen, 1958). He also called for services for well-child care, school-age children's health, immunizations, mental health, health education for all, and health planning. The **Shattuck Report** was revolutionary in its scope and vision for public health, but it was virtually ignored during Shattuck's lifetime. It was 19 years later, in 1869, that the first state board of health was formed (Kalisch & Kalisch, 1986).

The Industrial Revolution

During the mid-1700s in England, capitalism emerged as an economic system based on profit. This emerging system resulted in mass production, as contrasted with the previous system of individual workers and craftsmen. In the simplest terms, the Industrial Revolution was the application of machine power to processes formerly done by hand. Machinery was invented during this era and ultimately standardized quality; individual craftsmen were forced to give up their crafts and lands and become factory laborers for the capitalist owners. All types of industries were affected; this new-found efficiency produced profit for owners of the means of production. Because of this, the era of invention flourished, factories grew, and people moved in record numbers to the work in the cities. Urban areas grew, tenement housing projects emerged, and overcrowded cities became serious threats to well-being (Donahue, 1985).

Workers were forced to go to the machines, rather than the other way around. Such relocations meant giving up not only farming, but a way of life that had existed for centuries. The emphasis on profit over people led to child labor, frequent layoffs, and long work days filled with stressful, tedious, unfamiliar work. Labor unions did not exist, nor was there any legal protection against exploitation of workers, including children (Donahue, 1985). All these rapid changes and often threatening conditions created the world of Charles Dickens, where, as in his book *Oliver Twist,* children worked as adults without question.

According to Donahue (1985), urban life, trade, and industrialization contributed to these overwhelming health hazards, and the situation was confounded by the lack of an adequate means of social control. Reforms were desperately needed, and the social reform movement emerged in response to the unhealthy by-products of the Industrial Revolution. It was in this world of the 19th century that reformers such as John Stuart Mill (1806–1873) emerged. Although the Industrial Revolution began in England, it quickly spread to the rest of Europe and to the United States (Bullough & Bullough, 1978). The reform movement is critical to understanding the emerging health concerns that were later addressed by Florence Nightingale. Mill championed popular education, the emancipation of women, trade unions, and religious toleration. Other reform issues of the era included the abolition of slavery and, most important for nursing, more humane care of the sick, the poor, and the wounded (Bullough & Bullough, 1978). There was a renewed energy in the religious community with the reemergence of new religious orders in the Catholic Church that provided service to the sick and disenfranchised.

Epidemics had ravaged Europe for centuries, but they became even more serious with urbanization. Industrialization had brought people to cities, where they worked in close quarters (as compared with the isolation of the farm) and contributed to the social decay of the second half of the 1800s. Sanitation was poor or nonexistent, sewage disposal from the growing population was lacking, cities were filthy, public laws

> Epidemics had ravaged Europe for centuries, but they became even more serious with urbanization.

were weak or nonexistent, and congestion of the cities inevitably brought pests in the form of rats, lice, and bedbugs, which transmitted many pathogens. Communicable diseases continued to plague the population, especially those who lived in these unsanitary environments. For example, during the mid-1700s typhus and typhoid fever claimed twice as many lives each year as did the Battle of Waterloo (Hanlon & Pickett, 1984). Through foreign trade and immigration, infectious diseases were spread to all of Europe and eventually to the growing United States.

John Snow and the Science of Epidemiology

John Snow, a prominent physician, is credited with being the first epidemiologist by demonstrating in 1854 that cholera rates were linked with water pump use in London (Cartwright, 1972). Snow investigated the area around Golden Square in London and arrived at the conclusion that cholera was not carried by bad air, nor necessarily by direct contact. He formed the opinion that diarrhea, unwashed hands, and shared food somehow played a large part in spreading the disease.

People around Golden Square in London were not supplied with water by pipes but drew their water from surface wells by means of hand-operated pumps. A severe outbreak of cholera occurred at the end of August 1853, resulting in at least 500 deaths in just 10 days in Golden Square. By using rates of cholera, Snow for the first time linked the sources of the drinking water at the Broad Street pump to the outbreaks of cholera. This proved that cholera was a waterborne disease. Dr. Snow's epidemiological investigation started a train of events that eventually would end the great epidemics of cholera, dysentery, and typhoid.

When Snow attended the now-famous community meeting of Golden Square and gave his evidence, government officials asked him what measures were necessary. His reply was, "Take the handle off the Broad Street pump." The handle was removed the next day, and no more cholera cases occurred (Snow, 1855). Although he did not discover the true cause of the cholera—the identification of the organism—he came very close to the truth (Rosen, 1958).

And Then There Was Nightingale . . .

Florence Nightingale has become synonymous with modern nursing.

Florence Nightingale was named one of the 100 most influential persons of the last millennium by *Life* magazine (1997). She was one of only eight women identified as such. Of those eight women, such as Joan of Arc, Helen Keller, and Elizabeth I, Nightingale was identified as a true "angel of mercy," having reformed military health care in the Crimean War and having used her political savvy to forever change the way society views the health of the vulnerable, the poor, and the forgotten. She is probably one of the most written about women in history (Bullough & Bullough. 1978). Florence Nightingale has become synonymous with modern nursing.

Florence Nightingale was the second child born to the wealthy English family of William and Frances Nightingale on May 12, 1820, in her namesake city, Florence, Italy. As a young child, Florence displayed incredible curiosity and intellectual abilities not common to female children of the Victorian age. She mastered the fundamentals of Greek and Latin, and she studied history, art, mathematics, and philosophy. To her family's dismay, she believed that God had called her to be a nurse. Nightingale was keenly aware of the suffering that industrialization created; she became obsessed with the plight of the miserable and suffering. There existed conditions of general starvation that accompanied the Industrial Revolution, overflowing prisons and workhouses, and displaced persons in all sections of British life. She wrote in the spring of 1842, "My mind is absorbed with the sufferings of man; it besets me behind and before. . . . All that the poets sing of the glories of this world seem to me untrue. All the people that I see are eaten up with care or poverty or disease" (Woodham-Smith, 1951, p. 31).

For Nightingale, her entire life would be haunted by this conflict between the opulent life of gaiety that she enjoyed and the plight and misery of the world, which she was unable to alleviate. She was, in essence, an "alien spirit in the rich and aristocratic social sphere of Victorian England" (Palmer, 1977, p. 14). Nightingale remained unmarried, and at the age of 25, she expressed a desire to be trained as a nurse in an English hospital. Her parents emphatically denied her request, and for the next 7 years, she made repeated attempts to change their minds and allow her to enter nurse training. She wrote, "I crave for some regular occupation, for something worth doing instead of frittering my time away on useless trifles" (Woodham-Smith,

1951, p. 162). During this time, she continued her education through the study of math and science and spent 5 years collecting data about public health and hospitals (Dietz & Lehozky, 1963). During a tour of Egypt in 1849 with family and friends, Nightingale spent her 30th year in Alexandria with the Sisters of Charity of St. Vincent de Paul, where her conviction to study nursing was only reinforced (Tooley, 1910). While in Egypt, Nightingale studied Egyptian, Platonic, and Hermetic philosophy; Christian scripture; and the works of poets, mystics, and missionaries in her efforts to understand the nature of God and her "calling" as it fit into the divine plan (Calabria, 1996; Dossey, 1985).

The next spring, Nightingale traveled unaccompanied to the Kaiserwerth Institute in Germany and stayed there for 2 weeks, vowing to return to train as a nurse. In June 1851, Nightingale took her future into her own hands and announced to her family that she planned to return to Kaiserwerth and study nursing. According to Dietz and Lehozky (1963, p. 42), her mother had "hysterics" and scene followed scene. Her father "retreated into the shadows," and her sister, Parthe, expressed that the family name was forever disgraced (Cook, 1913).

In 1851, at the age of 31, Nightingale was finally permitted to go to Kaiserwerth, and she studied there for 3 months with Pastor Fliedner. Her family insisted that she tell no one outside the family of her whereabouts, and her mother forbade her to write any letters from Kaiserwerth. While there, Nightingale learned about the care of the sick and the importance of discipline and commitment of oneself to God (Donahue, 1985). She returned to England and cared for her then ailing father, from whom she finally gained some support for her intent to become a nurse—her lifelong dream.

In 1852, Nightingale wrote the essay *Cassandra,* which stands today as a classic feminist treatise against the idleness of Victorian women. Through her voluminous journal writings, Nightingale reveals her inner struggle throughout her adulthood with what was expected of a woman and what she could accomplish with her life. The life expected of an aristocratic woman in her day was one she grew to loathe; throughout her writings, she poured out her detestation of the life of an idle woman (Nightingale, 1979, p. 5). In *Cassandra,* Nightingale put her thoughts to paper, and many scholars believe that her eventual intent was to extend the essay to a novel. She wrote in *Cassandra,* "Why have women passion, intellect, moral activity—these three—in a place in society where no one of the three can be exercised?" (Nightingale, 1979, p. 37). Although uncertain about the meaning of the name *Cassandra,* many scholars believe that it came from the Greek goddess Cassandra, who was cursed by Apollo and doomed to see and speak the truth but never to be believed. Nightingale saw the conventional life of women as a waste of time and abilities. After receiving a generous yearly endowment from her father, Nightingale moved to London and worked briefly as the superintendent of the Establishment for Gentlewomen During Illness hospital, finally realizing her dream of working as a nurse (Cook, 1913).

The Crimean Experience: "I Can Stand Out the War with Any Man"

Nightingale's opportunity for greatness came when she was offered the position of female nursing establishment of the English General Hospitals in Turkey by the secretary of war, Sir Sidney Herbert. Soon after the outbreak of the Crimean War, stories of the inadequate care and lack of medical resources for the soldiers became widely known throughout England (Woodham-Smith, 1951). The country was appalled at the conditions so vividly portrayed in the *London Times*. Pressure increased on Sir Herbert to react. He knew of one woman who was capable of bringing order out of the chaos and wrote the following now-famous letter to Nightingale on October 15, 1854, as a plea for her service:

> There is but one person in England that I know of who would be capable of organising and superintending such a scheme. . . . The difficulty of finding women equal to a task after all, full of horrors, and requiring besides knowledge and good will, great energy and great courage, will be great. Your own personal qualities, your knowledge and your power of administration and among greater things your rank and position in Society give you advantages in such a work which no other person possesses. (Woodham-Smith, 1951, pp. 87–89)

Nightingale took the challenge from Sir Herbert and set sail with 38 self-proclaimed nurses with varied training and experiences, of whom 24 were Catholic and Anglican nuns. Their journey to the Crimea took a month, and on November 4, 1854, the brave nurses arrived at Istanbul and were taken to Scutari the same day. Faced with 3000 to 4000 wounded men in a hospital designed to accommodate 1700, the nurses went to work (Kalisch & Kalisch, 1986). The nurses were faced with 4 miles of beds 18 inches apart. Most soldiers were lying naked with no bedding or blanket. There were no kitchen or laundry facilities. The little light present took the form of candles in beer bottles. The hospital was literally floating on an open sewage lagoon filled with rats and other vermin (Donahue, 1985).

The barrack "hospital" was more of a death trap than a place for healing before Nightingale's arrival. In a letter to Sir Herbert, Nightingale, demonstrating her sense of humor, wrote, with tongue in cheek, that "the vermin might, if they had but unity of purpose, carry off the four miles of beds on their backs and march them into the War Office" (Stanmore, 1906, pp. 393–394).

By taking the newly arrived medical equipment and setting up kitchens, laundries, recreation rooms, reading rooms, and a canteen, Nightingale and her team of nurses proceeded to clean the barracks of lice and filth. Nightingale was in her element. She set out not only to provide humane health care for the soldiers but to essentially overhaul the administrative structure of the military health services (Williams, 1961). Nightingale and her nurses were faced with overwhelming odds and deplorable conditions. No accommodations had been made for their quarters, so they ended up in one of the hospital towers, 39 women crowded into six small rooms. In addition to having no furniture, one of the rooms even had a long-neglected, forgotten corpse swarming with vermin! Ever the disciplinarian, Nightingale insisted on strict adherence to a standard nurse uniform: gray tweed dresses, gray worsted jackets, plain white caps, short woolen cloaks, and brown scarves embroidered in red with the words "Scutari Hospital" (Bullough & Bullough, 1978).

Florence Nightingale and Sanitation

Although Nightingale never accepted the germ theory, she demanded clean dressings; clean bedding; well-cooked, edible, and appealing food; proper sanitation; and fresh air. After the other nurses were asleep, Nightingale made her famous solitary rounds with a lamp or lantern to check on the soldiers. Nightingale had a lifelong pattern of sleeping few hours, spending many nights writing, developing elaborate plans, and evaluating implemented changes. She seldom believed in the "hopeless" soldier, only one that needed extra attention. Nightingale was convinced that most of the maladies that the soldiers suffered and died from were preventable (Williams, 1961).

Many soldiers wrote about their experiences of the Angel of Mercy, Florence Nightingale. One soldier wrote perhaps one of the most revealing tributes to this "Lady with the Lamp":

> What a comfort it was to see her pass even. She would speak to one and nod and smile to as many more, but she could not do it all, you know. We lay there by hundreds, but we could kiss her shadow as it fell, and lay our heads on the pillow again content. (Tyrell, 1856, p. 310)

Before Nightingale's arrival and her radical and well-documented interventions based on sound public health principles, the mortality rate from the Crimean War was estimated to be from 42% to 73%. Nightingale is credited with reducing that rate to 2% within 6 months of her arrival at Scutari. She did this through careful, scientific epidemiological research (Dietz & Lehozky, 1963). Upon arriving at Scutari, Nightingale's first act was to order 200 scrubbing brushes. The death rate fell dramatically once Nightingale discovered that the hospital was built literally over an open, sewage lagoon. A dead horse was even retrieved from the sewer system under Scutari (Andrews, 2003).

According to Palmer (1982), Nightingale possessed the qualities of a good researcher: insatiable curiosity, command of her subject, familiarity with methods of inquiry, a good background of statistics, and the ability to discriminate and abstract. She used these skills to maintain detailed and copious notes and to codify observations. Nightingale relied on statistics and attention to detail to back up her conclusions about sanitation, management of care, and disease causation. Her now-famous "cox combs" are a hallmark of military health services management by which she diagrammed deaths in the Army from wounds and from other diseases and compared them with deaths that occurred in similar populations in England (Palmer, 1977).

Nightingale was first and foremost an administrator: She believed in a hierarchical administrative structure with ultimate control lodged in one person to whom all subordinates and offices reported. Within a matter of weeks of her arrival in the Crimea, Nightingale was the acknowledged administrator and organizer of a mammoth humanitarian effort. From her Crimean experience on, Nightingale involved herself primarily in organizational activities and health planning administration. Palmer contends that Nightingale "perceived the Crimean venture, which was set up as an experiment, as a golden opportunity to demonstrate the efficacy of female nursing" (Palmer, 1982, p. 4). Although Nightingale faced initial resistance from the unconvinced and oppositional medical officers and surgeons, she boldly defied convention and remained steadfastly focused on her mission to create a sanitary and highly structured environment for her "children"—the British soldiers who dedicated their lives to the defense of Great Britain. Through her resilience and insistence on absolute authority regarding nursing and the hospital environment, Nightingale was known to send nurses home to England from the Crimea for suspicious alcohol use and character weakness.

It was through this success at Scutari that she began a long career of influence on the public's health through social activism and reform, health policy, and the reformation of career nursing. Using her well-publicized successful "experiment" and supportive evidence from the Crimea, Nightingale effectively argued the case for the reform and creation of military health that would serve as the model for people in uniform to the present (D'Antonio, 2002). Nightingale's ideas about proper hospital architecture and administration influenced a generation of medical doctors and the entire world, in both military and civilian service. Her work in *Notes on Hospitals,* published in 1859, provided the template for the organization of military health care in the Union Army when the US Civil war erupted in 1861. Her vision for health care of soldiers and the responsibility of the governments who send them to war continues today; her influence can be seen throughout the previous century and into this century as health care for the women and men who serve their country is a vital part of the well-being of not only the soldiers but for society in general (D'Antonio, 2002).

Mary Grant Seacole, an African nurse from Jamaica, offered her services to Nightingale after hearing of the need in Scutari. Although Nightingale was unwilling to hire Seacole as part of the nursing staff, Seacole volunteered her services without pay. Seacole was so committed to providing care to the British military that she set up an inn with her own money that provided food and lodging for soldiers and their families near Scutari (Hine, 1989). Although Seacole is less well known than Nightingale, her contributions to nursing in wartime were significant in the history of minority nursing. The School of Nursing in Kingston, Jamaica, is today named in her honor.

Scores have been written about Nightingale—an almost mythic figure in history. She truly was a beloved legend throughout Great Britain by the time she left the Crimea in July 1856, four months after the war. Longfellow immortalized this "Lady with the Lamp" in his poem of "Santa Filomena" (Longfellow, 1857).

Returning Home a Heroine: The Political Reformer

When Nightingale returned to London, she found that her efforts to provide comfort and health to the British soldier succeeded in making heroes of both Nightingale and the soldiers (Woodham-Smith, 1951). Both had suffered from negative stereotypes: The soldier was often portrayed as a drunken oaf with little ambition or honor, the nurse as a tipsy, self-serving, illiterate, promiscuous loser. After the Crimean War and the efforts of Nightingale and her nurses, both returned with honor and dignity, never more the downtrodden and disrespected.

After her return from the Crimea, Florence Nightingale never made a public appearance, never attended a public function, and never issued a public statement (Bullough & Bullough, 1978). She single-handedly raised nursing from, as she put it, "the sink it was" into a respected and noble profession (Palmer, 1977). As an avid scholar and student of the Greek writer Plato, Nightingale believed that she had a moral obligation to work primarily for the good of the community. Because she believed that education formed character, she insisted that nursing must go beyond care for the sick; the mission of the trained nurse must include social reform to promote the good. This dual mission of nursing—caregiver and political reformer—has shaped the profession as we know it today. LeVasseur (1998) contends that Nightingale's insistence on nursing's involvement in a larger political ideal is the historical foundation of the field and distinguishes us from other scientific disciplines, such as medicine.

How did Nightingale accomplish this? You will learn throughout this text how nurses effect change through others. Florence Nightingale is the standard by which we measure our effectiveness. She effected change through her wide command of acquaintances: Queen Victoria was a significant admirer of her intellect and ability to effect change, and she used her position as national heroine to get the attention of elected officials in Parliament. She was tireless and had an amazing capacity for work. She used people. Her brother-in-law, Sir Harry Verney, was a member of Parliament and often delivered her "messages" in the form of legislation. When she wanted the public incited, she turned to the press, writing letters to the *London Times* and having others of influence write articles. She was not above threats to "go public" by certain dates if an elected official refused to establish a commission or appoint a committee. And when those commissions were formed, Nightingale was ready with her list of selected people for appointment (Palmer, 1982).

Nightingale and Military Reforms

The first real test of Nightingale's military reforms came in the United States during the Civil War. Nightingale was asked by the Union to advise on the organization of hospitals and care of the sick and wounded. She sent recommendations back to the

United States based on her experiences and analysis in the Crimea, and her advisement and influence gained wide publicity. Following her recommendations, the Union set up a sanitary commission and provided for regular inspection of camps. She expressed a desire to help with the Confederate military also but, unfortunately, had no channel of communication with them (Bullough & Bullough, 1978).

The Nightingale School of Nursing at St. Thomas: The Birth of Professional Nursing

The British public honored Nightingale by endowing 50,000 pounds sterling in her name upon her return to England from the Crimea. The money had been raised from the soldiers under her care and donations from the public. This Nightingale Fund eventually was used to create the Nightingale School of Nursing at St. Thomas, which was to be the beginning of professional nursing (Donahue, 1985). Nightingale, at the age of 40, decided that St. Thomas' Hospital was the place for her training school for nurses. While the negotiations for the school went forward, she spent her time writing *Notes on Nursing: What It Is and What It Is Not* (Nightingale, 1860). The small book of 77 pages, written for the British mother, was an instant success. An expanded library edition was written for nurses and used as the textbook for the students at St. Thomas. The book has since been translated into many languages although it is believed that Nightingale refused all royalties earned from the publication of the book (Tooley, 1910; Cook, 1913). The nursing students chosen for the new training school were handpicked; they had to be of good moral character, sober, and honest. Nightingale believed that the strong emphasis on morals was critical to gaining respect for the new "Nightingale nurse," with no possible ties to the disgraceful association of past nurses. Nursing students were monitored throughout their 1-year program both on and off the hospital grounds; their activities were carefully watched for character weaknesses, and discipline was severe and swift for violators. Accounts from Nightingale's journals and notes revealed instant dismissal of nursing students for such behaviors as "flirtation, using the eyes unpleasantly, and being in the company of unsavory persons." Nightingale contended that "the future of nursing depends on how these young women behave themselves" (Smith, 1934, p. 234). She knew that the experiment at St. Thomas to educate nurses and raise nursing to a moral and professional calling was a drastic departure from the past images of nurses and would take extraordinary women of high moral character and intelligence. Nightingale knew every nursing student, or probationer, personally, often having the students at her house for weekend visits. She devised a system of daily journal keeping for the probationers; Nightingale herself read the journals monthly to evaluate their character and work habits. Every nursing student admitted to St. Thomas had to submit an acceptable "letter of good character" and Nightingale herself placed graduate nurses in approved nursing positions.

One of the most important features of the Nightingale School was its relative autonomy. Both the school and the hospital nursing service were organized under the head matron. This was especially significant because it meant that nursing service began independently of the medical staff in selecting, retaining, and disciplining students and nurses (Bullough & Bullough, 1978).

Nightingale was opposed to the use of a standardized government examination and the movement for licensure of trained nurses. She believed that schools of nursing would lose control of educational standards with the advent of national licensure, most notably those related to moral character. Nightingale led a staunch opposition to the movement by the British Nurses Association (BNA) for licensure of trained nurses, one the BNA believed critical to protecting the public's safety by ensuring the qualification of nurses by licensure exam. Nightingale was convinced that qualifying a nurse by examination only tested the acquisition of technical skills, not the equally important evaluation of character. She believed nursing involved "divergencies too great for a single standard to be applied" (Woodham-Smith, 1951; Nutting & Dock, 1907).

Taking Health Care to the Community: Nightingale and Wellness

Early efforts to distinguish hospital from community health nursing are evidence of Nightingale's views on "health nursing," which she distinguished from "sick nursing." She wrote two influential papers, one in 1893, "Sick-Nursing and Health Nursing" (Nightingale, 1893), which was read in the United States at the Chicago Exposition, and the second, "Health Teaching in Towns and Villages" in 1894 (Monteiro, 1985). Both papers praised the success of prevention-based nursing practice. Winslow (1946) acknowledged Nightingale's influence in the United States by being one of the first in the field of public health to recognize the importance of taking responsibility for one's health. She wrote in 1891 that "There are more people to pick us up and help us stand on our own two feet" (Attewell, 1996). According to Palmer (1982), Nightingale was a leader in the wellness movement long before the concept was identified. Nightingale saw the nurse as the key figure in establishing a healthy society. She saw a logical extension of nursing in acute hospital settings to the broadest sense of community used in nursing today. Clearly, through her *Notes on Nursing,* she visualized the nurse as "the nation's first bulwark in health maintenance, the promotion of wellness, and the prevention of disease" (Palmer, 1982, p. 6).

William Rathbone, a wealthy ship owner and philanthropist, is credited with the establishment of the first visiting nurse service, which eventually evolved into district nursing in the community. He was so impressed with the private duty nursing care that his sick wife had received at home that he set out to develop a "district nursing service" in Liverpool, England. At his own expense, in 1859, he developed a corps of nurses trained to care for the sick poor in their homes (Bullough & Bullough, 1978). He divided the community into 16 districts; each was assigned a nurse and a social worker who provided nursing and health education. His experiment in district nursing was so successful that he was unable to find enough nurses to work in the districts. Rathbone contacted Nightingale for assistance. Her recommendation was to train more nurses, and she advised Rathbone to approach the Royal Liverpool Infirmary with a proposal for opening another training school for nurses (Rathbone, 1890; Tooley, 1913). The infirmary agreed to Rathbone's proposal, and district nursing soon spread throughout England as successful "health nursing" in the community for the sick poor through voluntary agencies (Rosen, 1958). Ever the visionary, Nightingale contended that "Hospitals are but an intermediate stage of civilization. The ultimate aim is to nurse the sick poor in their own homes (1893)" (Attewell, 1996). She also wrote in regard to visiting families at home, "We must not talk to them or at them but with them (1894)" (Attewell, 1996). A similar service, health visiting, began in Manchester, England, in 1862 by the Manchester and Salford Sanitary Association. The purpose of placing "health visitors" in the home was to provide health information and instruction to families. Eventually, health visitors evolved to provide preventive health education and district nurses to care for the sick at home (Bullough & Bullough, 1978).

Although Nightingale is best known for her reform of hospitals and the military, she was a great believer in the future of health care, which she anticipated should be preventive in nature and would more than likely take place in the home and community. Her accomplishments in the field of "sanitary nursing" extended beyond the walls of the hospital to include workhouse reform and community sanitation reform. In 1864, Nightingale and William Rathbone once again worked together to lead the reform of the Liverpool Workhouse Infirmary, where more than 1200 sick paupers were crowded into unsanitary and unsafe conditions. Under the British Poor Laws, the most desperately poor of the large cities were gathered into large workhouses. When sick, they were sent to the workhouse infirmary. Trained nursing care was all but nonexistent. Through legislative pressure and a well-designed public campaign describing the horrors of the Workhouse Infirmary, reform of the workhouse system was accomplished by 1867. Although not as complete as Nightingale had wanted, nurses were in place and being paid a salary (Seymer, 1954).

The Legacy of Nightingale

When Nightingale returned to London after the Crimean War, she remained haunted by her experiences related to the soldiers dying of preventable diseases. She was troubled by nightmares and had difficulty sleeping in the years that followed. She wrote in her journal: "Oh my poor men; I am a bad mother to come home and leave you in your Crimean graves. . . . I can never forget. . . . I stand at the altar of the murdered men and while I live, I fight their cause" (Woodham-Smith, 1983, pp. 178, 193). Nightingale became a prolific writer and a staunch defender of the causes of the British soldier, sanitation in England and India, and trained nursing.

As a woman, she was not able to hold an official government post, nor could she vote. Historians have had varied opinions about the exact nature of the disability that kept her homebound for the remainder of her life. Recent scholars have speculated that she experienced post-traumatic stress disorder from her experiences in the Crimea; there is also considerable evidence that she suffered from the painful disease brucellosis (Barker, 1989; Young, 1995). She exerted incredible influence through friends and acquaintances, directing from her sick room sanitation and poor law reform. Her mission to "cleanse" spread from the military to the British Empire; her fight for improved sanitation both at home and in India consumed her energies for the remainder of her life (Vicinus & Nergaard, 1990).

According to Monteiro (1985), two recurrent themes are found throughout Nightingale's writings about disease prevention and wellness outside the hospital. The most persistent theme is that nurses must be trained differently and instructed specifically in district and instructive nursing. She consistently wrote that the "health nurse" must be trained in the nature of poverty and its influence on health, something she referred to as the "pauperization" of the poor. She also believed that above all, health nurses must be good teachers about hygiene and helping families learn to better care for themselves (Nightingale, 1893). She insisted that untrained, "good intended women" could not substitute for nursing care in the home. Nightingale pushed for an extensive orientation and additional training, including prior hospital experience, before one was hired as a district nurse. She outlined the qualifications in her paper "On Trained Nursing for the Sick Poor," in which she called for a month's "trial" in district nursing, a year's training in hospital nursing, and 3 to 6 months training in district nursing (Monteiro, 1985). She said, "There is no such thing as amateur nursing."

The second theme that emerged from her writings was the focus on the role of the nurse. She clearly distinguished the role of the health nurse in promoting what we today call self-care. In the past, philanthropic visitors in the form of Christian charity would visit the homes of the poor and offer them relief (Monteiro, 1985). Nightingale believed that such activities did little to teach the poor to care for themselves and further "pauperized" them—dependent and vulnerable—keeping them unhealthy, prone to disease, and reliant on others to keep them healthy. The nurse then must help the families at home manage a healthy environment for themselves, and Nightingale saw a trained nurse as being the only person who could pull off such a feat. She stated, "Never think that you have done anything effectual in nursing in London, till you nurse, not only the sick poor in workhouses, but those at home."

My view you know is that the ultimate destination of all nursing is the nursing of the sick in their own homes. . . . I look to the abolition of all hospitals and workhouse infirmaries. But no use to talk about the year 2000.
Nightingale, 1894

By 1901, Nightingale lived in a world without sight or sound, leaving her unable to write. Over the next 5 years, Miss Nightingale lost her ability to communicate and most days existed in a state of unconsciousness. In November of 1907,

CRITICAL THINKING QUESTIONS

Some nurses believe that Florence Nightingale is holding nursing back and represents the negative and backward elements of nursing. This view cites as evidence that Nightingale supported the subordination of nurses to physician, opposed registration of nurses, and did not see mental health nurses as part of the profession. Wheeler has gone so far as to say, "The nursing profession needs to exorcise the myth of Nightingale, not necessarily because she was a bad person, but because the impact of her legacy has held the profession back too long." After reading this chapter, what do you think? Is Nightingale relevant in the 21st century to the nursing profession? Why or why not?

Source: Wheeler, W. (1999). Is Florence Nightingale holding us back? *Nursing 99, 29*(10), 22–23.

Nightingale was honored with the Order of Merit by King Edward VII, the first time ever given to a woman. After 50 years, in May of 1910, the Nightingale Training School of Nursing at St. Thomas celebrated its Jubilee. There were now over a thousand training schools for nurses in the United States alone (Tooley, 1910; Cook, 1913).

Nightingale died in her sleep around noon on August 13, 1910, and was buried quietly and without pomp near the family's home at Embley, her coffin carried by six sergeants of the British Army. Only a small cross marks her grave at her request: "FN. Born 1820. Died 1910." (Brown, 1988). The family refused a national funeral and burial at Westminster Abbey out of respect for Nightingale's last wishes. She had lived for 90 years and 3 months.

Early Nursing Education and Organization in the United States

In the United States, the first training schools for nursing were modeled after the Nightingale School of Nursing at St. Thomas in London. The earliest programs for trained nurses in the United States were the Bellevue Training School for Nurses in New York City; Connecticut Training School for Nurses in New Haven, Connecticut; and the Boston Training School for Nurses at Massachusetts General Hospital (Nutting & Dock, 1907; Christy, 1975). Based on the Victorian belief in the natural affinity for women to be sensitive, possess high morals, and be caregivers, early nursing training required that applicants be female. Sensitivity, high moral character, purity of character, subservience, and "ladylike" behavior became the associated traits of a "good nurse," thus setting the "feminization of nursing" as the ideal standard for a good nurse. These historical roots of gender- and race-based caregiving continued to exclude males and minorities from the nursing profession for many years to come and still influence career choices for men and women today. These early training schools provided a stable, subservient, white female workforce, as student nurses served as the primary nursing staff for these early hospitals.

A significant report, known simply as the **Goldmark Report**, *Nursing and Nursing Education in the United States,* was released in 1922 and advocated the establishment of university schools of nursing to train nursing leaders. The report, initiated by Nutting in 1918, was an exhaustive and comprehensive investigation into the state of nursing education and training resulting in a 500-page document. Josephine Goldmark, social worker and author of the pioneering research of nursing preparation in the United States, stated,

From our field study of the nurse in public health nursing, in private duty, and as instructor and supervisor in hospitals, it is clear that there is need of a basic undergraduate training for all nurses alike, which should lead to a nursing diploma. (Goldmark, 1923, p. 35)

The first university school of nursing was developed at the University of Minnesota in 1909. Although the new nurse training school was under the college of medicine and offered only a 3-year diploma, the Minnesota program was nevertheless a significant leap forward in nursing education. *Nursing for the Future* or the **Brown Report**, authored by Esther Lucille Brown in 1948 and sponsored by the Russell Sage Foundation, was critical of the quality and structure of nursing schools in the United States. The Brown Report became the catalyst for the implementation of educational nursing program accreditation through the National League for Nursing (NLN) (Brown, 1936, 1948). As a result of the post-World War II nursing shortage, an Associate Degree in Nursing (ADN) was established by Dr. Mildred Montag in 1952 as a 2-year program for registered nurses (Montag, 1959). In 1950, nursing became the first profession for which the same licensure exam, the State Board Test Pool, was used throughout the nation to license registered nurses. This increased mobility for the registered nurse resulted in a significant advantage for the relatively new profession of nursing (Board Test Pool Examination, 1952).

The Evolution of Nursing in the United States: The First Century of Professional Nursing

The Profession of Nursing Is Born in the United States

Early nurse leaders of the 20th century included **Isabel Hampton Robb**, who in 1896 founded the Nurses' Associated Alumnae, which in 1911 officially became known as the **American Nurses Association (ANA)**; and **Lavinia Lloyd Dock**, who became a militant suffragist linking women's roles as nurses to the emerging women's movement in the United States.

Mary Adelaide Nutting, Lavinia L. Dock, Sophia Palmer, and Mary E. Davis were instrumental in developing the first nursing journal, the *American Journal of Nursing (AJN)* in October of 1900. Through the ANA and the *AJN*, nurses then had a professional organization and a national journal with which to communicate with each other (Kalisch & Kalisch, 1986).

State licensure of trained nurses began in 1903 with the enactment of North Carolina's licensure law for nursing. Shortly thereafter, New Jersey, New York, and Virginia passed similar licensure laws for nursing. Over the next several years, professional nursing was well on its way to public recognition of practice and educational standards as state after state passed similar legislation.

Margaret Sanger worked as a nurse on the Lower East Side of New York City in 1912 with immigrant families. She was astonished to find widespread ignorance among these families about conception, pregnancy, and childbirth. After a horrifying experience with the death of a woman from a failed self-induced abortion, Sanger devoted her life to teaching women about birth control. A staunch activist in the early family planning movement, Sanger is credited with founding Planned Parenthood of America (Sanger, 1928).

The emerging new profession saw two significant events that propelled the need for additional trained nurses in the United States: World War I and the influenza epidemic.

By 1917, the emerging new profession saw two significant events that propelled the need for additional trained nurses in the United States: World War I and the influenza epidemic. Nightingale and the devastation of the Civil War had well established the need for nursing care in wartime. Mary Adelaide Nutting, now Professor of Nursing and Health at Columbia University, chaired the newly established Committee on Nursing in response to the need for nurses as the United States entered the war in Europe. Nurses in the United States realized early that World War I was unlike previous wars. It was a global conflict that involved coalitions of nations against nations involving vast amounts of supplies and demanding the organization of all the nations' resources for military purposes (Kalisch & Kalisch, 1986). Along with Lillian Wald and **Jane A. Delano**, Director of Nursing in the American Red Cross, Nutting initiated a national publicity campaign to recruit young women to enter nurses' training. The Army School of Nursing, headed by **Annie Goodrich** as Dean, and the Vassar Training Camp for Nurses prepared nurses for the war as well as home nursing and hygiene nursing through the Red Cross (Dock & Stewart, 1931). The committee estimated that there were at the most about 200,000 active "nurses" in the United States, both trained and untrained, which was inadequate for the military effort abroad (Kalisch & Kalisch, 1986).

At home, the influenza epidemic of 1917 to 1919 led to increased public awareness of the need for public health nursing and public education about hygiene and disease prevention. The successful campaign to attract nursing students focused heavily on patriotism, which ushered in the new era for nursing as a profession. By 1918, nursing school enrollments were up by 25%. In 1920, Congress passed a bill that provided nurses with military rank (Dock & Stewart, 1931). Following close behind, the passage of the Nineteenth Amendment to the US Constitution granted women the right to vote. According to Stewart in 1921:

> Probably the greatest contribution of the war experience to nursing lies in the fact that the whole system of nursing education was shaken for a little while out of its well-worn ruts and brought out of its comparative seclusion into the light of public discussion and criticism. When so many lives hung on the supply of nurses, people were aroused to a new sense of their dependence on the products of nursing schools, and many of them learned for the first time of the hopelessly limited resources which nursing educators have had to work with in the training of these indispensable public servants. Whatever the future may bring, it is unlikely that nursing schools will willingly sink back

again into their old isolation or that they will accept unquestionably the financial status which the older system imposed on them. (Stewart, 1918, p. 6)

The Emergence of Community and Public Health Nursing

The pattern for health visiting and district nursing practice outside the hospital was similar in the United States to that in England (Roberts, 1954). American cities were besieged by overcrowding and epidemics after the Civil War. The need for trained nurses evolved as in England, and schools throughout the United States developed along the Nightingale model. Visiting nurses were first sent to philanthropic organizations in New York City (1877), Boston (1886), Buffalo (1885), and Philadelphia (1886) to care for the sick at home. By the end of the century, most large cities had some form of visiting nursing program, and some headway was being made even in smaller towns (Heinrich, 1983). Industrial or occupational health nursing was first started in Vermont in 1895 by a marble company interested in the health and welfare of its workers and their families. Tuberculosis (TB) was a leading cause of death in the 1800s; nurses visited patients bedridden from TB and instructed persons in all settings about prevention of the disease (Abel, 1997).

Lillian Wald, Public Health Nursing, and Community Activism

Lillian Wald, a wealthy young woman with a great social conscience, graduated from the New York Hospital School of Nursing in 1891 and is credited with creating the title "public health nurse." After a year working in a mental institution, Wald entered medical school at Woman's Medical College in New York. While in medical school, she was asked to visit immigrant mothers on New York's Lower East Side and instruct them on health matters. Wald was appalled by the conditions there. During one now famous home visit, a small child asked Wald to visit her sick mother. And the rest, as they say, is history (Box 1-1).

What Wald found changed her life forever and secured a place for her in American nursing history. Wald said, "All the maladjustments of our social and economic relations seemed epitomized in this brief journey" (1915, p. 6). Wald was profoundly affected by her observations; she and her colleague, **Mary Brewster**, quickly established the Henry Street Settlement in this same neighborhood in 1893. She quit medical school and devoted the remainder of her life to "visions of a better world" for the public's health. According to Wald, "Nursing is love in action, and there is no finer manifestation of it than the care of the poor and disabled in their own homes" (Wald, 1915, p. 14).

The **Henry Street Settlement** was an independent nursing service where Wald lived and worked. This later became the Visiting Nurse Association of New York City, which laid the foundation for the establishment of public health nursing in the United States. The health needs of the population were met through addressing social, economic, and environmental determinants of health, in a pattern after

BOX 1-1   LILLIAN WALD TAKES A WALK

From the schoolroom where I had been giving a lesson in bed-making, a little girl led me one drizzling March morning. She had told me of her sick mother, and gathering from her incoherent account that a child had been born, I caught up the paraphernalia of the bed-making lesson and carried it with me.

The child led me over broken roadways ... between tall, reeking houses whose laden fire-escapes, useless for their appointed purpose, bulged with household goods of every description. The rain added to the dismal appearance of the streets and to the discomfort of the crowds which thronged them, intensifying the odors which assailed me from every side. Through Hester and Division Streets we went to the end of Ludlow; past odorous fish-stands, for the streets were a market-place, unregulated, unsupervised, unclean; past evil-smelling, uncovered garbage cans . . .

All the maladjustments of our social and economic relations seemed epitomized in this brief journey and what was found at the end of it. The family to which the child led me was neither criminal nor vicious. Although the husband was a cripple, one of those who stand on street corners exhibiting deformities to enlist compassion, and masking the begging of alms by a pretense of selling; although the family of seven shared their two rooms with boarders—who were literally boarders, since a piece of timber was placed over the floor for them to sleep on—and although the sick woman lay on a wretched, unclean bed, soiled with a hemorrhage two days old, they were not degraded human beings, judged by any measure of moral values.

In fact, it was very plain that they were sensitive to their condition, and when, at the end of my ministrations, they kissed my hands (those who have undergone similar experiences will, I am sure, understand), it would have been some solace if by any conviction of the moral unworthiness of the family I could have defended myself as a part of a society which permitted such conditions to exist. Indeed, my subsequent acquaintance with them revealed the fact that miserable as their state was, they were not without ideals for the family life, and for society, of which they were so unloved and unlovely a part.

That morning's experience was a baptism of fire. Deserted were the laboratory and the academic work of the college. I never returned to them. On my way from the sick-room to my comfortable student quarters my mind was intent on my own responsibility. To my inexperience it seemed certain that conditions such as these were allowed because people did not know, and for me there was a challenge to know and to tell. When early morning found me still awake, my naive conviction remained that, if people knew things—and "things" meant everything implied in the condition of this family—such horrors would cease to exist, and I rejoiced that I had a training in the care of the sick that in itself would give me an organic relationship to the neighborhood in which this awakening had come.

Source: Wald, L. D. (1915). *The House on Henry Street.* New York: Henry Holt and Company.

Nightingale. These nurses helped educate families about disease transmission and emphasized the importance of good hygiene. They provided preventive, acute, and long-term care. As such, Henry Street went far beyond the care of the sick and the prevention of illness: It aimed at rectifying those causes that led to the poverty and misery. Wald was a tireless social activist for legislative reforms that would provide a more just distribution of services for the marginal and disadvantaged in the United States (Donahue, 1985). Wald began with 10 nurses in 1893, which grew to 250 nurses serving 1300 clients a day by 1916. During this same period, the budget grew from nothing to more than $600,000 a year, all from private donations.

Wald hired African-American nurse **Elizabeth Tyler** in 1906 as evidence of her commitment to cultural diversity. Although unable to visit white clients, Tyler made her own way by "finding" African-American families who needed her service. In 3 months, Tyler had so many African-American families within her case-load that Wald hired a second African-American nurse, Edith Carter. Carter remained at Henry Street for 28 years until her retirement (Carnegie, 1991). During her tenure at Henry Street, Wald demonstrated her commitment to racial and cultural diversity by employing 25 African-American nurses over the years, and she paid them salaries equal to white nurses and provided identical benefits and recognition to minority nurses (Carnegie, 1991). This was exceptional during the early part of the 1900s, a time when African-American nurses were often denied admission to white schools of nursing and membership in professional organizations and were denied opportunities for employment in most settings. Because hospitals of this era often set quotas for African-American clients, those nurses who managed to graduate from nursing schools found themselves with few clients who needed or could afford their services. African-American nurses struggled for the right to take the registration examination available for white nurses.

Wald submitted a proposal to the city of New York after learning of a child's dismissal from a New York City school for a skin condition. Her proposal was for one of the Henry Street Settlement nurses to serve free for 1 month in a New York school. The results of her experiment were so convincing that salaries were approved for 12 school nurses. From this, school nursing was born in the United States and became one of many community specialties credited to Wald (Dietz & Lehozky, 1963). In 1909, Wald proposed a program to the Metropolitan Life Insurance Company to provide nursing visits to their industrial policyholders. Statistics kept by the company documented the lowered mortality rates of policyholders attributed to the nurses' public health practice and clinical expertise. The program demonstrated savings for the company and was so successful that it lasted until 1953 (Hamilton, 1988).

Wald's other significant accomplishments include the establishment of the Children's Bureau, set up in 1912 as part of the US Department of Labor. She also was an enthusiastic supporter of and participant in women's suffrage, lobbied for inspections of the workplace, and supported her employee, Margaret Sanger, in her efforts to give women the right to birth control. She was active in the American and International Red Cross and helped form the Women's Trade Union League to protect women from sweatshop conditions.

Wald first coined the phrase "public health nursing" and transformed the field of community health nursing from the narrow role of home visiting to the population focus of today's community health nurse (Robinson, 1946). According to Dock and Stewart (1931), the title of public health nurse was purposeful: The role designation was designed to link the public's health to governmental responsibility, not private funding. As state departments of health and local governments began to employ more and more public health nurses, their role increasingly focused on prevention of illness in the entire community. Discrimination developed between the visiting nurse, who was employed by the voluntary agencies primarily to provide home care to the sick, and the public health nurse, who concentrated on preventive measures (Brainard, 1922). Early public health nurses came closer than hospital-based nurses to the autonomy and professionalism that Nightingale advocated. Their work was conducted in the unconfined setting of the home and community, they were independent, and they enjoyed recognition as specialists in preventive health (Buhler-Wilkerson, 1985). Public health nurses from the beginning were much more holistic in their practice than their hospital counterparts. They were involved with the health of industrial workers, immigrants, and their families, and were concerned about exploitation of women and children. These nurses also played a part in prison reform and care of the mentally ill (Heinrich, 1983).

Considered the first African-American public health nurse, **Jessie Sleet Scales** was hired in 1902 by the Charity Organization Society, a philanthropic organization, to visit African-American families infected by TB. Scales provided district nursing care to New York City's African-American families and is credited with paving the way for African-American nurses in the practice of community health (Mosley, 1996).

Dorothea Linde Dix

Dorothea Linde Dix, a Boston schoolteacher, became aware of the horrendous conditions in prisons and mental institutions when asked to do a Sunday school class in the House of Correction at Cambridge, Massachusetts. She was appalled at what she saw and went about studying if the conditions were isolated or widespread; she took 2 years off to visit every jail and almshouse from Cape Cod to Berkshire (Tiffany, 1890, p. 76). Her report was devastating. Boston was scandalized by the reality that the most progressive state in the Union was now associated with such appalling conditions. The shocked legislature voted to allocate funds to build hospitals. For the rest of her life, Dorothea Dix stood out as a tireless zealot for the humane treatment of the insane and imprisoned. She had exceptional savvy in dealing with legislators. She acquainted herself with the legislators and their records and displayed the "spirit of a crusader." For her contributions, Dix is recognized as one of the pioneers of the reform movement for mental health in the United States, and her efforts are felt worldwide to the present day (Dietz & Lehozky, 1963).

Dix was also known for her work in the Civil War, having been appointed super-intendent of the female nurses of the Army by the secretary of war in 1861. Her tire-less efforts led to the recruitment of more than 2000 women to serve in the army during the Civil War. Officials had consulted with Nightingale concerning military hospitals and were determined not to make the same mistakes. Dix enjoyed far more sweeping powers than Nightingale in that she had the authority to organize hospitals, to appoint nurses, and to manage supplies for the wounded (Brockett & Vaughan, 1867). Among her most well-known nurses during the Civil War were the poet Walt Whitman and the author Louisa May Alcott (Donahue, 1985).

Clara Barton

The idea for the International Red Cross was the brainchild of a Swiss banker, J. Henri Dunant, who proposed the formation of a neutral international relief soci-ety that could be activated in time of war. The International Red Cross was ratified by the Geneva Convention on August 22, 1864. **Clara Barton**, through her work in the Civil War, had come to believe that such an organization was desperately needed in the United States. However, it was not until 1882 that Barton was able to convince Congress to ratify the Treaty of Geneva, thus becoming the founder of the American Red Cross (Kalisch & Kalisch, 1986). Barton also played a leadership role in the Spanish-American War in Cuba, where she led a group of nurses to provide care for both US and Cuban soldiers and Cuban civilians. At the age of 76, Barton went to President McKinley and offered the help of the Red Cross in Cuba. The President agreed to allow Barton to go with Red Cross nurses, but only to care for the Cuban citizens. Once in Cuba, the US military saw what Barton and her nurses were able to accomplish with the Cuban military, and American soldiers pressured military officials to allow Barton's help. Along with battling yellow fever, Barton was able to provide care to both Cuban and US military personnel and eventually expanded that care to Cuban citizens in Santiago. One of Barton's most famous clients was young Colonel Teddy Roosevelt, who led his Rough Riders and who later became the president of the United States. Barton became an instant heroine both in Cuba and in the United States for her bravery, tenaciousness, and for orga-nizing services for the military and civilians torn apart by war. On August 13, 1898, the Spanish-American War came to an end. The grateful people of Santiago, Cuba, built a statue to honor Clara Barton in the town square, where it stands to this day. The work of Barton and her Red Cross nurses spread through the newspapers of the United States and in the schools of nursing. A congressional committee inves-tigating the work of Barton's Red Cross staff applauded the work of these nurses and recommended that the US Medical Department create a permanent reserve corps of trained nurses. These reserve nurses became the Army Nurse Corps in

1901. Clara Barton will always be remembered both as the founder of the American Red Cross and the driving force behind the creation of the Army Nurse Corps (Frantz, 1998).

Birth of the Midwife in the United States

Women have always assisted other women in the birth of babies. These "lay midwives" were considered by communities to possess special skills and somewhat of a "calling." With the advent of professional nursing in England, registered nurses became associated with safer and more predictable childbirth practices. In England and in other countries where Nightingale nurses were prevalent, most registered nurses were also trained as midwives with a 6-month specialized training period. In the United States, the training of registered nurses in the practice of midwifery was prevented primarily by physicians. US physicians saw midwives as a threat and intrusion into medical practice. Such resistance indirectly led to the proliferation of "granny wives" who were ignorant of modern practices, were untrained, and were associated with high maternal morbidity (Donahue, 1985).

The first organized midwifery service in the United States was the **Frontier Nursing Service** founded in 1925 by **Mary Breckenridge**. Breckenridge graduated from the St. Luke's Hospital Training School in New York in 1910 and received her midwifery certificate from the British Hospital for Mothers and Babies in London in 1925. She had extensive experience in the delivery of babies and midwifery systems in New Zealand and Australia. In rural Appalachia, babies had been delivered for decades by granny midwives, who relied mainly on tradition, myths, and superstition as the bases of their practice. For example, they might use ashes for medication and place a sharp axe, blade up, under the bed of a laboring woman to "cut" the pain. The people of Appalachia were isolated because of the terrain of the hollows and mountains, and roads were limited to most families. They had one of the highest birth rates in the United States. Breckenridge believed that if a midwifery service could work under these conditions, it could work anywhere (Donahue, 1985).

Breckenridge had to use English midwives for many years and only began training her own midwives in 1939 when she started the Frontier Graduate School of Nurse Midwifery in Hyden, Kentucky, with the advent of World War II. The nurse midwives accessed many of their families on horseback. In 1935, a small 12-bed hospital was built at Hyden and provided delivery services. The nurse midwives under the direction of Breckenridge were successful in lowering the highest maternal mortality rate in the United States (in Leslie County, Kentucky) to substantially below the national average. These nurses, as at Henry Street Settlement, provided health care for everyone in the district for a small annual fee. A delivery had an additional small fee. Nurse midwives provided primary care, prenatal care, and postnatal care, with an emphasis on prevention (Wertz & Wertz, 1977).

Armed with the right to vote, the Roaring Twenties ushered American women into the new freedom of the "flapper era"—shrinking dress hemlines, shortened hairstyles, and the increased use of cosmetics. Hospitals were used by greater numbers of people, and the scientific basis of medicine became well established as most surgical procedures were done in hospitals. Penicillin was discovered in 1928, creating a revolution in the prevention of infectious disease deaths (Kalisch & Kalisch, 1986; Donahue, 1985). The previously mentioned Goldmark Report recommended the establishment of college- and university-based nursing programs.

Mary D. Osborne, who functioned as supervisor of public health nursing for the state of Mississippi from 1921 to 1946, had a vision for a collaboration with community nurses and granny midwives, who delivered 80% of the African-American babies in Mississippi. The infant and maternal mortality rates were both exceptionally high among African-American families, and these granny midwives, who were also African-American, were untrained and had little education.

Osborne took a creative approach to improving maternal and infant health among African-American women. She developed a collaborative network of public health nurses and granny midwives in which the nurses implemented training programs for the midwives, and the midwives in turn assisted the nurses in providing a higher standard of safe maternal and infant health care. The public health nurses used Osborne's book, *Manual for Midwives,* which contained guidelines for care and was used in the state until the 1970s. They taught good hygiene, infection prevention, and compliance with state regulations. Osborne's innovative program is credited with reducing the maternal and infant mortality rates in Mississippi and in other states where her program structure was adopted (Sabin, 1998).

The Nursing Profession Responds to the Great Depression and World War II

With the stock market crash of 1929 came the Great Depression resulting in widespread unemployment of private duty nurses, the closing of nursing schools while simultaneously creating the increasing need for charity health services for the population. Nursing students who had previously been the primary source to staff hospitals declined. Unemployed graduate nurses were hired to replace them for minimal wages, a trend which was to influence the profession for years to come (MacEachern, 1932). Other nurses found themselves accompanying troops to Europe as the United States entered World War II. Military nurses were a critical presence at the invasion of Normandy in 1938, as well as in North Africa, Italy, France, and the Philippines, while Navy nurses provided care aboard hospital ships. Over 100,000 nurses volunteered and were certified for military service in the Army and Navy Nurse Corps. The resulting severe shortage of nurses on the home front resulted in the development of the **Cadet Nurse Corps. Frances Payne Bolton**, congressional representative from Ohio, is credited with the founding of the Cadet Nurse Corps through the Bolton Act of 1945. By the end of the war, over 180,000 nursing students had been trained through this act, while advanced practice graduate nurses in psychiatry and public health nursing had received graduate education to increase the numbers of nurse educators (Kalisch & Kalisch, 1986; Donahue, 1985). Ernie Pyle, a famous war correspondent in World War II, offered Americans a "front-seat view" through his detailed journalistic accounts of daily life on the war front. Pyle was the first journalist who put his own life in danger by reporting from the battlefront; he spent a great deal of time with soldiers during active combat and was killed during a sniper attack in Ie Shima, Japan. Chaplin Nathan Baxter Saucier was assigned to retrieve his body, conduct his service, and assist the soldiers with building his coffin. The funeral service lasted only about 10 minutes. Pyle was buried with his helmet on, at Chaplin Saucier's request. The Navy, Marine Corps, and Army were all represented at the service. Pyle, who died during the Battle of Okinawa in 1945, was a highly regarded and humanistic voice for those serving America during World War II. Here is an example of Pyle's accounts of life for nurses in a field hospital in Europe:

> The officers and nurses live two in a tent on two sides of a company street—nurses on one side, officers on the other. . . . The nurses wear khaki overalls because of the mud and dust. Pink female panties fly from a line among the brown warlike tents. On the flagpole is a Red Cross flag made from a bed sheet and a French soldier's red sash. The American nurses—and there were lots of them turned out just as you would expect: wonderfully. Army doctors and patients too were unanimous in their praise of them. Doctors told me that in the first rush of casualties they were calmer than the men. For the first ten days they had to live like animals, even using open ditches for toilets but they never complained. One nurse was always on duty in each tentful of 20 men. She had medical orderlies to help her. The touch of femininity, the knowledge that a woman was around, gave the wounded man courage and confidence and a feeling of security. (Pyle, 1942)

During the midst of the Depression, many nurses found the expansion and advances in aviation as a new field for nurses. In efforts to increase the public's confidence in the safety of transcontinental air travel, nurses were hired in the promising new role of "nurse-stewardess" (Kalisch & Kalisch, 1986). Congress created an additional relief program, the Civil Works Administration (CWA), in 1933 that provided jobs to the unemployed, including placing nurses in schools, public hospitals and clinics, public health departments, and public health education community surveys and campaigns. The Social Security Act of 1935 was passed by Congress to provide old-age benefits, rehabilitation services, unemployment compensation administration, aid to dependent and/or disabled children and adults, and monies to state and local health services. The Social Security Act included Title VI, which authorized the use of federal funds for the training of public health personnel. This led to the placement of public health nurses in state health departments and the expansion of public health nursing as a viable career path. While nursing was forging new paths for itself in various fields, Hollywood began featuring nurses in films during the 1930s. The only feature-length films to ever focus entirely on the nursing profession were released during this decade. *War Nurse* (1930), *Night Nurse* (1931), *Once to Every Woman* (1934), *The White Parade* (1934 Academy Award nominee for Best Picture), *Four Girls in White* (1939), *The White Angel* (1936), and *Doctor and Nurse* (1937) all used nurses as major characters. During the bleak years of the economic depression, young women found these nurse heroines who promoted idealism, self-sacrifice, and the profession of nursing over personal desires particularly appealing. No longer were nurses depicted as subservient handmaidens who worked as nurses only as a temporary pastime before marriage (Kalisch & Kalisch, 1986).

Science and Health Care, 1945–1960: Decades of Change

Dramatic technological and scientific changes characterized the decades following World War II, including the discovery of sulfa drugs, new cardiac drugs, surgeries, and treatment for ventricular fibrillation (Howell, 1996). The Hill Burton Act passed in 1946 provided funds to increase the construction of new hospitals. A significant change in the healthcare system was the expansion of private health insurance coverage and the dramatic increase in the birth rate, coined the "baby boom" generation. Clinical research, both in medicine and in nursing, became an expectation of health providers and more nurses sought advanced degrees. The *Journal of Nursing Research* was first published, heralding the arrival of nursing scholarship in the United States. Due to increased numbers of hospital beds, additional financial resources for health care, and the post–World War II economic resurgence, nursing faced an acute shortage and nurses faced increasingly stressful working conditions. Nurses began showing signs of the strain through debates about strikes and collective bargaining demands. The American Nurses Association (ANA) accepted African-American nurses for membership, consequently ending racial discrimination in the dominant nursing organizations. The National Association of Colored Graduate Nurses was disbanded in 1951. Males entered nursing schools in record number, often as a result of previous military experience as medics. Prior to the 1950s and 1960s, male nurses also suffered minority status and were discouraged from nursing as a career. Seemingly forgotten by modern society, including Florence Nightingale and early US nursing leaders, more than one-half of the nurses were male during medieval times. The Knights Hospitalers, Teutonic Knights, Franciscans, and many other male nursing orders had provided excellent nursing care for their societies. Saint Vincent de Paul had first conceived of the idea of social service. Pastor Theodor Fliedner, teacher and mentor of Florence Nightingale at Kaiserwerth in Germany; Ben Franklin; and Walt Whitman during the Civil War all either served as nurses or were strong advocates for male nurses (Kalisch & Kalisch, 1986).

> Dramatic technological and scientific changes characterized the decades following World War II, including the discovery of sulfa drugs, new cardiac drugs, surgeries, and treatment for ventricular fibrillation.

Years of Revolution, Protest, and the New Order, 1961–2000

During the social upheaval of the 1960s, nursing was influenced by many changes in society, such as the women's movement, the organized protest against the Vietnam conflict, civil rights movement, President Lyndon Johnson's "Great Society" social reforms, and increased consumer involvement in health care. Specialization in nursing, such as cardiac ICU, nurse anesthetist training, and the clinical specialist role for nursing became trends that affected both education and practice in the healthcare system. Medicare and Medicaid, enacted in 1965 under Title XVIII of the Social Security Act, provided access to health care for the elderly, the poor, and disabled. The American Nurses Association took a courageous and controversial stand in that same year (1965) by approving its first position paper on nursing education, advocating for all nursing education for professional practice to take place in colleges and universities (American Nursing Association, 1965). Nurses returning from Vietnam faced emotional challenges through the recognition of post-traumatic stress disorder (PTSD) affecting their postwar lives.

With increased specialization in medicine, the demand for primary care healthcare providers exceeded the supply (Christman, 1971). As a response to this need for general practitioners, Dr. Henry Silver (MD) and Dr. Loretta Ford (RN) collaborated to develop the first nurse practitioner program in the United States at the University of Colorado (Ford & Silver, 1967). Nurse practitioners (NPs) were initially prepared in pediatrics with advanced role preparation in common childhood illness management and well-child care. Ford and Silver (1967) found that NPs could manage as much as 75% of the pediatric patients in community clinics, leading to the widespread use of and educational programs for nurse practitioners. The first state in 1971 to recognize diagnosis and treatment as part of the legal scope of practice for NPs was Idaho. Alaska and North Carolina were among the first states to expand the NP role to include prescriptive authority (Ford, 1979). By the new century, nurse practitioner programs were offered at the MSN level in family nursing; gerontology; adult, neonatal, mental health, and maternal-child areas and have expanded to include the acute care practitioner as well (Huch, 2001). Certification of nurse practitioners now occurs at the national level through the American Nurses Association, by many specialty organizations, and NPs are licensed throughout the United States by state boards of nursing.

Escalating healthcare costs resulting from the explosion of advanced technology and the increased life span of Americans led to the demand for healthcare reform in the late 1980s. The nursing profession heralded healthcare reform with an unprecedented collaboration of more than 75 nursing associations, led by the American Nurses Association and the National League for Nursing, in the publication of *Nursing's Agenda for Health Care Reform*. In this document, the challenge of managed care was addressed in the context of cost containment and quality assurance of healthcare service for the nursing profession (American Nurses Association, 1991).

Managed care is a market approach based on managed competition as a major strategy to contain healthcare costs, which is still the dominant approach today (Lundy, Janes, & Hartman, 2001).

The New Century: An Era of Managed Care

The Institute of Medicine's (IOM) report *The Future of the Public's Health in the 21st Century* (2003) builds upon the 1988 report and is anticipated to have a major impact on health policy development. There are several specific recommendations contained within the report on strengthening the relationship between the vital sectors charged with protecting the public's health. The report proposes an ecological model upon which to base health professional education, including nursing, clinical activities, and research with a population focus. Multiple determinants of health form the basis for an ecological model, which operates on the assumption that health is affected on several levels by these factors. Since nursing comprises the largest single workforce within the health system, the report recommendations and the potential use of an ecological model for a population-focused practice have significant potential for creating new paths in nursing practice, education, and research. A companion study, *Who Will Keep the Public Healthy?*, builds upon an ecological model and considers factors likely to affect public health in this century such as globalization, technological and scientific advances, and demographic shifts in the US population.

Although healthcare reform continues to be debated, it is unlikely that there will be significant changes at the national level in the immediate future. The US healthcare system today continues to focus on federal coverage, access, and controlling healthcare costs. Healthcare organizations in a managed care environment, such as preferred provider organizations (PPOs) and health maintenance organizations (HMOs), now see the economic and quality outcome benefits of caring for patients and managing their care over a continuum of possible settings and needs. Patients are followed more closely within the system, both during illness and wellness. Hospital stays are shorter, and more and more healthcare services are being provided in outpatient facilities and through community-based settings, such as home health, occupational health, and school health (Lundy, Janes, & Hartman, 2008).

> **CRITICAL THINKING QUESTION**
>
> What do you think would be the response of historical nursing leaders such as Florence Nightingale, Lillian Wald, or Mary Breckinridge if they could see what the profession of nursing looks like today?

Conclusion

Since September 11, 2001, terrorism is a constant threat to our nation and to the global community. War, bioterrorism, and emerging epidemics are just some of the challenges for today's nurses. Hurricane Katrina further reminded us of our inadequate disaster and public health resources for vulnerable populations. Although Hurricane Katrina hit the Mississippi Gulf Coast and New Orleans,

Louisiana, in August of 2005, populations in those areas continue to face serious health consequences from inadequate economic and social resources. Although billions have been spent to date on the recovery, health officials predict at least a decade of unmet population needs.

Consensus regarding basic education and the entry level of registered nurses has not occurred. Changes in the advanced practice role will challenge the educational and healthcare system as the primary healthcare needs of the US population compete with acute care for scarce resources. Relating to the global community as well as our own diverse population demands that nurses remain committed to cultural sensitivity in care delivery.

The history of health care and nursing provides us with ample examples and the wisdom of our forbears in the advocacy of nursing in these challenging settings and the unknown future. Nurses today, by considering the lessons of the past, find a profession well prepared to provide care with the direction needed to focus on providing the full range of quality, cost-effective services in the promotion of health throughout this century.

CLASSROOM ACTIVITY 1

There have been many theories about the cause of Nightingale's chronic illness, which led her to being an invalid for most of her adult life. Many people have interpreted this as hypochondriacal, something of a melodrama of the Victorian times. Nightingale was rich and could take to her bed. Rumors have floated around among nursing students for years that she suffered from tertiary syphilis. She became ill during the Crimean War in May of 1855 and was diagnosed with a severe case of Crimean fever. Today Crimean fever is recognized as Mediterranean fever and is categorized as brucellosis. She developed spondylitis, or inflammation of the spine. For the next 34 years, she managed to continue her writing and advocacy, often predicting her imminent death. Even others have claimed that she suffered from a bipolar disorder, causing her to experience long periods of depression and remarkable bursts of productivity. Read about the various theories of her chronic disabling condition and reflect on your own conclusions about her mysterious illness. Based on supporting evidence, what are your conclusions about Nightingale's health condition?

Sources: Dossey, B. (2000). *Florence Nightingale: Mystic, visionary, healer.* Philadelphia: Lippincott, Williams & Wilkins. Nightingale suffered bipolar disorder. (2004). *Australian Nursing Journal, 12,* 2.

CLASSROOM ACTIVITY 2

What would Florence Nightingale's résumé or vita look like?
Check out Nightingale's vita at http://www.countryjoe.com/nightingale/cv.htm.

References

Abel, E. K. (1997). Take the cure to the poor: Patients' responses to New York City's tuberculosis program, 1894–1918. *American Journal of Public Health, 87,* 11.

American Nurses Association. (1965). *Educational preparation for nurse practitioners and assistants to nurses: A position paper.* New York: Author.

American Nurses Association. (1991). *Nursing's agenda for health care reform: Executive summary.* Washington, DC: Author.

Andrews, G. (2003). Nightingale's geography. *Nursing Inquiry, 10*(4), 270–274.

Attewell, A. (1996). Florence Nightingale's health-at-home visitors. *Health Visitor, 6.9*(10), 406.

Barker, E. R. (1989). Care givers as casualties. *Western Journal of Nursing Research, 11*(5), 628–631.

Boorstin, D. J. (1985). *The discoverers: A history of man's search to know his world and himself.* New York: Vintage.

Brainard, A. M. (1922). *The evolution of public health nursing.* Philadelphia: W. B. Saunders.

Brockett, L. P., & Vaughan, M. C. (1867). *Women's work in the Civil War: A record of heroism: Patriotism and patience.* Philadelphia: Seigler McCurdy.

Brooke, E. (1997). *Medicine women: A pictorial history of women healers.* Wheaton, IL: Quest Books.

Brown, E. L. (1936). *Nursing as a profession.* New York: Russell Sage Foundation.

Brown, E. L. (1948). *Nursing for the future.* New York: Russell Sage Foundation.

Brown, P. (1988). *Florence Nightingale.* Hats, UK: Exley Publications.

Buhler-Wilkerson, K. (1985). Public health nursing: In sickness or in health? *American Journal of Public Health, 75,* 1155–1156.

Bullough, V. L., & Bullough, B. (1978). *The care of the sick: The emergence of modern nursing.* New York: Prodist.

Calabria, M. D. (1996). *Florence Nightingale in Egypt and Greece: Her diary and visions.* Albany: State University of New York Press.

Carnegie, M. E. (1991). *The path we tread: Blades in nursing 1854–1990* (2nd ed.). New York: National League for Nursing Press.

Cartwright, F. F. (1972). *Disease and history.* New York: Dorset Press.

Christman, L. (1971). The nurse specialist as a professional activist. *Nursing Clinics of North America, 6*(2), 231–235.

Christy, T. E. (1975). The fateful decade: 1890–1900. *American Journal of Nursing, 75*(7), 1163–1165.

Cohen, M. N. (1989). *Health and the rise of civilization.* New Haven, CT: Yale University Press.

Cook, E. (1913). *The life of Florence Nightingale* (Vols. 1 and 2). London: Macmillan.

D'Antonio, P. (2002). Nurses in war. *Lancet, 360*(9350), 7–12.

Diamond, J. (1997). *Guns, germs, and steel: The fates of human societies.* New York: W. W. Norton.

Dickens, C. (1844). *Martin Chuzzlewit.* New York: Macmillan.

Dietz, D. D., & Lehozky, A. R. (1963). *History and modern nursing.* Philadelphia: F. A. Davis.

Dock, L., & Stewart, I. (1931). *A short history of nursing from the earliest times to the present day* (3rd ed.). New York: G. P. Putman's Sons.

Donahue, M. P. (1985). *Nursing: The finest art.* St. Louis: Mosby.

Dossey, B. M. (1999). *Florence Nightingale: Mystic, visionary, healer.* Springhouse, PA: Springhouse.

Ford, L. C. (1979). A nurse for all seasons: The nurse practitioner. *Nursing Outlook, 27*(8), 516–521.

Ford, L. C., & Silver, H. K. (1967). The expanded role of the nurse in child care. *Nursing Outlook, 15*(8), 43–45.

Frantz, A. K. (1998). Nursing pride: Clara Barton in the Spanish American War. *American Journal of Nursing, 98*(10), 39–41.

Goldmark, J. C. (1923). *Nursing and nursing education in the United States.* New York: Macmillan.

Hamilton, D. (1988). Clinical excellence, but too high a cost: The Metropolitan Life Insurance Company Visiting Nurse Service (1909–1953). *Public Health Nursing, 5,* 235–240.

Hanlon, J. J., & Pickett, G. E. (1984). *Public health administration and practice* (8th ed.). St. Louis: Mosby.

Heinrich, J. (1983). Historical perspectives on public health nursing. *Nursing Outlook, 32*(6), 317–320.

Hine, D. C. (1989). *Black women in white: Racial conflict and cooperation in the nursing profession 1889–1950.* Bloomington: Indiana University Press.

Howell, J. (1996). *Technology in the hospital.* Baltimore, MD: Johns Hopkins University Press.

Huch, M. (2001). Advanced practice nursing in the community. In K. S. Lundy & S. Janes (Eds.), *Community health nursing: Caring for the public's health* (pp. 968–980). Sudbury, MA: Jones and Bartlett Publishers.

Institute of Medicine. (1988). *The future of public health.* Washington, DC: National Academy Press.

Institute of Medicine. (2003). *The future of the public's health in the 21st century.* Washington, DC: National Academy Press.

Kalisch, P. A., & Kalisch, B. J. (1986). *The advance of American nursing* (2nd ed.). Boston: Little, Brown.

LeVasseur, J. (1998). Plato: Nightingale and contemporary nursing. *Image: Journal of Nursing Scholarship, 30*(3), 281–285.

Longfellow, H. W. (1857). Santa Filomena. *Atlantic Monthly, 1,* 22–23.

Lundy, K. S., Janes, S., & Hartman, S. (2001). Opening the door to health care in the community. In K. S. Lundy & S. Janes (Eds.), *Community health nursing: Caring for the public's health* (pp. 5–29). Sudbury, MA: Jones and Bartlett.

MacEachern, M. T. (1932). Which shall we choose: Graduate or student service? *Modern Hospital, 38,* 97–98, 102–104.

Montag, M. L. (1959). *Community college education for nursing: An experiment in technical education for nursing.* New York: McGraw-Hill.

Monteiro, L. A. (1985). Florence Nightingale on public health nursing. *American Journal of Public Health, 75*(2), 181–185.

Mosley, M. O. P. (1996). Satisfied to carry the bag: Three black community health nurses' contribution to health care reform, 1900–1937. *Nursing History Review, 4,* 65–82.

Nightingale, F. (1860). *Notes on nursing: What it is and what it is not.* London: Harrison.

Nightingale, F. (1893). Sick-nursing and health-nursing. In B. Burdett-Coutts (Ed.), *Women's mission* (pp. 184–205). London: Sampson, Law, Marston and Co.

Nightingale, F. (1894). *Health teaching in towns and villages.* London: Spottiswoode & Co.

Nightingale, F. (1979). Cassandra. In M. Stark (Ed.), *Florence Nightingale's Cassandra.* Old Westbury, NY: Feminist Press.

Nutting, M. A., & Dock, L. L. (1907). *A history of nursing: The evolution of nursing systems from the earliest times to the foundation of the first English and American training schools for nurses.* New York: G. P. Putnam's Sons.

The 100 people who made the millennium. (1997). *Life Magazine, 20*(10a).

Palmer, I. S. (1977). Florence Nightingale: Reformer, reactionary, researcher. *Nursing Research, 26*(2), 13–18.

Palmer, I. S. (1982). *Through a glass darkly: From Nightingale to now.* Washington, DC: American Association of College of Nursing.

Pyle, E. (1944). *Here is your war: The story of G.I. Joe.* Cleveland, OH: World Publishing Co.

Rathbone, W. (1890). *A history of nursing in the homes of the poor.* Introduction by Florence Nightingale. London: Macmillan.

Richardson, B. I. W. (1887). *The health of nations: A review of the works of Edwin Chadwick* (Vol. 2). London: Longmans, Green and Company.

Roberts, M. (1954). *American nursing: History and interpretation.* New York: Macmillan.

Robinson, V. (1946). *White caps: The story of nursing.* Philadelphia: J. B. Lippincott.

Rosen, G. (1958). *A history of public health.* New York: M.D. Publications.

Sabin, L. (1998). *Struggles and triumphs: The story of Mississippi nurses 1800–1950.* Jackson: Mississippi Hospital Association Health, Research and Educational Foundation.

Sanger, M. (1928). *Motherhood in bondage.* New York: Brentano's.

Seymer, L. (1954). *Selected writings of Florence Nightingale.* New York: Macmillan.

Shryock, R. H. (1959). *The history of nursing: An interpretation of the social and medical factors involved.* Philadelphia: W. B. Saunders.

Smith, E. (1934). *Mississippi special public health nursing project made possible by federal funds.* Paper presented at the 1934 annual Mississippi Nurses Association meeting, Jackson, MS.

Snow, J. (1855). *On the mode of communication of cholera* (2nd ed.). London: Churchill Publishers.

Stanmore, A. H. G. (1906). *Sidney Herbert of Lea: A memoir.* New York: E. P. Dutton.

State board test pool examination. (1952). *American Journal of Nursing, 52,* 613.

Stewart, I. M. (1921). Developments in nursing education since 1918. *U.S. Bureau of Education Bulletin, 20*(6), 3–8.

Taylor, H. O. (1922). *Greek biology and medicine.* Boston: Marshall Jones.

Tiffany, R. (1890). *The life of Dorothea Linda Dix.* Boston: Houghton, Mifflin.

Tooley, S. A. (1910). *The life of Florence Nightingale.* London: Cassell and Co.

Tyrell, II. (1856). *Pictorial history of the war with Russia 1854–1856.* London: W. and R. Chambers.

Vicinus, M., & Nergaard, B. (1990). *Ever yours: Florence Nightingale: Selected letters.* Cambridge, MA: Harvard University Press.

Wald, L. D. (1915). *The house on Henry Street.* New York: Henry Holt.

Wertz, R. W., & Wertz, D. C. (1977). *Lying-in: A history of childbirth in America.* New Haven, CT: Yale University Press.

Wheeler, W. (1999). Is Florence Nightingale holding us back? *Nursing 99, 29*(10), 22–23.

Williams, C. B. (1961). Stories from Scutari. *American Journal of Nursing, 61,* 88.

Winslow, C.-E. A. (1946). Florence Nightingale and public health nursing. *Public Health Nursing, 38,* 330–332.

Woodham-Smith, C. (1951). *Florence Nightingale.* New York: McGraw-Hill.

Woodham-Smith, C. (1983). *Florence Nightingale.* New York: Athenaeum.

Young, D. A. (1995). Florence Nightingale's fever. *British Medical Journal, 311,* 1697–1700.

chapter 2

Framework for Professional Nursing Practice

Kathleen Masters

LEARNING OBJECTIVES

After completing this chapter, the student should be able to:
1. Identify the four metaparadigm concepts of nursing.
2. Identify and describe several theoretical works in nursing.
3. Begin the process of identifying theoretical frameworks of nursing that are consistent with a personal belief system.

Key Terms and Concepts

- Concept
- Conceptual model
- Propositions
- Assumptions
- Theory
- Metaparadigm
- Person
- Environment
- Health
- Nursing
- Philosophies

Although the beginning of nursing theory development can be traced to Florence Nightingale, it was not until the second half of the 1900s that nursing theory caught the attention of nursing as a discipline. During the decades of the 1960s and 1970s, theory development was a major topic of discussion and publication. During the 1970s, much of the discussion was related to the development of one global theory for nursing. However, in the 1980s, attention turned from the development of a global theory for nursing as scholars began to recognize multiple approaches to theory development in nursing.

Because of the plurality in nursing theory, this information must be organized in order to be meaningful for practice, research, and further knowledge development. The goal of this chapter is to present an organized and practical overview of the major concepts, models, philosophies, and theories that are essential in professional nursing practice.

It may be helpful to define some of the terms that are used that may be unfamiliar. A concept is a term or label that describes a phenomenon (Meleis, 2004). The phenomenon described by a **concept** may be either empirical or it may be abstract. An empirical concept is one that can be either observed or experienced through the senses. An abstract concept is one that is not observable, such as hope or caring (Hickman, 2002).

A **conceptual model** is defined as a set of concepts and statements that integrate the concepts into a meaningful configuration (Lippitt, 1973; as cited in Fawcett, 1994). **Propositions** are statements that describe relationships between events, situations, or actions (Meleis, 2004). **Assumptions** also describe concepts or connect two concepts and represent values, beliefs, or goals. When assumptions are challenged, they become propositions (Meleis, 2004).

Conceptual models are composed of abstract and general concepts and propositions that provide a frame of reference for members of a discipline. This frame of reference determines how the world is viewed by members of a discipline and guides the members as they propose questions and make observations relevant to the discipline (Fawcett, 1994).

"A **theory** is an organized, coherent, and systematic articulation of a set of statements related to significant questions in a discipline that are communicated in a meaningful whole" (Meleis, 2004). According to Fawcett (1994), "The primary distinction between a conceptual model and a theory is the level of abstraction. A conceptual model is a highly abstract system of global concepts and linking statements. A theory, in contrast, deals with one or more specific, concrete concepts and propositions."

A **metaparadigm** is the most global perspective of a discipline and "acts as an encapsulating unit, or framework, within which the more restricted . . . structures develop" (Eckberg & Hill, 1979, p. 927). Each discipline singles out phenomena of interest that it will deal with in a unique manner. The concepts and propositions that identify and interrelate these phenomena are even more abstract than those in the conceptual models. These are the concepts that comprise the metaparadigm of the discipline (Fawcett, 1994).

The conceptual models and theories of nursing represent various paradigms derived from the metaparadigm of the discipline of nursing. Therefore, although each of the conceptual models may link and define the four metaparadigm concepts differently, the four metaparadigm concepts are present in each of the models.

The central concepts of the discipline of nursing are **person**, **environment**, **health**, and **nursing**. These four concepts of the metaparadigm of nursing are more specifically, "The person receiving the nursing, the environment within which the person exits, the health-illness continuum within which the person falls at the time of the interaction with

The conceptual models and theories of nursing represent various paradigms derived from the metaparadigm of the discipline of nursing.

the nurse, and, finally, nursing actions themselves" (Flaskerud & Holloran, 1980, cited in Fawcett, 1994, p. 5).

Because concepts are so abstract at the metaparadigm level, many conceptual models have developed from the metaparadigm of nursing. Subsequently, multiple theories have been developed from each conceptual model in an effort to describe, explain, and predict the phenomena within the model.

Overview of Selected Nursing Theories

To apply nursing theory in practice, the nurse must have some knowledge of the theoretical works of the nursing profession. This chapter is not intended to provide an in-depth analysis of each of the theoretical works in nursing but rather to provide an introductory overview of selected theoretical works in order to give you a launching point for further reflection and study as you begin your journey into professional nursing practice.

Theoretical works in nursing are generally categorized either as philosophies, conceptual models, or theories depending on the level of abstraction. We begin with the most abstract of these theoretical works, the philosophies of nursing.

Selected Philosophies of Nursing

Philosophies set forth the general meaning of nursing and nursing phenomena through reasoning and the logical presentation of ideas. Philosophies are broad and address general ideas about nursing. Because of their breadth, nursing philosophy contributes to the discipline by providing direction, clarifying values, and forming a foundation for theory development (Alligood, 2006).

Nightingale's Environmental Theory

Nightingale's philosophy includes the four metaparadigm concepts of nursing (Table 2-1), but the focus is primarily on the patient and the environment, with the nurse manipulating the environment to enhance patient recovery. Nursing

---

TABLE 2-1   METAPARADIGM CONCEPTS AS DEFINED IN NIGHTINGALE'S MODEL

Person   Recipient of nursing care

Environment   External (temperature, bedding, ventilation) and internal (food, water, and medications)

Health   Health is "not only to be well, but to be able to use well every power we have to use" (Nightingale, 1969, p. 24)

Nursing   Alter or manage the environment to implement the natural laws of health

interventions using Nightingale's philosophy are centered on her 13 canons, which include the following (Nightingale, 1969):

- Ventilation and warmth: The interventions subsumed in this canon include keeping the patient and the patient's room warm and keeping the patient's room well ventilated and free of odors. Specific instructions included "keep the air within as pure as the air without" (Nightingale, 1969, p. 10).
- Health of houses: This canon includes the five essentials of pure air, pure water, efficient drainage, cleanliness, and light.
- Petty management: Continuity of care for the patient when the nurse is absent is the essence of this canon.
- Noise: Instructions include the avoidance of sudden noises that startle or awaken patients and keeping noise in general to a minimum.
- Variety: This canon refers to an attempt at variety in the patient's room to avoid boredom and depression.
- Food intake: Interventions include the documentation of the amount of food and liquids that the patient ingested.
- Food: Instructions include trying to include patient food preferences.
- Bed and bedding: The interventions in this canon include comfort measures related to keeping the bed dry and wrinkle free.
- Light: The instructions contained in this canon relate to adequate light in the patient's room.
- Cleanliness of rooms and walls: This canon focuses on keeping the environment clean.
- Personal cleanliness: This canon includes measures such as keeping the patient clean and dry.
- Chattering hopes and advises: Instructions in this canon include the avoidance of talking without reason or giving advice that is without fact.
- Observation of the sick: This canon includes instructions related to making observations and documenting observations.

The 13 canons were central to Nightingale's theory but were not all inclusive. Nightingale believed that nursing was a calling and that the recipients of nursing care were holistic individuals with a spiritual dimension; thus, the nurse was expected to care for the spiritual needs of the patients in spiritual distress. Nightingale also believed that nurses should be involved in health promotion and health teaching with the sick and with those who were well (Bolton, 2006).

Although Nightingale's theory was developed long ago in response to a need for environmental reform, the nursing principles are still relevant today. Although some of Nightingale's rationales have been modified or disproved by advances in medicine and science, many of the concepts in her theory have not only endured, but have been used to provide general guidelines for nurses for over 150 years (Pfettscher, 2006).

Virginia Henderson: Definition of Nursing and 14 Components of Basic Nursing Care

Henderson made such significant contributions to the discipline of nursing during her more-than-60-year career as a nurse, teacher, author, and researcher that she has been referred to by some as the Florence Nightingale of the 20th century (Tomey, 2006). She is perhaps best known for her definition of nursing, which was first published in 1955 (Harmer & Henderson, 1955) and then published in 1966 with minor revisions. According to Henderson,

> The unique function of the nurse is to assist the individual, sick or well, in the performance of those activities contributing to health or its recovery (or to a peaceful death) that he would perform unaided if he had the necessary strength, will, or knowledge and to do this in such a way as to help him gain independence as rapidly as possible. (Henderson, 1966, p. 15)

In her work Henderson emphasized the art of nursing as well as empathetic understanding, stating that the nurse must "get inside the skin of each of her patients in order to know what he needs" (Henderson, 1964, p. 63). She believed that "the beauty of medicine and nursing is the combination of your heart, your head and your hands and where you separate them, you diminish them . . ." (McBride, 1997, as cited by Gordon, 2001).

Henderson identified 14 basic needs upon which nursing care is based. These needs include the following:

- Breathe normally.
- Eat and drink adequately.
- Eliminate bodily wastes.
- Move and maintain desirable postures.
- Sleep and rest.
- Select suitable clothes; dress and undress.
- Maintain body temperature within normal range by adjusting clothing and modifying the environment.
- Keep the body clean and well groomed and protect the integument.
- Avoid dangers in the environment, and avoid injuring others.
- Communicate with others in expressing emotions, needs, fears, or opinions.
- Worship according to one's faith.
- Work in such a way that there is a sense of accomplishment.
- Play or participate in various forms of recreation.
- Learn, discover, or satisfy the curiosity that leads to normal development and health and use the available health facilities (Henderson, 1966, 1991).

Although Henderson did not consider her work a theory of nursing, and did not explicitly state assumptions or define each of the domains of nursing, it is possible to identify and describe the metaparadigm concepts of nursing (Furukawa & Howe, 2002) in her work (Table 2-2).

TABLE 2-2 METAPARADIGM CONCEPTS AS DEFINED IN HENDERSON'S PHILOSOPHY AND ART OF NURSING

Person Recipient of nursing care who is composed of biological, psychological, sociological, and spiritual components

Environment External environment (temperature, dangers in environment); some discussion of impact of community on the individual and family

Health Based upon the patient's ability to function independently (as outlined in 14 components of basic nursing care)

Nursing Assist the person, sick or well, in performance of activities (14 components of basic nursing care) and help the person gain independence as rapidly as possible (Henderson, 1966, p. 15)

Jean Watson: Philosophy and Science of Caring

According to Watson's theory (1996), the goal of nursing is to help persons attain a higher level of harmony within the mind–body–spirit. Attainment of that goal can potentiate healing and health (Table 2-3). This goal is pursued through transpersonal caring guided by carative factors.

Watson's Theory for Nursing Practice is based on 10 carative factors (1979). These carative factors as refined by Watson include (Jesse, 2006):

- Practice of loving kindness and equanimity with context of caring consciousness
- Being authentically present and enabling and sustaining the deep belief system and subjective life world of self and the one being cared for
- Cultivation of one's own spiritual practices and transpersonal self, going beyond ego self; being sensitive to self and other
- Developing and sustaining a helping–trusting, authentic caring relationship
- Being present to and supportive of the expression of positive and negative feelings as a connection with a deeper spirit of self and the one being cared for

---

TABLE 2-3 METAPARADIGM CONCEPTS AS DEFINED IN WATSON'S PHILOSOPHY AND SCIENCE OF CARING

Person A "unity of mind–body–spirit/nature" (Watson, 1996, p. 147)

Environment A "field of connectedness" at all levels (Watson, 1996, p. 147)

Health (healing) Harmony, wholeness, and comfort

Nursing Reciprocal transpersonal relationship in caring moments guided by carative factors

- Creative use of self and all ways of knowing as part of the caring process and engagement in artistry of caring–healing practices
- Engaging in a genuine teaching–learning experience that attends to unity of being and meaning and attempts to stay within others' frame of reference
- Creating a healing environment at all levels whereby wholeness, beauty, comfort, dignity, and peace are potentiated
- Assisting with basic needs, with an intentional caring consciousness; administering human care essentials, which potentiate alignment of the mind–body–spirit, wholeness, and unity of being in all aspects of care; attending to both embodied spirit and evolving emergence
- Opening and attending to spiritual–mysterious and existential dimensions of one's own life–death; soul care for self and the one being cared for

Regarding the value system that is blended with these 10 curative factors Watson (1985) stated:

> Human care requires high regard and reverence for a person and human life. . . . There is high value on the subjective–internal world of the experiencing person and how the person (both patient and nurse) is perceiving and experiencing health–illness conditions. An emphasis is placed upon helping a person gain more self-knowledge, self control, and readiness for self-healing. (pp. 34, 35)

The carative factors described by Watson provide guidelines for nurse–patient interactions; however, the theory does not furnish instructions about what to do to achieve authentic caring–healing relationships. Watson's theory is more about being than doing, but it provides a useful framework for the delivery of patient-centered nursing care (Neil & Tomey, 2006).

Selected Conceptual Models and Grand Theories of Nursing

Conceptual models provide a comprehensive view and guide for nursing practice. They are organizing frameworks that guide the reasoning process in professional nursing practice (Alligood, 2006).

Martha Rogers's Science of Unitary Human Beings

According to Rogers (1994), nursing is a learned profession, both a science and an art. The art of nursing is the creative use of the science of nursing for human betterment.

Rogers's theory asserts that human beings are dynamic energy fields integral with environmental energy fields. Both human energy fields and environmental fields are open systems, pandimensional in nature and in a constant state of change. Pattern is the identifying characteristic of energy fields (Table 2-4).

Rogers identified the principles of helicy, resonancy, and integrality to describe the nature of change within human and environmental energy fields. Together,

TABLE 2-4 METAPARADIGM CONCEPTS AS DEFINED IN ROGERS'S THEORY

Person   An irreducible, irreversible, pandimensional, negentropic energy field identified by pattern; a unitary human being develops through three principles: helicy, resonancy, and integrality (Rogers, 1992)

Environment   An irreducible, pandimensional, negentropic energy field, identified by pattern and manifesting characteristics different from those of the parts and encompassing all that is other than any given human field (Rogers, 1992)

Health   Health and illness as part of a continuum (Rogers, 1970)

Nursing   Seeks to promote symphonic interaction between human and environmental fields, to strengthen the integrity of the human field, and to direct and redirect patterning of the human and environmental fields for realization of maximum health potential (Rogers, 1970)

these principles are known as the principle of homeodynamics. The helicy principle describes the unpredictable but continuous, nonlinear evolution of energy fields, as evidenced by a spiral development that is a continuous, nonrepeating, and innovative patterning that reflects the nature of change. Resonancy is depicted as a wave frequency and an energy field pattern evolution from lower to higher frequency wave patterns and is reflective of the continuous variability of the human energy field as it changes. The principle of integrality emphasizes the continuous mutual process of person and environment (Rogers, 1970, 1992).

Rogers (1970) identified five assumptions that support and connect the concepts within her conceptual model:

- Man is a unified whole possessing his own integrity and manifesting characteristics more than and different from the sum of his parts (p. 47).
- Man and environment are continuously exchanging matter and energy with one another (p. 54).
- The life process evolves irreversibly and unidirectionally along the space-time continuum (p. 59).
- Pattern and organization identify man and reflect his innovative wholeness (p. 65).
- Man is characterized by the capacity for abstraction and imagery, language and thought, sensation, and emotion (p. 73).

Rogers's model is an abstract system of ideas but is applicable to practice, with nursing care focused on pattern appraisal and patterning activities. Pattern appraisal involves a comprehensive assessment of environmental field patterns and human field patterns of communication, exchange, rhythms, dissonance, and harmony through the use of cognitive input, sensory input, intuition, and language. Patterning activities may include interventions such as meditation, imagery, journaling, or modifying surroundings. Evaluation is ongoing and requires a repetition of the appraisal process (Gunther, 2006).

Dorothea Orem's General Theory of Nursing

Orem describes her theory as a general theory that is made up of three related theories that include the Theory of Self-Care, the Theory of Self-Care Deficit, and the Theory of Nursing Systems. The Theory of Self-Care describes why and how people care for themselves. The Theory of Self-Care Deficit describes and explains why people can be helped through nursing. The Theory of Nursing Systems describes and explains relationships that must exist and be maintained for nursing to occur. These three theories in relationship constitute Orem's general theory of nursing known as the Self-Care Deficit Theory of Nursing (Taylor, 2006).

Orem identified three types of self-care requisites. Universal self-care requisites are those found in all human beings and are associated with life processes. These requisites include items such as the maintenance of air, water, and food intake. Developmental self-care requisites are related to different stages in the human life cycle and might include issues related to adolescence or aging. Health-deviation self-care requisites are related to deviations in structure or function of a human being. There are six categories of health-deviation requisites (Orem, 1995):

- Seeking and securing appropriate medical assistance
- Being aware of and attending to the effects and results of illness states
- Effectively carrying out medically prescribed treatments
- Being aware of and attending to side effects of treatment
- Modifying self-concept in accepting oneself in a particular state of health
- Learning to live with the effects of illness and medical treatment

There are eight general propositions for the Self-Care Deficit Theory of Nursing (although each of the three individual theories also has its own set of propositions) (Meleis, 2004):

- Human beings have capabilities to provide their own self-care or care for dependents to meet universal, developmental, and health-deviation self-care requisites. These capabilities are learned and recalled.
- Self-care abilities are influenced by age, developmental state, experiences, and sociocultural background.
- Self-care deficits should balance between self-care demands and self-care capabilities.
- Self-care or dependent care is mediated by age, developmental stage, life experience, sociocultural orientation, health, and resources.
- Therapeutic self-care includes actions of nurses, patients, and others that regulate self-care capabilities and meet self-care needs.

- Nurses assess the abilities of patients to meet their self-care needs and their potential of not performing their self-care.
- Nurses engage in selecting valid and reliable processes, technologies, or actions for meeting self-care needs.
- Components of therapeutic self-care are wholly compensatory, partly compensatory, and supportive–educative.

In addition to these other concepts, the four metaparadigm concepts of nursing are identified in Orem's theory (Table 2-5). Orem's theory clearly differentiates the focus of nursing and is one of the nursing theories that is most commonly used in practice.

Callista Roy's Adaptation Model

The Roy Adaptation Model presents the person as an adaptive system in constant interaction with the internal and the external environment. The main task of the human system is to maintain integrity in the face of environmental stimuli (Phillips, 2006). The goal of nursing is to foster successful adaptation (Table 2-6).

According to Roy and Andrews (1999), adaptation refers to "the process and outcome whereby thinking and feeling persons, as individuals or in groups, use conscious awareness and choice to create human and environmental integration" (p. 54). Adaptation leads to optimum health and well-being, to quality of life, and to death with dignity (Andrews & Roy, 1991).

The propositions of Roy's theory include the following:

- Nursing actions promote a person's adaptive responses.
- Nursing actions can decrease a person's ineffective adaptive responses.

TABLE 2-5 METAPARADIGM CONCEPTS AS DEFINED BY OREM'S THEORY

Person (patient) A person under the care of a nurse; a total being with universal, developmental needs, and capable of self-care

Environment Physical, chemical, biologic, and social contexts within which human beings exist; environmental components include environmental factors, environmental elements, environmental conditions, and developmental environment (Orem, 1985)

Health "A state characterized by soundness or wholeness of developed human structures and of bodily and mental functioning" (Orem, 1995, p. 101)

Nursing Therapeutic self-care designed to supplement self-care requisites. Nursing actions fall into one of three categories: wholly compensatory, partly compensatory, or supportive–educative system (Orem, 1985)

TABLE 2-6   METAPARADIGM CONCEPTS AS DEFINED IN ROY'S MODEL

Person   "A whole with parts that function as a unity" (Roy & Andrews, 1999, p. 31)

Environment   Internal and external stimuli; "the world within and around humans as adaptive systems" (Roy & Andrews, 1999, p. 51)

Health   "A state and process of being and becoming an integrated and whole human being" (Roy & Andrews, 1999, p. 54)

Nursing   Manipulation of stimuli to foster successful adaptation

---

- People interact with the changing environment in an attempt to achieve adaptation and health.
- Nursing actions enhance the interaction of persons with the environment.
- Enhanced interactions of persons with the environment promote adaptation (Meleis, 2004).

The Roy Adaptation Model is commonly used in nursing practice. To use the model in practice, the nurse follows Roy's six-step nursing process, which includes (Phillips, 2006):

- Assessing the behaviors manifested from the four adaptive modes (physiological–physical mode, self-concept–group identity mode, role function mode, and interdependence mode)
- Assessing and categorizing the stimuli for those behaviors
- Making a nursing diagnosis based on the person's adaptive state
- Setting goals to promote adaptation
- Implementing interventions aimed at managing stimuli to promote adaptation
- Evaluating achievement of adaptive goals

Andrews and Roy (1986) pointed out that by manipulating the stimuli rather than the patient, the nurse enhances "the interaction of the person with their environment, thereby promoting health" (p. 51).

Betty Neuman's Systems Model

The Neuman Systems Model is a wellness model based on general systems theory in which the client system is exposed to stressors from within and without the system. The focus of the model is on the client system in relationship to stressors. The client system is protected by a circular series of buffers known as lines of defense that minimize the impact of stressors. Progressing inward, there are three lines of defense that include the flexible line of defense, the normal line of defense, and lines

---

TABLE 2-7   METAPARADIGM CONCEPTS AS DEFINED IN NEUMAN'S MODEL

Person   A composite of physiological, psychological, sociocultural, developmental, and spiritual variables in interaction with the internal and external environment; represented by central structure, lines of defense, and lines of resistance

Environment   All internal and external factors of influences surrounding the client system

Health   A continuum of wellness to illness

Nursing   Prevention as intervention; concerned with all potential stressors

---

of resistance (Table 2-7). The greater the quality of the client system's health, the greater protection is provided by the various lines of defense (Geib, 2006).

Basic assumptions of the Neuman Systems Model include the following (Meleis, 2004; Neuman, 1995):

- Nursing clients have both unique and universal characteristics and are constantly exchanging energy with the environment.
- The relationships between client variables influence a client's protective mechanisms and determine the client's response.
- Clients present a normal range of responses to the environment that represent wellness and stability.
- Stressors attack flexible lines of defense and then normal lines of defense.
- Nurses' actions are focused on primary, secondary, and tertiary prevention.

The Neuman Systems Model is health oriented, with an emphasis on prevention as intervention, and has been used in a wide variety of settings. Perhaps one of the greatest attractions to this model is the ease with which it can be used for families, groups, and communities as well as the individual patient. The use of the model in practice requires only moderate adaptation of the nursing process with a focus on assessment of stressors and client system perceptions.

Imogene King's Interacting Systems Framework and Theory of Goal Attainment

King, in her Interacting Systems Framework, conceptualizes three levels of dynamic interacting systems that include personal systems (individuals), interpersonal systems (groups), and social systems (society). Individuals exist within personal systems, and concepts relevant to this system include body image, growth and development, perception, self, space, and time. Interpersonal systems are formed when two or more individuals interact. The concepts important to understanding this system include communication, interaction, role, stress, and transaction. Examples of social systems may include religious systems, educational systems, and healthcare systems. Concepts important to understanding the social system include authority, decision making, organization, power, and status (King, 1981; Sieloff, 2006).

King's Theory of Goal Attainment was derived from her Interacting Systems Framework (Sieloff, 2006) and addresses nursing as a process of human interaction (Norris & Frey, 2006). The theory focuses on the interpersonal system interactions in the nurse–client relationship (Table 2-8). During the nursing process, the nurse and the client each perceive one another, make judgments, and take action that results in reaction. Interaction results, and if perceptual congruence exists, transactions occur (Sieloff, 2006).

The propositions of King's Theory of Goal Attainment include the following (King, 1981):

- If perceptual accuracy is present in nurse–client interactions, transactions will occur.
- If the nurse and client make transactions, goals will be attained.
- If goals are attained, satisfactions will occur.
- If goals are attained, effective nursing care will occur.
- If transactions are made in the nurse–client interactions, growth and development will be enhanced.
- If role expectations and role performance as perceived by the nurse and client are congruent, transactions will occur.
- If role conflict is experienced by nurse and client or both, stress in nurse–client interactions will occur.
- If nurses with special knowledge and skills communicate appropriate information to clients, mutual goal setting and goal attainment will occur.

TABLE 2-8 METAPARADIGM CONCEPTS AS DEFINED IN KING'S MODEL

Person   A personal system that interacts with interpersonal and social systems

Environment   A context "within which human beings grow, develop, and perform daily activities" (King, 1981, p. 18). The internal environment of human beings transforms energy to enable them to adjust to continuous external environmental changes (King, 1981, p. 5)

Health   "Dynamic life experiences of a human being, which implies continuous adjustment to stressors in the internal and external environment through optimum use of one's resources to achieve maximum potential for daily living" (King, 1981, p. 5)

Nursing   A process of human interaction; the goal of nursing is to help patients achieve their goals.

The use of King's theory in practice may be approached using the nursing process where assessment focuses on the perceptions of the nurse and client, communication of the nurse and client, and interaction of the nurse and client. Planning involves a decision about goals and agreement as to how to attain goals. Implementation focuses on transactions made and evaluation focuses on goals attained using King's theory (King, 1992).

Johnson's Behavioral System Model in Nursing Practice

Johnson's model for nursing presents the client as a living open system that is a collection of behavioral subsystems that interrelate to form a behavioral system (Table 2-9). The seven subsystems of behavior proposed by Johnson include achievement, affiliative, aggressive, dependence, sexual, eliminative, and ingestive. Motivational drives direct the activities of the subsystems that are constantly changing because of maturation, experience, and learning (Johnson, 1980).

The achievement subsystem functions to control or master an aspect of self or environment to achieve a standard. This subsystem encompasses intellectual, physical, creative, mechanical, and social skills. The affiliative or attachment subsystem forms the basis for social organization. Its consequences are social inclusion, intimacy, and the formation and maintenance of strong social bonds. The aggressive or protective subsystem functions to protect and preserve the system. The dependency subsystem promotes helping or nurturing behaviors. The consequences include approval, recognition, and physical assistance. The sexual subsystem has the function of procreation and gratification and includes development of gender role identity and gender role behaviors. The eliminative subsystem addresses "when, how, and under what conditions we eliminate," whereas the ingestive subsystem "has to do with when, how, what, how much, and under what conditions we eat" (Johnson, 1980, p. 213).

If using Johnson's model in practice, the focus of the assessment process is obtaining information to evaluate current behavior in terms of past patterns,

---

TABLE 2-9   METAPARADIGM CONCEPTS AS DEFINED IN JOHNSON'S THEORY

Person   A biopsychosocial being who is a behavioral system with seven subsystems of behavior

Environment   Includes internal and external environment

Health   Efficient and effective functioning of system; behavioral system balance and stability

Nursing   An external regulatory force that acts to preserve the organization and integrity of the patient's behavior at an optimal level under those conditions in which the behavior constitutes a threat to physical or social health or in which illness is found (Johnson, 1980, p. 214)

determining the impact of the current illness on behavioral patterns, and establishing the maximum level of health. The assessment is specifically related to gathering information related to the structure and function of the seven behavioral subsystems as well as the environmental factors that impact the behavioral subsystems (Holaday, 2006).

Selected Theories and Middle-Range Theories of Nursing

Rosemary Parse's Human Becoming Theory

The Human Becoming Theory consists of three major themes: meaning, rhythmicity, and transcendence (Parse, 1998). The three major principles of the Human Becoming Theory flow from these themes.

The first principle of the Human Becoming Theory states, "Structuring meaning multidimensionally is cocreating reality through the languaging of valuing and imaging" (Parse, 1998, p. 35). This principle proposes that persons structure or choose the meaning of their realities and that the choosing occurs at levels that are not always known explicitly (Mitchell, 2006). This means that one person cannot decide the significance of something for another person and does not even understand the meaning of the event unless that person shares the meaning through the expression of his or her views, concerns, and dreams.

The second principle states, "Cocreating rhythmical patterns of relating is living the paradoxical unity of revealing–concealing and enabling–limiting while connecting–separating" (Parse, 1998, p. 42). This principle means that persons create patterns in life, and these patterns tell about personal meanings and values. The patterns of relating that persons create involve complex engagements and disengagements with other persons, ideas, and preferences (Mitchell, 2006). According to Parse (1998), persons change their patterns when they integrate new priorities, ideas, hopes, and dreams.

The third principle of the Human Becoming Theory states, "Cotranscending with the possibles is powering unique ways of originating in the process of transforming" (Parse, 1998, p. 46). This principle means that persons are always engaging with and choosing from infinite possibilities. The choices reflect the person's ways of moving and changing in the process of becoming (Mitchell, 2006).

Three processes for practice have been developed from the concepts and principles in the Human Becoming Theory, including the following (Parse, 1998, pp. 69, 70):

- Illuminating meaning is explicating what was, is, and will be. Explicating is making clear what is appearing now through language.
- Synchronizing rhythms is dwelling with the pitch, yaw, and roll of the human–universe process. Dwelling with is immersing with the flow of connecting–separating.
- Mobilizing transcendence is moving beyond the meaning moment with what is not yet. Moving beyond is propelling with envisioned possibles of transforming.

> ### TABLE 2-10 METAPARADIGM CONCEPTS AS DEFINED IN PARSE'S THEORY
>
> **Person** An open being, more than and different than the sum of parts in mutual simultaneous interchange with the environment who chooses from options and bears responsibility for choices (Parse, 1987, p. 160)
>
> **Environment** In mutual process with the person
>
> **Health** Continuously changing process of becoming
>
> **Nursing** Use of true presence to facilitate the becoming of the participant

In practice, nurses guided by the Human Becoming Theory prepare to be truly present (Table 2-10) with others through focused attentiveness on the moment at hand through immersion (Parse, 1998).

Madeleine Leininger's Cultural Diversity and Universality Theory

Leininger (1995) identified the main features of the Theory of Cultural Diversity and Universality Theory:

> Transcultural nursing is a substantive area of study and practice focused on comparative cultural care (caring) values, beliefs, and practices of individuals or groups of similar or different cultures with the goal of providing culture-specific and universal nursing care practices in promoting health or well-being or to help people face unfavorable human conditions, illness, or death in culturally meaningful ways. (p. 58)

Consistent with the focus of her theory, Leininger defined the metaparadigm concepts of nursing in a manner that causes the nurse to specifically consider culture in the delivery of competent nursing care (Table 2-11).

> ### TABLE 2-11 METAPARADIGM CONCEPTS AS DEFINED IN LEININGER'S THEORY
>
> **Person** Human being, family, group, community, or institution
>
> **Environment** Totality of an event, situation, or experience that gives meaning to human expressions, interpretations, and social interactions in physical, ecological, sociopolitical, and/or cultural settings (Leininger, 1991)
>
> **Health** A state of well-being that is culturally defined, valued, and practiced (Leininger, 1991, p. 46)
>
> **Nursing** Activities directed toward assisting, supporting, or enabling with needs in ways that are congruent with the cultural values, beliefs, and lifeways of the recipient of care (Leininger, 1996)

According to Leininger (2001), three modalities guide nursing judgments, decisions, and actions in order to provide culturally congruent care that is beneficial, satisfying, and meaningful to the persons the nurse serves. These three modes include cultural care preservation and/or maintenance, cultural care accommodation and/or negotiation, and cultural care repatterning or restructuring.

The nurse using Leininger's theory plans and makes decisions with clients with respect to these three modes of action. All three care modalities require coparticipation of the nurse and client working together to identify, plan, implement, and evaluate nursing care with respect to the cultural congruence of the care (Leininger, 2001).

Hildegard Peplau's Theory of Interpersonal Relations

In her theory, Peplau addresses all of nursing's metaparadigm concepts (Table 2-12), but she is primarily concerned about one aspect of nursing: how persons relate to one another. According to Peplau, the nurse–patient relationship is the center of nursing (Young, Taylor, & McLaughlin-Renpenning, 2001).

Peplau (1952) describes four phases in nurse–patient relationships that overlap and occur over the time of the relationship: orientation, identification, exploitation, and resolution. During the orientation phase, a health problem has emerged resulting in a "felt need," and professional assistance is sought (p. 18). In the phase of identification, the patient identifies those who can help, and the nurse permits exploration of feelings by the patient. While experiencing the exploitation phase, the patient "makes full use of the services offered" (p. 37). During this phase, the nurse can begin to focus the patient on the achievement of new goals. The phase of identification and exploitation is also known as the "working phase" of the nurse–patient relationship. The resolution phase is the time when the patient gradually adopts new goals and frees the self from identification with the nurse (Peplau, 1952).

TABLE 2-12   METAPARADIGM CONCEPTS AS DEFINED IN PEPLAU'S THEORY

Person   Encompasses the patient (one who has problems for which expert nursing services are needed or sought) and the nurse (a professional with particular expertise) (Peplau, 1992, p. 14)

Environment   Includes culture as important to the development of personality

Health   "Implies forward movement of personality and other ongoing human processes in the direction of creative, constructive, productive, personal, and community living" (Peplau, 1992, p. 12)

Nursing   The therapeutic, interpersonal process between the nurse and the patient

Peplau (1952) also described six nursing roles that emerge during the phases of the nurse–patient relationship: the role of the stranger, the role of the resource person, the teaching role, the leadership role, the surrogate role, and the counseling role.

Peplau (1952) also described four psychobiological experiences: needs, frustration, conflict, and anxiety. According to Peplau, these experiences "all provide energy that is transformed into some form of action" (p. 71) and provide a basis for goal formation and nursing interventions (Howk, 2002).

Peplau (1952) made the implicit assumption that "the nursing profession has legal responsibility for the effective use of nursing and for its consequences to patients" (p. 6). Peplau (1952, p. xii) also identifies two explicit assumptions in her theory:

- "The kind of person that the nurse becomes makes a substantial difference in what each patient will learn as he or she receives nursing care."
- "Fostering personality development toward maturity is a function of nursing and nursing education. Nursing uses principles and methods that guide the process toward resolution of interpersonal problems."

> **CRITICAL THINKING QUESTION**
>
> Think about the definitions of the metaparadigm concepts and the assumptions or propositions of each of the theories presented. Which of the theories most closely matches your beliefs?

Peplau, as one of the first theorists since Nightingale to present a theory for nursing, is considered a pioneer in the area of theory development in nursing. Although her book was first published in 1952, her model continues to be used extensively by clinicians and continues to provide direction to educators, researchers, as well as clinicians (Howk, 2002).

Relationship of Theory to Professional Nursing Practice

The use of a theoretical framework provides a systematic and knowledgeable approach to your nursing practice.

How will theory affect your nursing practice? Using a theoretical framework to guide your nursing practice will assist you as you organize patient data, understand and analyze patient data, make decisions related to nursing interventions, plan patient care, predict outcomes of care, and evaluate patient outcomes (Alligood & Tomey, 2002). Why? The use of a theoretical framework provides a systematic and knowledgeable approach to your nursing practice. The framework also becomes a tool that will assist you to think critically as you plan and provide nursing care.

How do you begin? Now that you know why nursing theory is important to your nursing practice, it is time to identify a theoretical framework that fits you and your practice. Alligood (2006) presented guidelines for selecting a framework for theory-based nursing practice. The steps include:

- Consider the values and beliefs that you truly hold in nursing.
- Write a philosophy of nursing that clarifies your beliefs related to person, environment, health, and nursing.

- Survey definitions of person, environment, health, and nursing in nursing models
- Select two or three frameworks that best fit with your beliefs related to the concepts of person, environment, health, and nursing.
- Review the assumptions of the frameworks that you have selected.
- Make applications of those frameworks in a selected area of nursing practice.
- Compare the frameworks on client focus, nursing action, and client outcome.
- Review the nursing literature written by persons who have used the frameworks.
- Select a framework and develop its use in your nursing practice.

Conclusion

As demonstrated by the descriptions of the philosophies, conceptual models, and theories presented in this chapter, there is a wide variety of perspectives and frameworks from which to practice nursing. There is no one right or wrong answer. Begin with whichever one seems to "fit," and then practice using it as you provide nursing care. "The full realization of nursing theory-guided practice is perhaps the greatest challenge that nursing as a scholarly discipline has ever faced" (Cody, 2006). So, be patient; developing your nursing practice guided by nursing theory will take time and practice. All nursing theories require in-depth study over time to master fully (this chapter has provided only a brief introduction), but the incorporation of theory into your practice will transform your nursing practice. The end result of this process will be seen in the excellent nursing care that you are able to provide to patients over the course of your professional nursing career.

CLASSROOM ACTIVITY 1

Divide into small groups and give each group a copy of the same case study. Assign a different nursing theory to each group, and ask the groups to develop a plan of care with the assigned nursing theory as the basis for practice. Each group should share the plan of care with the class. Discuss the differences and similarities in the foci of care based upon each of the selected theories.

CLASSROOM ACTIVITY 2

Think about the metaparadigm concepts of nursing. Draw each of the concepts in relation to the other concepts to show your ideas of how each of the concepts interfaces with one another. Present your "conceptual model" to the class, and discuss your ideas about each of the concepts represented.

This activity works best if colored pencils, crayons, or markers and a large piece of paper are provided for students. Actual student examples are presented in Figure 2-1 and Figure 2-2.

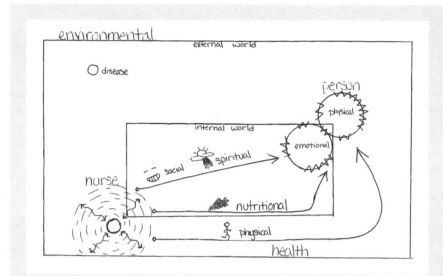

Figure 2-1
Student Conceptual
Model: Example 1

Source: Used with
permission of Heather
Grush.

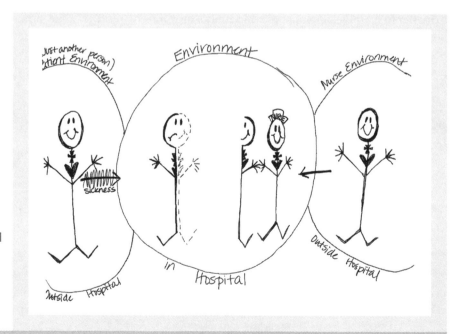

Figure 2-2
Student Conceptual
Model: Example 2

Source: Used with
permission of Linzee
McGinnis.

References

Alligood, M. R. (2006). Philosophies, models, and theories: Critical thinking structures. In M. R. Alligood & A. M. Tomey (Eds.), *Nursing theory: Utilization & application* (3rd ed., pp. 43–65). St. Louis, MO: Mosby.

Alligood, M. R., & Tomey, A. M. (2002). Significance of theory for nursing as a discipline and profession. In A. M. Tomey & M. R. Alligood (Eds.), *Nursing theorists and their work* (5th ed., pp. 14–31). St. Louis, MO: Mosby.

Andrews, H. A., & Roy, C., Sr. (1986). *Essentials of the Roy adaptation model.* Norwalk, CT: Appleton-Century-Crofts.

Andrews, H. A., & Roy, C., Sr. (1991). Essentials of the Roy adaptation model. In Sr. C. Roy & H. A. Andrews (Eds.), *The Roy adaptation model: The definitive statement* (pp. 2–25). Norwalk, CT: Appleton & Lange.

Bolton, K. (2006). Nightingale's philosophy in nursing practice. In M. R. Alligood & A. M. Tomey (Eds.), *Nursing theory: Utilization & application* (3rd ed., pp. 89–102). St. Louis, MO: Mosby.

Cody, W. K. (2006). Nursing theory-guided practice: What it is and what it is not. In W. K. Cody (Ed.), *Philosophical and theoretical perspectives for advanced nursing practice* (4th ed., pp. 119–121). Sudbury, MA: Jones and Bartlett.

Eckberg, D. L., & Hill, L., Jr. (1979). The paradigm concept and sociology: A critical review. *American Sociological Review, 44,* 925–937.

Fawcett, J. (1994). *Analysis and evaluation conceptual models of nursing.* Philadelphia: F. A. Davis.

Flaskerud, J. H., & Halloran, E. J. (1980). Areas of agreement in nursing theory development. *Advances in Nursing Science, 3*(1), 1–7.

Furukawa, C. Y., & Howe, J. S. (2002). Definition and components of nursing: Virginia Henderson. In J. B. George (Ed.), *Nursing theories: The base for professional nursing practice* (5th ed., pp. 83–109). Upper Saddle River, NJ: Prentice Hall.

Geib, K. M. (2006). Neuman's systems model in nursing practice. In M. R. Alligood & A. M. Tomey (Eds.), *Nursing theory: Utilization & application* (3rd ed., pp. 229–254). St. Louis, MO: Mosby.

Gordon, S. C. (2001). Virginia Avenel Henderson: Definition of nursing. In M. Parker (Ed.), *Nursing theories and nursing practice.* Philadelphia: F. A. Davis.

Gunther, M. (2006). Rogers' science of unitary human beings in nursing practice. In M. R. Alligood & A. M. Tomey (Eds.), *Nursing theory: Utilization & application* (3rd ed., pp. 283–306). St. Louis, MO: Mosby.

Harmer, B., & Henderson, V. (1955). *Textbook of the principles and practice of nursing.* New York: Macmillan.

Henderson, V. (1964). The nature of nursing. *American Journal of Nursing, 64,* 62–68.

Henderson, V. (1966). *The nature of nursing: A definition and its implications for practice, research, and education.* New York: Macmillan.

Henderson, V. (1991). *The nature of nursing: Reflections after 25 years.* New York: National League for Nursing Press.

Hickman, J. S. (2002). An introduction to nursing theory. In J. B. George (Ed.), *Nursing theories: A base for professional nursing practice* (5th ed., pp. 1–20). Upper Saddle River, NJ: Prentice Hall.

Holaday, B. (2006). Johnson's behavioral system model in nursing practice. In M. R. Alligood & A. M. Tomey (Eds.), *Nursing theory: Utilization & application* (3rd ed., pp. 157–180). St. Louis, MO: Mosby.

Howk, C. (2002). Hildegard E. Peplau: Psychodynamic nursing. In A. M. Tomey & M. R. Alligood (Eds.), *Nursing theorists and their work* (5th ed., pp. 379–398). St. Louis, MO: Mosby.

Jesse, E. (2006). Watson's philosophy in nursing practice. In M. R. Alligood & A. M. Tomey (Eds.), *Nursing theory: Utilization & application* (3rd ed., pp. 103–129). St. Louis, MO: Mosby.

Johnson, D. (1980). The behavioral systems model for nursing. In J. Riehl & C. Roy (Eds.), *Conceptual models for nursing practice* (2nd ed., pp. 207–216). New York: Appleton-Century-Crofts.

King, I. M. (1981). *A theory of nursing: Systems, concepts, process.* New York: John Wiley & Sons.

King, I. M. (1992). King's theory of goal attainment. *Nursing Science Quarterly, 5*(1), 19–26.

Leininger, M. (1995). Transcultural nursing perspectives: Basic concepts, principles, and culture care incidents. In M. M. Leininger (Ed.), *Transcultural nursing: Concepts, theories, research, and practices* (2nd ed., pp. 57–92). New York: McGraw-Hill.

Leininger, M. (2001). *Culture care diversity and universality: A theory of nursing.* Sudbury, MA: Jones and Bartlett.

Lippitt, G. L. (1973). *Visualizing change: Model building and the change process.* Fairfax, VA: NTL Learning Resources.

McBride, A. B. (Narrator). (1997). *Celebrating Virginia Henderson* (Video). (Available from Center for Nursing Press, 550 West North Street, Indianapolis, IN 46202).

Meleis, A. I. (2004). *Theoretical nursing: Development & progress* (4th ed.). Philadelphia: J. B. Lippincott.

Mitchell, G. J. (2006). Rosemarie Rizzo Parse: Human becoming. In A. M. Tomey & M. R. Alligood (Eds.), *Nursing theorists and their work* (6th ed., pp. 522–559). St. Louis, MO: Mosby.

Neil, R. M., & Tomey, A. M. (2006). Jean Watson: Philosophy and science of caring. In A. M. Tomey & M. R. Alligood (Eds.), *Nursing theorists and their work* (6th ed., pp. 91–115). St. Louis, MO: Mosby.

Neuman, B. (1995). *The Neuman systems model* (3rd ed.). Norwalk, CT: Appleton & Lange.

Nightingale, F. (1969). *Notes on nursing: What it is and what it is not.* New York: Dover.

Norris, D., & Frey, M. A. (2006). King's system framework and theory in nursing practice. In M. R. Alligood & A. M. Tomey (Eds.), *Nursing theory: Utilization & application* (3rd ed., pp. 181–205). St. Louis, MO: Mosby.

Orem, D. (1985). *Nursing: Concepts of practice* (3rd ed.). St. Louis, MO: Mosby.

Orem, D. (1995). *Nursing: Concepts of practice* (5th ed.). St. Louis, MO: Mosby.

Parse, R. R. (1987). *Nursing science: Major paradigms, theories, and critiques.* Philadelphia: Saunders.

Parse, R. R. (1998). *The human becoming school of thought: A perspective for nurses and other health professionals.* Thousand Oaks, CA: Sage.

Peplau, H. (1952). *Interpersonal relations in nursing.* New York: G. P. Putnam's Sons.

Pfettscher, S. A. (2006). Florence Nightingale: Modern nursing. In A. M. Tomey & M. R. Alligood (Eds.), *Nursing theorists and their work* (6th ed., pp. 71–90). St. Louis, MO: Mosby.

Phillips, K. D. (2006). Sister Callista Roy: Adaptation model. In A. M. Tomey & M. R. Alligood (Eds.), *Nursing theorists and their work* (6th ed., pp. 355–385). St. Louis, MO: Mosby.

Rogers, M. E. (1970). *An introduction to the theoretical basis of nursing.* Philadelphia: F. A. Davis.

Rogers, M. E. (1992). Nursing science and the space age. *Nursing Science Quarterly, 5,* 27–34.

Rogers, M. E. (1994). The science of unitary human beings: Current perspectives. *Nursing Science Quarterly, 7,* 33–35.

Roy, C., Sr., & Andrews, H. A. (1999). *The Roy adaptation model* (2nd ed.). Stamford, CT: Appleton & Lange.

Sieloff, C. L. (2006). Imogene King: Interacting systems framework and middle range theory of goal attainment. In A. M. Tomey & M. R. Alligood (Eds.), *Nursing theorists and their work* (6th ed., pp. 297–317). St. Louis, MO: Mosby.

Taylor, S. G. (2006). Self-care deficit theory of nursing. In A. M. Tomey & M. R. Alligood (Eds.), *Nursing theorists and their work* (6th ed., pp. 267–296). St. Louis, MO: Mosby.

Tomey, A. M. (2006). Nursing theorists of historical significance. In A. M. Tomey & M. R. Alligood (Eds.), *Nursing theorists and their work* (6th ed., pp. 54–67). St. Louis, MO: Mosby.

Watson, J. (1979). *Nursing: The philosophy and science of caring.* Boston: Little, Brown.

Watson, J. (1985). *Nursing: Human science and human care: A theory of nursing.* Sudbury, MA: Jones and Bartlett.

Watson, J. (1996). Watson's philosophy and theory of human caring in nursing. In J. P. Riehl-Sisca (Ed.), *Conceptual models for nursing practice* (pp. 219–235). Norwalk, CT: Appleton & Lange.

Young, A., Taylor, S. G., & McLaughlin-Renpenning, K. (2001). *Connections: Nursing research, theory, and practice.* St. Louis, MO: Mosby.

Philosophy of Nursing

Mary W. Stewart

LEARNING OBJECTIVES

After completing this chapter, the student should be able to:

1. Identify various philosophical views of truth.
2. Differentiate between values and beliefs.
3. Discuss the process of value clarification.
4. Explain the major components of nursing philosophy.
5. Articulate the purpose for having a personal philosophy of nursing.
6. Begin the development of a personal philosophy of nursing.

Key Terms and Concepts

- Philosophy
- Paradigm
- Realism
- Idealism
- Beliefs
- Person
- Environment
- Health
- Nursing
- Values
- Values clarification

What is truth? Where do our ideas about truth originate? Why does truth matter?

In a previous chapter, information was presented about the four principal domains of nursing: person, environment, health, and nursing. These concepts are the building blocks for all philosophies of nursing. As you are learning about these ideas, you are also learning that many nurses develop nursing theories or models. Think about it . . . nurses creating theory! Yet, who better to describe our profession than professional nurses? All right, so maybe you are not that excited about this reality. Still, you have to admit that the ability to articulate nursing values and beliefs to guide us in our understanding of professional nursing is impressive. More than impressive, nursing theory is necessary.

In this chapter, we look more closely at nursing philosophy and its significance to professional nursing. We study the difference between beliefs and values and investigate the importance of values clarification. Finally, we examine guidelines for creating a personal philosophy of nursing.

Philosophy

Though no single definition of **philosophy** is uncontroversial, philosophy is the discipline concerned with questions of how one should live; what sorts of things exist and what are their essential natures; what counts as genuine knowledge; and what are the correct principles of reasoning (Philosophy, 2007). The *American Heritage Dictionary of the English Language* (2000) provides the following definitions of philosophy:

- Love and pursuit of wisdom by intellectual means and moral self-discipline
- Investigation of the nature, causes, or principles of reality, knowledge, or values, based on logical reasoning rather than empirical methods
- A system of thought based on or involving such inquiry: the philosophy of Hume
- The critical analysis of fundamental assumptions or beliefs
- The disciplines presented in university curriculums of science and the liberal arts, except medicine, law, and theology
- The discipline comprising logic, ethics, aesthetics, metaphysics, and epistemology
- A set of ideas or beliefs relating to a particular field or activity; an underlying theory: an original philosophy of advertising
- A system of values by which one lives: has an unusual philosophy of life

Examples of philosophies can be found in university catalogs, clinical agency manuals, and nursing school handbooks—and they are prolific on the Internet. Needless to say, people have strong values and beliefs about many topics. A written statement of philosophy is a good way to communicate to others what you see as truth.

Some people are anxious to prescribe their own system of values to others by implying what "should be." However, each person or group of persons is responsible for delineating their particular philosophy. At the same time, how the insider's philosophy fits with the outsider's view is also important, particularly in situations such as nursing. Because nursing is inextricably linked to society, those of us within the profession must consider how society defines the values and beliefs within nursing.

So, how do we please everyone all the time? The answer is simple: We don't. We do, however, consider our own values and beliefs, which are interdependent of society, as we convey our professional philosophy of nursing. Does the philosophy ever change? Absolutely. As society and individuals change, our philosophy of nursing changes to be congruent with new and renewed understanding. How did we ever get started on this journey? A brief look at the beginnings of philosophy may help answer that question.

Early Philosophy

> As society and individuals change, our philosophy of nursing changes to be congruent with new and renewed understanding.

In the beginning, the Greeks moved from seeking supernatural to natural explanations. One assumption by the early Greek philosophers was that "something" had always existed. They did not question how something could come from nothing. Rather, they wanted to know what the "something" was. The pre-Socratics took the first step toward science in that they abandoned mythological thought and sought reason to answer their questions.

Heraclitus, a pre-Socratic philosopher, is well known for his thesis, Everything Is in Flux. He moved from simply looking at "being," to "becoming." A popular analogy he used was that of a river, saying, "You cannot step into the same river twice, for different and again different waters flow." More emphasis was placed on the senses versus reasoning.

On the other hand, Parmenides, who followed Heraclitus, said these two things: (1) nothing can change, and (2) our sensory perceptions are unreliable. He is called the first metaphysician, a "hard-core philosopher." Metaphysics is the study of reality as a whole, including beyond the natural senses. What is the nature of reality? The universe? He starts with what it means and then moves to how the world must ultimately be. He does not go with his sense or experience. Parmenides thought that everything in the world had always been and that there was no such thing as change. He did, of course, sense that things changed, but his reason told him otherwise. He believed that our senses give us incorrect information and that we can only rely on our reason for acquiring knowledge about the world. This is called rationalism.

Probably a name more familiar to us is Socrates (469–399 BC), famous for the "know thyself" philosophy that focused on man, not nature. Plato wrote about his teacher, "Socrates . . . believed in the immortal soul—all natural phenomena are merely shadows of the eternal forms or ideas. The soul, which existed before the body, longs to return to the world of ideas." Plato was a rationalist—we know with our reason.

Aristotle (384–322 BC) followed Socrates and Plato. His father was a physician, apparently framing his own interest in the natural world. He is known for his contribution to logic. Aristotle believed that the highest degree of reality is what we perceive with our senses. Unlike Plato, Aristotle did not believe in forms as separate from the real objects! When an object has both form and matter, it is called a substance. Aristotle said happiness was man's goal and came through balance of the following: life of pleasure and enjoyment, life as a free and responsible citizen, and life as a thinker and philosopher.

During the Neoplatonism age in the third century, philosophy became known as the soul's vehicle to return to its intelligible roots. There was an extrarational approach to reach union with the One. Thinking was that truth, and certainty was not found in this world. This was a revival of the "other worldliness" thinking of Plato.

The birth of Christianity and Western philosophy came at the death of classicism. Augustine of Hippo (AD 354–430) became a Christian and was attracted to Neoplatonism, where existence is divine. In that period, evil was defined as an absence or incompleteness. Saint Thomas Aquinas (AD 1225–1274) is credited with bringing theology and philosophy together.

Throughout the centuries, from the Greeks to the present day, people have debated the same questions: What is man? What is God? How do God and man relate? How does man relate to man? One can become dizzy thinking about the possibilities. Humans have been asking questions for a very long time, and thankfully, that practice is not about to change. People have searched for truth and will continue to do so. Therefore, we should not strive to find absolute answers; rather, we should endeavor to be comfortable with the questioning. Table 3-1 provides an overview of the perspectives of truth through the ages. From the pre-Socratics to the poststructuralists and postmodern thinkers, ways of knowing and finding truth have changed.

Now, back to the real world: What is the purpose for this dialogue in a text on professional nursing? One of the critical theorists, Habermas, would say, "Communication is the way to truth." We have this discussion because it leads us to truth. In this case, the dialogue leads us to truth about nursing. What we hold as truth does not come through mere reading, studying, or debating. The truth comes through dialogue. Let's continue.

Paradigms

How do you see the world? Whether you know it or not, you have an established worldview or **paradigm**. A paradigm is the lens through which you see the world. Paradigms are also philosophical foundations that support our approaches to research (Weaver & Olson, 2006). The continuum of **realism** and **idealism** explains bipolar paradigms (Box 3-1). Most people today would agree that "somewhere in the middle" of these dichotomies lies truth.

Our philosophies are established from a lifelong process of learning and show us how we find truth. In other words, a philosophy is our method of knowing. The experiences we have with ourselves, others, and the environment provide structure to our thinking. Ultimately, our philosophies are demonstrated in the outcomes of our day-to-day living. Nurses' values and beliefs about the profession come from observation and experience (Buresh & Gordon, 2000).

> ### CRITICAL THINKING QUESTION
>
> Where do you see yourself and your understanding of truth on the continuum of realism and idealism?

TABLE 3-1 OVERVIEW OF THE PERSPECTIVES OF TRUTH THROUGH THE AGES

School of Thought	Meaning of Truth (Philosophers)
Classical philosophers	Truth corresponds with reality, and reality is achieved through our perceptions of the world in which we live. Truth could be found in the natural world—through our sensory experiences. (Heraclitus, Aristotle) Truth can be found in the natural world—through our rational intellect. (Parmenides, Plato) Truth is found when one knows self. (Socrates) Truth is not of this world. (Plotinus)
Theocratics	Truth comes through an understanding of God. Truth can be found through both the senses and the intellect. (St. Thomas Aquinas)
Empiricists	Truth is based on experience and relating to our experiences. (Bacon, Locke, Hume, Mill)
Rationalists	All things are knowable by man's deductive reasoning. (Descartes, Spinoza)
Idealists	Truth exists only in the mind. (Berkeley, Hegel, Kant)
Positivists	Truth is science and the facts that science discovers. (Comte, Mill, Spencer)
Early existentialists	Truth is found through man's faith in his existence as it relates to God. (Kierkegaard)
Pragmatists	Truth is relative and practical—if it works, then it is truth. (James, Peirce, Dewey)
Relativists	Truth is always dependent on the knower and the knower's context. (Kuhn, Laudan)
Phenomenologists	Truth is in human consciousness. (Husserl, Heidegger)
Existentialists	If truth can be found, it can only be found through man's search for self. (Sartre, Merleau-Ponty, Gadamer)
Poststructuralists/ Postmodernists	Truth (if there is truth) is not singular and is always historical. Truth can be found in the deconstruction of language. (Derrida) Truth is (evolves from) the outcome of events. (Foucault) Truth is created through dialogue with a purpose of emancipatory action. (Habermas, Freire) Truth is unique to gender. (Feminists)

BOX 3-1   THE CONTINUUM OF REALISM AND IDEALISM

Realism

- ❏ The world is static.
- ❏ Seeing is believing.
- ❏ The social world is a given.
- ❏ Reality is physical and independent.
- ❏ Logical thinking is superior.

Idealism

- ❏ The world is evolving.
- ❏ There is more than meets the eye.
- ❏ The social world is created.
- ❏ Reality is a conception perceived in the mind.
- ❏ Thinking is dynamic and constructive.

Your worldview of nursing began long before you enrolled in nursing school. As far as you can remember, think back on your understanding of nursing. What did you think you would do as a nurse? Did you know a nurse? Did you have an experience with a nurse? What images of the nurse did you see on television or in the movies? Since that time, your worldview of nursing has changed. What experiences in school have changed your perspective of nursing? Undoubtedly, how you see nursing now will differ from your worldview in a few years—or even a few months.

Beliefs

A chief goal in this chapter is to provide a starting point for writing a personal philosophy of nursing. To do that, we must have a discussion of beliefs and values. **Beliefs** indicate what we value, and according to Steele (1979), beliefs have a faith component. Rokeach (1973) identified three categories of beliefs: existential, evaluative, and prescriptive/proscriptive beliefs. Existential beliefs can be shown to be true or false. An example is the belief that the sun will come up each morning. Evaluative beliefs describe beliefs that make a judgment about whether something is good or bad. The belief that social drinking is immoral is an evaluative belief. Prescriptive and proscriptive beliefs refer to what people should (prescriptive) or should not (proscriptive) do. An example of a prescriptive or desirable belief is that everyone should vote. An example of an undesirable or proscriptive belief is that people should not be dishonest. Beliefs demonstrate a personal confidence in the validity of a person, object, or idea.

How would you define **person**? Look at the following attributes given to a person: (1) the ability to think and conceptualize, (2) the capacity to interact with others, (3) the need for boundaries, and (4) the use of language (Doheny, Cook, & Stopper, 1997). Would you agree? What about Maslow's description of humanness in terms of a hierarchy of needs with self-actualization at the top? Another possibility is that persons are the major focus of nursing. Do you see humans as good or evil?

CRITICAL THINKING QUESTION

What are your beliefs about the major concepts in nursing—person, environment, health, nursing?

Consider a second concept in nursing: **environment**. How do you define the internal (within the person) and external (outside the person) environments? Is it important that nurses look beyond the individual toward the surroundings and structures that influence quality of human life? If yes, then how do you see the relationship between the internal and external environments? Is one dimension more important than the other? How do they interact with each other? Martha Rogers, a grand theorist in nursing, described the environment as continuous with the person, no boundaries, in constant exchange of energy. Would you agree?

Health is the third domain of nursing to ponder. Is health the same as the absence of illness? Is health perception? A person who is living and surviving may be described as "healthy." Would you support that as a comprehensive definition of health? Doheny et al. (1997) referred to health in the following way: "Health is dynamic and ever changing, not a stagnant state. Health can be measured only in relative terms. No one is absolutely healthy or ill. In addition, health applies to the total person, including progression toward the realization and fulfillment of one's potential as well as maintaining physical, psychosocial health" (p. 19). Maybe that definition is sufficient, but probably not. All definitions—including yours—have limitations. Definitions merely give us a way to express our beliefs.

Finally, consider common beliefs about **nursing**. Clarke (2006) posed that question in "So What Exactly Is a Nurse?" a recent article addressing the problematic nature of defining nursing. The American Nurses Association (ANA) provided a much used definition of nursing in 1980: "Nursing is the diagnosis and treatment of human responses to actual and potential health problems" (p. 9). Fifteen years later, the ANA (1995, p. 6) expanded its basic definition of nursing to include four fundamental aspects. Nursing is the following:

- Attention to the full range of human experiences and responses to health and illness without restriction to a problem-focused orientation
- Integration of objective data with an understanding of the subjective experience of the patient
- Application of scientific knowledge to the processes of diagnosis and treatment
- Provision of a caring relationship that facilitates health and healing

How would you define nursing? Understanding our beliefs and articulating them in definitions are beginning steps for developing a personal philosophy. Definitions tell us what things are. Our philosophy tells us how things are. One other piece must be addressed before we begin writing our personal philosophy: the topic of values.

Values

Values refer to what the normative standard should be, not necessarily to how things actually are. Values are the principles and ideals that give meaning and direction to our social, personal, and professional life. Steele (1979) defined value as "an affective disposition towards a person, object, or idea" (p. 1). The values of nursing have been articulated by groups such as the ANA in the Code of Ethics (2001) and the American Association of Colleges of Nursing's (AACN) (1998) competencies for baccalaureate nursing education. The AACN's (1998) curriculum guidelines call for integration of professional nursing values in baccalaureate education; they are altruism, autonomy, human dignity, integrity, and social justice. As expected with time and evolved understanding, AACN is currently undergoing revisions of their guidelines and essentials, yet these five core values remain consistent in the drafts of the revised document (AACN, 2007). Ways of teaching these values have been addressed in recent literature (Fahrenwald, 2003).

Nursing values have been identified as the fundamentals that guide our standards, influence practice decisions, and provide the framework used for evaluation (Kenny, 2002). Nevertheless, nursing has been criticized as not clearly articulating what our values are (Kenny, 2002). If nursing is to engage in the move to "interprofessional working," which is beyond uniprofessional and multiprofessional relationships, we have to define our values clearly. Interprofessional working validates what others provide in health care, and the relationships depend on mutual input and collaboration. Values in nursing need to be clearly articulated so that they can be discussed in the context of interprofessional partnership. We can then work together across traditional boundaries for the good of patients. Nursing offers something to health care that no one else does, but that *something* must first be clear to those of us in nursing. "It is not enough just to argue that caring is never value-free, and that values are a fundamental aspect of nursing. What is required is greater precision and clarity so that values can be identified by those within the profession and articulated beyond it" (Kenny, 2002, p. 66). Statements such as those by the ANA and the AACN mentioned earlier are a step in the right direction.

Nursing offers something to health care that no one else does, but that *something* must first be clear to those of us in nursing.

Others have identified nursing values using different language. Antrobus (1997) saw nursing values as humanistic and included (1) a nurturing response to someone in need, (2) a view of the whole individual, (3) an emphasis on the individual's perspective, (4) concentration on developing human potential, (5) an aim of well-being, and (6) maintenance of the nurse–patient relationship at the heart of the helping situation. Nursing values have also been listed as caregiving, accountability, integrity, trust, freedom, safety, and knowledge (Weis & Schank, 2000).

Rokeach (1973) made the following assertions about values:

- Each person has a few.
- All humans possess the same values.
- People organize values into systems.
- Values are developed in response to culture, society, and personality.
- Behaviors are manifestations or consequences of values.

The process of valuing involves three steps: (1) choosing values, (2) prizing values, and (3) acting on values (Chitty, 2001). To choose a value is an intellectual stage in which a person selects a value from identified alternatives. Second, prizing values involves the emotional or affective dimension of valuing. When we "feel" a certain way about our values, it is because we have reached this second step. Finally, we have to act on our intellectual choice and emotion. This third step includes behavior or action that demonstrates our value. Ideally, a genuine value is evidenced by consistent behavior.

Steele (1979) distinguished between intrinsic and extrinsic values. An intrinsic value is required for living (e.g., food and water), whereas an extrinsic value is not required for living and is originated external to the person. According to Simon and Clark (1975), the following criteria must be met in acquiring values:

- Must be freely chosen
- Must be selected from a list of alternatives
- Must have thoughtful consideration of each of the outcomes of the alternatives
- Must be prized and cherished
- Must involve a willingness to make values known to others
- Must precipitate action
- Must be integrated into lifestyle

Value acquisition refers to when a new value is assumed, and value abandonment is when a value is relinquished. Value redistribution occurs when society changes views about a particular value. Values are more dynamic than attitude because values include motivation as well as cognitive, affective, and behavioral components. Therefore, people have fewer values than attitudes (feelings or dispositions toward a person, object, or idea). In the end, values determine our choices.

According to Steele (1979), values may compete with each other on our "hierarchy of values." We typically have values that we hold about education, politics, gender, society, occupations, culture, religion, and so on. The values that are higher in the hierarchy receive more time, energy, resources, and attention. For change to occur there must be conflict among the value system. For example, if a patient values both freedom from pain and long life but is diagnosed with bone cancer, a conflict in values will occur. If professional responsibilities and religious beliefs conflict, the solution is not as simple as "right versus wrong." Rather, it is the choice between two goods. For example, suppose you have strong religious views about abortion.

During your rotation, you are assigned to care for someone who elects to have an abortion. As a nurse, you must balance the value of the patient's choice with your personal value about elective abortions. These decisions are not easy.

Dowds and Marcel (1998) conducted a study involving 40 female nursing students who were taking a psychology class. The students completed the World Hypothesis Scale, which provided 12 items, each with four possible explanations of an event. Each of the four explanations represented a distinct way of thinking. A list of definitions and descriptions of the different ways of thinking would include the following:

- Contextualism: Understanding is embedded in context; meaning is subjective and open to change and dependent on the moment in time and the person's perspective.
- Formism: Understanding events in relationship to their similarity to an ideal or objective standard comes from categorization (e.g., the classification of plants and animals in biology).
- Mechanism: Understanding is in terms of cause and effect relationships, the common approach used by modern medicine.
- Organicism: Understanding comes from patterns and relationships; must understand the whole to understand the parts (e.g., cannot look at a child's language development without looking at his or her overall development history).

The students ranked the explanations in terms of their preferences for understanding the event. Nursing students chose mechanistic thinking significantly more than all other ways of thinking and chose contextualistic thinking significantly less than the other worldviews. No other comparisons were significant among or between the four worldviews. In other words, the nursing students did not choose options that allowed for more than one right answer. They resisted the options that allowed for ambiguity. What this tells us in relationship to values is that we may say that we value human response and the whole individual, but do we really? Human situations are dynamic, fluid, and open for multiple options. Nursing claims to respond to these contextual needs, but do we?

CRITICAL THINKING QUESTION

Do you believe there is more than one right answer to situations? How do you value the whole individual? What barriers prevent us from responding to the contextual needs of our patients?

Values Clarification

Clarifying our values is an eye-opening experience. The process of **values clarification** can occur in a group or individually and helps us understand who we are and what is most important to us. The outcome of values clarification is positive because the outcome is growth. If the process occurs in a group, there must be trust within the group. No one should be embarrassed or intimidated. Everyone is respected.

Values clarification exercises help people discern their individual values. A simple approach to begin the process is considering your responses to statements such as "Patients have a right to know everything that is in the medical record." What is your immediate reaction? How do you feel about the options available in this situation? Have you acted on these beliefs in the past? Another statement to consider is this: "Everyone should have equal access to health care—regardless of income." Ask yourself the same questions. Other exercises involve real or hypothetical clinical situations. For example, a 19-year-old male with HIV disease is totally dependent. His parents remain at his bedside but do not say a word. Another example is a single mom who has recently been diagnosed with multiple sclerosis. What about a 70-year-old man who loses his wife of 42 years, only to remarry a woman who is soon diagnosed with dementia? Reflect. What questions do you have? Why are these people in these situations? Does that matter? What in the patient's life choices conflicts with your choices? Share this with your peers, your friends, and your teachers. In values clarification, one should consider the steps identified earlier as necessary for value acquisition: (1) choosing freely from among alternatives, (2) experiencing an emotional connection, and (3) demonstrating actions consistent with a stated value.

We act on values as the climax of the values clarification process. We are more aware, more empathetic to others, and have greater insight to ourselves and those around us for having gone through this process. Our words and actions are not so different, and we become more content with the individuals we are (i.e., self-actualization). Values clarification also allows us to be more open to accepting others' choice of values.

We must keep in mind that values vary from person to person. Returning to the concept of health, if we asked several people "What is health?" we would get different responses because it means different things to different people. Most likely we would find that others do not place health as high in their hierarchy of values as we do. This helps explain why some people go to the physician for every little ailment, whereas others wait until the situation is critical. Maintaining a nonjudgmental attitude about the values of others is crucial to the nurse–patient relationship.

In health care, we need to clarify values for both the consumer and provider in society. Referring once again to health, we recognize that although the majority of our society states that health is a right, not a privilege, everyone does not have health care. Is health positioned at the top of society's hierarchy of values? We also have to assess the individual's values for congruency with the societal values. As research gives us new options to consider, continual reassessment of values is essential. A questioning attitude is healthy and necessary.

As a profession, nursing is responsible for clarifying our values on a regular basis. Just as society places a value on health, society also determines the value of nursing in the provision of health. Additionally, nurses need to be involved in all levels

CRITICAL THINKING QUESTION

Do I believe in health care for everyone? Does health care for everyone have value to me as a person? Does it have value to me as a nurse? What value does universal health care have to my patients?

where decisions based on values are made, particularly with ethical decisions. The values that nursing supports need to be clearly communicated to those making the policies that affect the health of our society.

Values clarification is done for the purpose of understanding self—to discover what is important and meaningful (Steele, 1979). Throughout life, the process continues as it gives direction to life. As you work through the course of values clarification, keep in mind that personal and professional values are not necessarily the same.

Developing a Personal Philosophy of Nursing

Before we begin writing our individual nursing philosophies, consider the following comments about philosophy. According to Doheny et al. (1997), philosophy is defined as "beliefs of a person or group of persons" and "reveals underlying values and attitudes regarding an area" (p. 259). In this concise definition, these authors mentioned the building blocks of philosophy that we have discussed thus far: attitudes, beliefs, and values. Another definition that is not as concise reads, "Nursing philosophy is a statement of foundational and universal assumptions, beliefs, and principles about the nature of knowledge and truth (epistemology) and about the nature of the entities—nursing practice and human healing processes—represented in the metaparadigm (ontology)" (Reed, 1999, p. 483). Finally, philosophy "looks at the nature of things and aims to provide the meaning of nursing phenomena" (Blais, Hayes, Kozier, & Erb, 2002, p. 90).

In *Nursing's Agenda for the Future*, the ANA (2002) identified the need for nurses to "believe, articulate, and demonstrate the value of nursing" (p. 15). To do that, each professional nurse is responsible for clearly articulating a personal philosophy of nursing. Suggestions for developing personal professional philosophies have been presented in the literature (Brown & Gillis, 1999). The overall purpose of personal philosophy is to define how one finds truth. Because there are different ways of knowing, each person has a unique way of finding truth, in other words, identifying our individual philosophy. Therefore, your philosophy of nursing will be unique.

How do you start writing? A suggested guide for writing your personal philosophy of nursing is in Box 3-2.

When defining nursing, you may refer to definitions by professional individuals or groups. You may also choose to write an original definition, which is certainly acceptable. A final challenge would be this: Once you have used words to describe your personal philosophy, try drawing it. This exercise may enlighten you to gaps in your understanding and further clarify the picture for you.

Writing a philosophy does not have to be a difficult exercise. In fact, you have one already—you just need to practice putting it on paper. Keep in mind that your

BOX 3-2   GUIDE FOR WRITING A PERSONAL PHILOSOPHY OF NURSING

1. Introduction
   a. Who are you?
   b. Where do you practice nursing?
2. Define nursing.
   a. What is nursing?
   b. Why does nursing exist?
   c. Why do you practice nursing?
3. What are your assumptions or underlying beliefs about:
   a. Nurses?
   b. Patients?
   c. Other healthcare providers?
   d. Communities?
4. Define the major domains of nursing and provide examples:
   a. Person
   b. Health
   c. Environment
5. Summary
   a. How are the domains connected?
   b. What is your vision of nursing for the future?
   c. What are the challenges that you will face as a nurse?
   d. What are your goals for professional development?

philosophy will change over time. In addition, composing a nursing philosophy will help you see yourself as an active participant in the profession.

Consider the scene if no one in nursing had a philosophy. What would happen? Unfortunately, we would find ourselves doing tasks without considering the rationale and performing routines in the absence of purpose. Most likely, we would find ourselves devalued by our patients and fellow care providers. Although our individual philosophies vary, there are similarities that link us in our universal philosophy as a profession. As a whole, we are kept on track by continually evaluating our attitudes, beliefs, and values. We are able to evaluate our efforts by reflecting on our philosophies. In the process of personal and professional reflection, we are challenged to reach global relevancy and to begin the development of a global nursing philosophy (Henry, 1998).

CRITICAL THINKING QUESTION

How does my personal philosophy fit with the context of nursing? Does it fit? What areas, if any, need assessing?

Conclusion

In this chapter, we have discussed one of the most ambiguous concepts in professional disciplines—nursing philosophy. The history of philosophy helps us to see that asking questions about humans, environment, health, and nursing is a continual process that leads to a better understanding of truth in our profession. Our own values and beliefs must be clarified in order to authentically respond to the healthcare needs of our patients and to society as a whole. All along the way, our philosophies are changing. Therefore, we must constantly question the values of our profession, our society, and ourselves—aiming to better the health of all people worldwide.

Hegel, an early philosopher, said, "History is the spirit seeking freedom." On this path of searching for truth, we ask the same question, but in different contexts and with distinct experiences. The answers for one person do not provide the same satisfaction for another person. Through our individual and collective searching, we become *truth knowers*. Habermas, the supporter of dialogue, would suggest that the journey does not end with communication and questioning alone. When truth is revealed, oppressive forces are acknowledged, and the truth knowers are then responsible to move to action. Through that action comes a change in the social structure and the hope of rightness in the world.

CLASSROOM ACTIVITY 1

Take about 15 minutes after the discussion related to developing a philosophy of nursing to begin answering the questions in Box 3-2. Jot down answers to the questions in Box 3-2. Ask questions as necessary while still in the classroom. This simple activity will make it easier when writing a personal philosophy of nursing.

CLASSROOM ACTIVITY 2

After thinking about your answers to the questions in Box 3-2 related to the metaparadigm concepts (person, health, environment, and nursing), draw each of these concepts as you define them on a separate piece of paper. Save your drawings, and think about them and refine them as you develop your philosophy of nursing.

This activity works best if colored pencils, crayons, or markers and paper are provided for students. An example is presented in Figure 3-1.

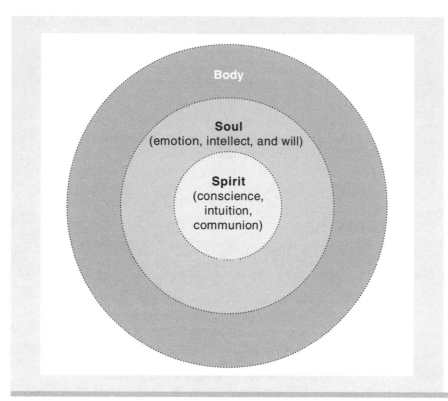

Figure 3-1
Drawing of the
Concept of Person

Source: Masters, 2006,
as adapted from Nee,
1968.

References

American Association of Colleges of Nursing. (1998). *The essentials of baccalaureate educa-tion for professional nursing practice.* Washington, DC: Author.

American Association of Colleges of Nursing. (2007). *Revision of the essentials of baccalau-reate education for professional nursing practice* (Draft Document, December 18, 2007). Washington, DC: Author.

American Heritage Dictionary of the English Language (4th ed.). (2000). Boston: Houghton Mifflin.

American Nurses Association. (1980). *Nursing: A social policy statement.* Washington, DC: Author.

American Nurses Association. (1995). *Nursing's social policy statement.* Washington, DC: Author.

American Nurses Association. (2001). *Code of ethics for nurses with interpretive statements.* Washington, DC: Author.

American Nurses Association. (2002, May). *Nursing's agenda for the future: A call to the nation.* Retrieved April 3, 2008, from http://www.nursingworld.org/MainMenuCategories/ HealthcareandPolicyIssues/Reports/AgendafortheFuture.aspx

Antrobus, S. (1997). An analysis of nursing in context: The effects of current health policy. *Journal of Advanced Nursing, 45,* 447–453.

Blais, K. K., Hayes, J. S., Kozier, B., & Erb, G. (2002). *Professional nursing practice: Concepts and perspectives* (4th ed.). Upper Saddle River, NJ: Prentice Hall.

Brown, S. C., & Gillis, M. A. (1999). Using reflective thinking to develop personal professional philosophies. *Journal of Nursing Education, 38,* 171–176.

Buresh, B., & Gordon, S. (2000). *From silence to voice: What nurses know and must communicate to the public.* New York: Cornell University Press.

Chitty, K. K. (2001). Philosophies of nursing. In K. K. Chitty (Ed.), *Professional nursing: Concepts and challenges* (pp. 199–217). Philadelphia: W. B. Saunders.

Clarke, L. (2006). So what exactly is a nurse? *Journal of Psychiatric and Mental Health Nursing, 13,* 388–394.

Doheny, M. O., Cook, C. B., & Stopper, M. C. (1997). *The discipline of nursing: An introduction* (4th ed.). Stamford, CT: Appleton & Lange.

Dowds, B. N., & Marcel, B. B. (1998). Students' philosophical assumptions and psychology in the classroom. *Journal of Nursing Education, 37,* 219–222.

Fahrenwald, N. L. (2003). Teaching social justice. *Nurse Educator, 28,* 222–226.

Henry, B. (1998). Globalization, nursing philosophy, and nursing science. *Image: Journal of Nursing Scholarship, 30,* 302.

Kenny, G. (2002). The importance of nursing values in interprofessional collaboration. *British Journal of Nursing, 11*(1), 65–68.

Masters, K. (2006). *Drawing of concept of person.* Unpublished classroom exercise.

Nee, W. (1968). *The spiritual man.* New York: Christian Fellowship Publishers.

Philosophy. (2007). In *Wikipedia, The Free Encyclopedia.* Retrieved November 21, 2007, from http://en.wikipedia.org/w/index.php?title=Philosophy&oldid=172913478

Reed, P. G. (1999). A treatise on nursing knowledge development for the 21st century: Beyond postmodernism. In E. C. Polifroni & M. Welch (Eds.), *Perspectives on philosophy of science in nursing* (pp. 478–490). Philadelphia: Lippincott.

Rokeach, M. (1973). *The nature of human values.* New York: Free Press.

Simon, S. B., & Clark, J. (1975). *Beginning values clarification: A guidebook for the use of values clarification in the classroom.* San Diego, CA: Pennant Press.

Steele, S. (1979). *Values clarification in nursing.* New York: Appleton-Century-Crofts.

Weaver, K., & Olson, J. K. (2006). Understanding paradigms used for nursing research. *Journal of Advanced Nursing, 53,* 459–469.

Weis, D., & Schank, M. J. (2000). An instrument to measure professional nursing values. *Journal of Nursing Scholarship, 32,* 201–204.

Foundations of Ethical Nursing Practice

Karen Rich and Janie B. Butts

LEARNING OBJECTIVES

After completing this chapter, the student should be able to:

1. Discuss the meaning of key terms associated with ethical nursing practice.
2. Compare and contrast ethical theories and approaches that may be used in nursing practice.
3. Discuss each of the popular bioethical principles as they relate to nursing practice: autonomy, beneficence, nonmaleficence, and justice.
4. Justify the importance of the *Code of Ethics for Nurses* for professional nursing practice.
5. Explain how nurses can identify and analyze dilemmas that occur in nursing practice.

Key Terms and Concepts

- Ethics
- Morals
- Bioethics
- Nursing ethics
- Moral reasoning
- Values
- Wholeness of character
- Integrity
- Basic dignity
- Personal dignity
- Virtues
- Deontology
- Utilitarianism
- Ethic of care
- Ethical principlism
- Autonomy
- Beneficence
- Paternalism
- Nonmaleficence
- Justice
- Ethical dilemma
- Moral suffering

Scientific and technological advances, economic realities, pluralistic world-views, and global communication make it impossible for nurses to ignore important ethical issues in the world community, their individual lives, and their work. As controversial and sensitive ethical issues continue to challenge nurses and other healthcare professionals, many professionals have begun to develop an appreciation for personal philosophies of ethics and the diverse viewpoints of others.

Mature ethical sensitivities are critical to professional nursing practice.

Ethical directives often are not clearly evident, which leads some people to argue that ethics can be based merely on personal opinions. However, if nurses are to enter into the global dialogue about ethics, they must do more than practice ethics based simply on their personal opinions, their intuition, or the unexamined beliefs that are proposed by other people. It is important for nurses to have a basic understanding of the various concepts, theories, approaches, and principles used in ethics throughout history and to identify and analyze ethical issues and dilemmas that are relevant to nurses in this century. Mature ethical sensitivities are critical to professional nursing practice.

Ethics in Everyday Life

Ethics, a branch of philosophy, means different things to different people. When the term is narrowly defined according to its original use, **ethics** is the study of ideal human behavior and ideal ways of being. The approaches to ethics and the meanings of ethically related concepts have varied over time among philosophers and ethicists. As a philosophical discipline of study, ethics is a systematic approach to understanding, analyzing, and distinguishing matters of right and wrong, good and bad, and admirable and deplorable as they exist along a continuum and as they relate to the well-being of and the relationships among sentient beings. Ethical determinations are applied through the use of formal theories, approaches, and codes of conduct. As contrasted with the term *ethics,* **morals** are specific beliefs, behaviors, and ways of being based on personal judgments derived from one's ethics. One's morals are judged to be good or bad through systematic ethical analysis. Because the word *ethics* is used when one may literally be referring to a situation of morals, the process-related conception of ethics is sometimes overlooked today. People often use the word *ethics* when referring to a collection of actual beliefs and behaviors, thereby using the terms *ethics* and *morals* in essentially synonymous ways.

Bioethics

The terms *bioethics* and *healthcare ethics* are sometimes used interchangeably in the literature. **Bioethics** is a specific domain of ethics that is focused on moral issues in the field of health care. Callahan (1995) called it "the intersection of ethics and the life sciences—but also an academic discipline" (p. 248). Bioethics has evolved into a discipline all its own as a result of life-and-death moral dilemmas encountered by physicians, nurses, other healthcare professionals, patients, and families.

In his book *The Birth of Bioethics,* Albert Jonsen (1998) designated a span of 40 years, from 1947 to 1987, as the era when bioethics was evolving as a discipline. This era began with the Nuremberg Tribunal in 1947, when Nazi physicians were charged and convicted for the murderous and tortuous war crimes that these physicians labeled as scientific experiments during the early 1940s. The 10 judgments in the final court ruling of the Nazi trial provided the basis for the worldwide Nuremberg Code of 1947. This code became a document to protect human subjects during research and experimentation.

The 1950s and 1960s were preliminary years before the actual birth of bioethics. A transformation was occurring during these years as technology advanced. In this era, a new ethic was emerging about life and extension of life through technology. The development of the polio vaccine, organ transplantation, life support, and many other advances occurred. Scientists and physicians were forced to ask questions: "Who should live?" "Who should die?" "Who should decide?" (Jonsen, 1998, p. 11). Many conferences and workshops during the 1960s and 1970s addressed issues surrounding life and death.

By 1970, the public, physicians, and researchers were referring to these phenomena as bioethics (Johnstone, 1999). Today, bioethics is a vast interdisciplinary venture that has engrossed the public's interest from the time of its conception. The aim of bioethicists today is to continue to search for answers to deep philosophical questions about life, death, and the significance of human beings and to help guide and control public policy (Kuhse & Singer, 1998).

Nursing Ethics

"It is the real-life, flesh-and-blood cases that raise fundamental ethical questions" (Fry & Veatch, 2000, p. 1) in nursing. **Nursing ethics** sometimes is viewed as a subcategory of the broader domain of bioethics, just as medical ethics is a subcategory of bioethics. However, controversy continues about whether nursing has unique moral problems in professional practice. Nursing ethics, similar to all healthcare ethics, usually begins with cases or problems that are practice based.

Many nursing ethicists distinguish issues of nursing ethics from broader bioethical issues that nurses encounter. These nursing ethicists view nursing ethics as a separate field because of the unique variety of ethical problems that surface in relationships between nurses and patients, families, physicians, and other professionals who are a part of the healthcare team. The key criteria for distinguishing issues of nursing ethics from bioethics are that nurses are the primary agents in the scenario, and ethical issues are viewed from a nursing rather than a medical perspective.

The key criteria for distinguishing issues of nursing ethics from bioethics are that nurses are the primary agents in the scenario, and ethical issues are viewed from a nursing rather than a medical perspective.

Moral Reasoning

In general, reasoning involves using abstract thought processes to solve problems and to formulate plans (Angeles, 1992). More specifically, **moral reasoning** pertains to making decisions about how humans ought to be and act. Deliberations about moral reasoning go back to the days of the ancient Greeks when Aristotle (Broadie, 2002), in *Nichomachean Ethics,* discussed the intellectual virtue of wisdom as being necessary for deliberation about what is good and advantageous in terms of moving toward worthy ends (Broadie, 2002).

Moral reasoning can be described by what Aristotle (Broadie, 2002) called the intellectual virtue of wisdom (*phronesis*), also known as prudence. Virtue is an excellence of intellect or character. The virtue of wisdom is focused on the good achieved from being wise, that is, knowing how to act in a particular situation, practicing good deliberation, and having a disposition consistent with excellence of character (Broadie, 2002). Therefore, prudence involves more than having good intentions or meaning well. It includes knowing "what is what" but also transforming that knowledge into well-reasoned decisions. Deliberation, judgment, and decision are the steps in transforming knowledge into action. Prudence becomes truth in action (Pieper, 1966).

In more recent times, Lawrence Kohlberg, in 1981, reported his landmark research about moral reasoning based on 84 boys who he had followed for over 20 years. Kohlberg defined six stages ranging from immature to mature moral development. Interestingly, Kohlberg did not include any women in his research but expected that his six-stage scale could be used to measure moral development in both males and females. When the scale was applied to women, they seemed to score only at the third stage of the sequence, a stage in which Kohlberg described morality in terms of interpersonal relationships and helping others. Kohlberg viewed this third stage of development as deficient in regard to mature moral reasoning.

In light of Kohlberg's exclusion of females in his research and the negative implications of women being placed within the third stage of moral reasoning, Carol Gilligan raised the concern of gender bias. Gilligan, in turn, published an influential book in 1982, *In a Different Voice,* in which she argued that women's moral reasoning is different but is not deficient (Gilligan, 1993; Grimshaw, 1993; Thomas, 1993). The distinction that is usually made between the ethics of Kohlberg and Gilligan is that Kohlberg's is a male-oriented ethic of justice and Gilligan's is a more feminine ethic of care. The Kohlberg–Gilligan justice–care debate is still at the heart of feminist ethics.

Often the work of nurses does not involve independent moral reasoning and decision making in regard to the well-publicized issues in bioethics, such as withdrawing life support. Independent moral reasoning and decision making for nurses usually occurs more in the day-to-day care and relationships between nurses and their patients and between nurses and their coworkers. Nurses' moral reasoning is similar to the findings of Gilligan and is often based on caring and the needs of good interpersonal relationships. However, this does not negate what nurses can learn from studying Aristotle and his virtue of *phronesis.* Nurses' moral reasoning needs to be deliberate and practically wise in order to facilitate patients' well-being.

Values in Nursing

Values are emphasized in the American Nurses Association (ANA, 2001) *Code of Ethics for Nurses with Interpretive Statements.* **Values** refer to a group's or individual's evaluative judgments about what is good or what makes something desirable. Professional values are integral to moral reasoning. Values in nursing encompass appreciating what is important for both the profession and nurses personally, as well as what is important for patients.

Values in nursing encompass appreciating what is important for both the profession and nurses personally, as well as what is important for patients.

In the *Code of Ethics for Nurses with Interpretive Statements* (discussed in more detail later in this chapter), the ANA (2001) included statements about **wholeness of character**, which pertains to knowing the values of the nursing profession and one's own authentic moral values, integrating these two belief systems, and expressing them appropriately. Integrity is an important feature of wholeness of character. According to the code, maintaining **integrity** involves acting consistently with personal values and the values of the profession. In a healthcare system often burdened with constraints and self-serving groups and organizations, threats to integrity can be a serious pitfall for nurses. When nurses are asked and pressured to do things that conflict with their values, such as to falsify records, deceive patients, or accept verbal abuse from others, emotional and moral suffering may occur. A nurse's values must guide moral reasoning and actions, even when other people challenge the nurse's beliefs. When compromise is necessary, the compromise must not be such that it compromises personal or professional values.

Recognizing the essential dignity of oneself and each patient is another value that is basic to nursing and is given priority in moral reasoning. Pullman (1999) described two conceptions of dignity. One type, called **basic dignity**, is intrinsic, or inherent, and dwells within all humans, with all humans being ascribed this moral worth. The other type, called **personal dignity**, often mistakenly equated with autonomy, is an evaluative type. Judging others and describing behaviors as dignified or undignified are of an evaluative nature. Personal dignity is a socially constructed concept that fluctuates in value from community to community, as well as globally. Most often, however, personal dignity is highly valued.

Ethical Theories and Approaches

Within each ethical theory or approach, a normative framework exists that includes foundational statements. Individuals who apply a particular theory or approach know what beliefs and values are right and wrong and what is and is not acceptable according to the particular ethical system. Normative ethical theories function as moral guides in answering the question: "What

Theory helps to provide guidance in moral thinking and reasoning and justification for moral actions.

ought I do or not do?" Theory helps to provide guidance in moral thinking and reasoning and justification for moral actions. Optimally, ethical theories and approaches should help people to discern commonplace morality and strengthen moral judgments "in the face of moral dilemmas" (Mappes & DeGrazia, 2001, p. 5).

Virtue Ethics

Since the time of Aristotle (384–322 BC), **virtues**, *arête* in Greek, refer to excellences of intellect or character. Aristotle, the Greek philosopher, was one of the most influential thinkers in regard to virtue ethics. Virtue ethics pertains to questions of "What sort of person must I be to achieve my life's purpose?" and "What makes one a good or excellent person?" rather than "what is right or good to do based on my duty or to achieve good consequences?" Virtues are intellectual and character traits or habits that are developed throughout one's life. The idea behind virtue ethics is that when people are faced with complex moral dilemmas or situations, they will choose the right course of action because doing the right thing comes from a virtuous person's basic character. Aristotle believed that in order for a person to develop moral character, personal effort, training, and practice must occur. Examples of virtues include benevolence, compassion, courage, justice, generosity, truthfulness, wisdom, and patience.

Natural Law Theory

St. Thomas Aquinas (1225–1274), who had a great influence on natural law theory as disseminated by Roman Catholic writers of that century, was himself influenced by Aristotle's work. Most versions of natural law theory today have their basis in Aquinas's basic philosophy. According to natural law theory, the rightness of actions is self-evident from the laws of nature, which in most cases is orchestrated by a law-giver God. Morality is determined not by customs and human preferences but is commanded by the law of reason, which is implanted in nature and human intellect. Natural law ethicists believe that behavior that is contrary to their views of the laws of nature is immoral. Examples include artificial means of birth control and homosexual relationships.

Deontology

Deontology refers to actions that are duty based, not based on their rewards, happiness, or consequences. One of the most influential philosophers for the deontologic way of thinking was Immanuel Kant, an 18th-century German philosopher. In his classic work, *Groundwork of the Metaphysics of Morals,* Kant (1785/2003) attempted to define a person as a rational human being with freedom, moral worth, and ideally having a good will, meaning that a person should act from a sense of duty. Because of their rationality, Kant believed that humans have the freedom to make moral judgments. Therefore, Kant argued that people ought to follow a universal framework of moral maxims, or rules, to guide right actions, because it is only through performing dutiful actions that people have moral worth. Even when individuals do not want to act from duty, Kant stated that they are required to do so if they want to be ethical. Maxims apply to everyone universally and become the laws for guiding conduct. According to Kant, moral actions should be ends in themselves, not the means to ends. In fact, when people use others as a means to an end, such as deliberately using another person to reach one's personal goals, they are not treating other people with the dignity that they deserve.

Kant made a distinction between two types of duties: hypothetical imperatives and categorical imperatives. Hypothetical imperatives are duties or rules that people ought to observe if certain ends are to be achieved. Hypothetical imperatives are sometimes called "if–then" imperatives, which are conditional: for instance, "If I want to pass my nursing course, then I should be diligent in my studies."

However, Kant stated that moral actions must be based on unconditional reasoning. Where moral actions are concerned, duties and laws are absolute and universal. Kant called these moral maxims, or duties, categorical imperatives. When acting according to a categorical imperative, one should ask this question: "If I perform this action, would I will that it becomes a universal law?" No action can ever be judged as right, according to Kant, if the action cannot have the potential to become a binding law for all people. For example, Kant's ethics would impose the categorical imperative that one can never tell a lie for any reason because if a person lies in any instance, the person cannot rationally wish that permission to lie should universally become a law for everyone.

Utilitarianism

Contrasted with deontology, the ethical approach of **utilitarianism** is to promote the greatest good that is possible in situations (i.e., the greatest good for the greatest number). British utilitarianism was promoted by Jeremy Bentham (1789/1988) in his book *An Introduction to the Principles of Morals and Legislation.* Bentham's thoughts on utilitarianism were that each form of happiness is equal and that each situation or action should be evaluated according to its production of happiness, good, or pleasure. John Stuart Mill (1863/2002) challenged Bentham's view when in his book, *Utilitarianism,* he clearly pointed out that experiences of pleasure and happiness do have different qualities and are not equal. For example, Mill stated that intellectual pleasures of humans have more value than physical pleasures of nonhuman animals.

Utilitarians place great emphasis on what is best for groups, not individual people. In doing so, the focus is on moral acts that produce the most good in terms of the most happiness. By aiming for the most happiness, this theory focuses on good consequences, utility (usefulness), or good ends. Although happiness is the goal, it should be kept in mind that utilitarianism is not based merely on subjective preferences or judgments of happiness. Commonsense ethical directives agreed upon by groups of people are usually applied.

Ethic of Care

The ethic of care has a history in feminist ethics, which has a focus in the moral experiences of women. In the **ethic of care** approach, personal relationships and relationship responsibilities are emphasized. Important concepts in this approach are compassion, empathy, sympathy, concern for others, and caring for others. Carol Gilligan with her study on gender differences in moral development (see the Moral Reasoning section in this chapter) has had an influence on the ethic of care approach.

People who uphold the ethic of care think in terms of particular situations and individual contexts, not in terms of impersonal universal rules and principles. In resolving moral conflicts and understanding a complex situation, a person must use critical thinking to inquire about relationships, circumstances, and the problem at hand. The situation must be brought to light with "caring, consideration, understanding, generosity, sympathy, helpfulness, and a willingness to assume responsibility" (Munson, 2004, p. 788).

> **CRITICAL THINKING QUESTION**
>
> Think about the ethical theories and approaches discussed in this section and think about moral conflicts you have experienced in the past. Have you used one of these approaches to resolve a conflict? Which approach or approaches have you used?

Ethical Principlism

The four principles that are most commonly used in bioethics are autonomy, beneficence, nonmaleficence, and justice.

Ethical principlism, a popular approach to ethics in health care, involves using a set of ethical principles that is drawn from the common or widely shared conception of morality. The four principles that are most commonly used in bioethics are autonomy, beneficence, nonmaleficence, and justice. In 1979, Tom Beauchamp and James Childress published the first edition of *Principles of Biomedical Ethics*, which featured these four principles. Currently, the book is in its fifth edition, and the four principles have become an essential foundation for analyzing and resolving bioethical problems.

These principles, which are closely associated with rule-based ethics, provide a framework to support moral behavior and decision making. However, the principles neither form a theory nor provide a well-defined decision-making model. The framework of principlism provides a prima facie model. As a prima facie model, principles are applied based on rules and justifications for moral behavior. Often, more than one principle is relevant in ethical situations, and no conflict occurs. However, if relevant principles conflict in any situation, judgment must be used in weighing which principle should take precedence in guiding actions.

Autonomy

The word *autonomy* is a derivative of "the Greek *autos* (self) and *nomos* (rule, governance, or law)" (Beauchamp & Childress, 2001, p. 57). **Autonomy** then involves one's ability to self-rule and to generate personal decisions independently. Some people argue that autonomy has a top priority among the four principles. However, there is no general consensus about this issue, and many people argue that other principles, such as beneficence, should take priority. Ideally, when using a framework of principlism, no one principle should automatically be assumed to rule supreme.

The principle of autonomy sometimes is described as respect for autonomy (Beauchamp & Childress, 2001). In the domain of health care, respect for a patient's autonomy includes situations such as obtaining informed consent for treatment; facilitating patient choice regarding treatment options; accepting patients' refusal of treatment; disclosing medical information, diagnoses, and treatment options to patients; and maintaining confidentiality. It is important to note that a patient's right to respect for autonomy is not unqualified. In cases of endangering or harming others, for example, through communicable diseases or acts of violence, people lose their basic rights to self-determination.

Beneficence

The principle of **beneficence** consists of deeds of "mercy, kindness, and charity" (Beauchamp & Childress, 2001, p. 166). Beneficence in nursing implies that nurses take actions to benefit patients and to facilitate their well-being. Beneficent nursing actions include obvious interventions such as lifting side rails on the patient's bed to prevent falls. More subtle actions also may be considered to be beneficent and kind actions, such as taking time to make phone calls for a frail, older patient who is unable to do so herself.

Occasionally, nurses may experience ethical conflicts when confronted with having to make a choice between respecting a patient's right to self-determination (autonomy) and the principle of beneficence. Nurses may decide to act in ways that they believe are for a patient's "own good" rather than allowing patients to exercise their autonomy. The deliberate overriding of a patient's autonomy in this way is called **paternalism**. An example of a paternalistic action is for a nurse to decide that a patient must try to ambulate in the hall, even though the patient moaned and complained of being too tired from his morning whirlpool treatment. In that case, the nurse was aware that the patient wanted to wait until a later time but insisted otherwise. Nurses must weigh carefully the value of paternalistic actions and determine whether they are truly in the patient's best interest. Justified paternalism often involves matters of patient safety.

> Nurses may decide to act in ways that they believe are for a patient's "own good" rather than allowing patients to exercise their autonomy. The deliberate overriding of a patient's autonomy in this way is called paternalism.

Nonmaleficence

Nonmaleficence, the injunction to "do no harm," is often paired with beneficence, but a difference exists between the two principles. Beneficence requires taking action to benefit others, whereas nonmaleficence involves refraining from action that might harm others. Nonmaleficence has a wide scope of implications in health care that includes most notably avoiding negligent care, as well as making decisions regarding withholding or withdrawing treatment and regarding the provision of extraordinary or heroic treatment.

Justice

The fourth major principle, justice, is a principle in healthcare ethics, a virtue, and the foundation of a duty-based ethical framework of moral reasoning. In other words, the concept of justice is quite broad in the field of ethics. **Justice** refers to the fair distribution of benefits and burdens. In regard to principlism, justice most often refers to the distribution of scarce healthcare resources. Most of the time, difficult resource allocation decisions are based on attempts to answer questions regarding who has a right to health care and who will pay for healthcare costs.

Professional Ethics and Codes

Professional nursing began in England in the 1800s at the school Florence Nightingale founded, where profession-shaping ethical precepts were communicated (Kuhse & Singer, 1998). Nightingale's achievement was a landmark in nursing even though graduates in the early days of the school were below average (Dossey, 2000). For the first 30 to 40 years in Nightingale's school, male physicians trained the probationers because not enough educated women were available to teach nursing. Because of this strong medical influence, early nursing education was focused on technical training rather than on the art and science of nursing as Nightingale would have preferred.

By the end of the 1800s, modern nursing was established, and by the early 1890s, ethics in nursing was seriously being discussed (Dossey, 2000; Kuhse & Singer, 1998). The Nightingale Pledge, first administered in 1893, was written under the chairmanship of Lystra Gretter, the principal of a Detroit nursing school, and the origination of the pledge helped to establish nursing as an art and a science (Dossey, 2000). The International Council of Nurses (ICN), which has been a pioneer in developing a code of nursing ethics, was established in 1899. By 1900, the first book on nursing ethics, *Nursing Ethics: For Hospital and Private Use,* was written by the American nursing leader Isabel Hampton Robb (Kuhse & Singer).

Historically, a primary consideration in nursing ethics has been the determination of who is the focus of nurses' work. Until the 1960s, this focus was on the physician, which is not surprising based on the fact that over the years most nurses have been women and most doctors have been men (Kuhse & Singer, 1998). The focus on nurses' obedience to physicians remained at the forefront of nursing responsibilities into the 1960s with this assumption still being reflected in the *ICN Code of Nursing Ethics* in 1965. By 1973, however, the focus of nurses' primary responsibility within the ICN's code changed from the physician to the patient, where it remains to this day.

No code can provide absolute or complete rules that are free of conflict and ambiguity. Because codes are unable to provide exact directives for ethical decision making and action in all situations, some ethicists believe that virtue ethics provides a better approach to ethics because the emphasis is on an agent's character rather than on rules, principles, and laws (Beauchamp & Childress, 2001). Proponents of virtue ethics consider that if a nurse's character is not virtuous, the nurse cannot be depended on to act in good or moral ways even with a professional code as a guide. Professional codes do serve a useful purpose in providing direction to healthcare professionals. Ultimately, one must remember that codes do not eliminate moral dilemmas and are of no use without professionals' motivation to act morally.

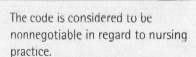

Ultimately, one must remember that codes do not eliminate moral dilemmas and are of no use without professionals' motivation to act morally.

The Code of Ethics for Nurses

The ANA first adopted its code in 1950 (Daly, 2002). Although it has always been implied that the code reflected ethical provisions, the word *ethics* was not added to the title until the 1985 code was replaced with its sixth and latest revision in 2001 (Fowler & Benner, 2001). The ANA's (2001) *Code of Ethics for Nurses* contains general moral provisions and standards for nurses to follow, but specific guidelines for clinical practice, education, research, and administration are contained within the accompanying interpretive statements. See Appendix B for ANA's *Code of Ethics for Nurses.*

The code is considered to be nonnegotiable in regard to nursing practice. Some of the significant positions and changes in the 2001 code include a return to the use of the word *patient,* rather than *client;* an application of the code to nurses in all roles, not just clinical roles; conceding that research is not the only method that contributes to professional development; reaffirming a stance against nurses' participation in euthanasia; emphasizing that nurses owe the same duties to self as to others; and recommending that members who represent nursing associations are responsible for expressing nursing values, maintaining professional integrity, and participating in public policy development (ANA, 2001; Fowler & Benner, 2001).

The code is considered to be nonnegotiable in regard to nursing practice.

Fowler (Fowler & Benner, 2001) and Daly (2002), nursing leaders involved in revising the code completed in 2001, have proposed that the new code is clearly patient focused whether the patient is considered to be "an individual, family, group, or community" (Daly, 2002, p. 98). The nurse's loyalty must be foremost to the patient even though institutional politics is a frequent influence in today's nursing environment.

With the expanding role of nurse administrators and advanced practice nurses, each nurse must be cognizant of conflicts of interest that could potentially have a negative effect on relationships with patients and patient care. Often nurses have overlooked the responsibility to the patient by nurses who are not in clinical roles. Nurse researchers, administrators, and educators are indirectly but still involved in affecting patient care. According to Fowler and Benner (2001), "It is not the possession of nursing credentials, degrees, and position that makes a nurse a nurse; rather it is this very commitment to the patient" (p. 435). Therefore, the code applies to all nurses regardless of their role.

One issue that created a vigorous debate with the 2001 revision of the code involved the ethical implications of collective bargaining in nursing (Daly, 2002). Ultimately, the nurses who formulated the revisions decided that it was important for the code to contain provisions supporting nurses who work to ensure that the environment in which they work is conducive to quality patient care and that nurses are able to fulfill their moral requirements. Collective bargaining was determined to be an appropriate avenue for more than just negotiating for better salaries and benefits. It also can be used to improve the moral level of the environment in which nurses work.

The ICN Code of Ethics for Nurses

In 1953, the International Council of Nurses (ICN) adopted its first *Code of Ethics for Nurses*. The most recent revision and review of the code occurred in 2006. The code has been revised and reaffirmed many times. The four principal elements contained within the ICN code involve standards related to nurses and people, practice, the profession, and coworkers. These elements form a framework to guide nursing conduct and are elaborated within the code with practice applications for practitioners and managers, educators and researchers, and national nurses' associations. The *ICN Code of Ethics for Nurses* is available online at http://www.icn.ch/icncode.pdf.

A Common Theme of ANA and ICN Codes

A theme common to the codes of the ANA (2001) and ICN (2006) is a focus on the importance of nurses delivering compassionate patient care aimed at alleviating suffering.

A theme common to the codes of the ANA (2001) and ICN (2006) is a focus on the importance of nurses delivering compassionate patient care aimed at alleviating suffering. This emphasis is threaded throughout the codes but begins with the patient being the central focus of a nurse's work. Nurses are to support patients in self-determination and are to protect the moral environment in which patients receive care. The interests of various nursing associations and healthcare institutions must not be placed above those of patients. Although opportunities in the healthcare environment to exhibit compassion are not unique to nurses, nurses must always uphold the moral agreement that they make with communities when they join the nursing profession. Nursing care includes the important responsibilities of promoting health and preventing illness, but the heart of nursing care has always involved caring for patients who are experiencing varying degrees of physical, psychologic, and spiritual suffering.

In the *Code of Ethics for Nurses with Interpretative Statements,* the ANA (2001) emphasized the importance of moral respect for all human beings, including nurses' respect for themselves. Self-respect also can be thought of as personal regard. Personal regard involves nurses extending attention and care to their own requisite needs. Nurses who do not regard themselves as worthy of care usually cannot fully care for others.

Ethical Analysis and Decision Making in Nursing

Ethical issues and dilemmas are ever present in healthcare settings. Many times, ethical issues are so prevalent in practice that nurses do not even realize that they are making minute-by-minute ethical decisions (Kelly, 2000; Chambliss, 1996). Whether or not they are cognizant of the ethical matters at the time that the decisions are made, nurses use their critical thinking skills to respond to many of these everyday decisions. Personal values, professional values and competencies, ethical principles, and ethical theories and approaches are variables

Many times, ethical issues are so prevalent in practice that nurses do not even realize that they are making minute-by-minute ethical decisions.

that must be considered when an ethical decision is made. Answers to the questions "What is the right thing to do for my patient?" and "What sort of nurse do I want to be?" are important to professional nursing practice.

Ethical Dilemmas and Conflicts

An **ethical dilemma** is a situation in which an individual is compelled to make a choice between two actions that will affect the well-being of a sentient being and both actions can be reasonably justified as being good, neither action is readily justifiable as good, or the goodness of the actions is uncertain. One action must be chosen, thereby generating a quandary for the person or group who must make the choice.

In addition to general, situational ethical dilemmas, dilemmas may arise from conflicts between nurses, other healthcare professionals, the healthcare organization, and the patient and family. A dilemma might involve nurses making a choice between staying to work an extra shift during a situation of inadequate staffing and going home to rest after a very tiring 8 hours of work. Nurses in this situation may believe that patients will not receive safe or good care if they do not stay to work the extra shift, but these nurses also might not provide safe care if they stay at the hospital because of already being tired from a particularly hard day of work.

Moral Suffering

Many times nurses experience disquieting feelings of anguish or uneasiness consistent with what might be called **moral suffering**. Moral suffering can be experienced when nurses attempt to sort out their emotions when they find themselves in situations that are morally unsatisfactory or when forces beyond their control prevent them from influencing or changing these perceived unsatisfactory moral situations. Suffering may occur because nurses believe that situations must be changed in order to bring well-being to themselves and others or to alleviate the suffering of themselves and others.

Moral suffering may arise, for example, from disagreements with institutional policy, such as a mandatory overtime or on-call policy that nurses believe does not allow adequate time for their psychological well-being. Nurses also may disagree with physicians' orders that the nurses believe are not in patients' best interest, or they may disagree with the way a family treats a patient or makes patient care decisions. These are but a few examples of the many types of encounters that nurses may have with moral suffering.

Another important, but often unacknowledged, source of moral suffering involves nurses freely choosing to act in ways in which they, themselves, know is not morally commendable. A difficult situation that may cause moral suffering for a nurse would be covering up a patient care error made by a valued nurse best friend. On the other hand, nurses may experience moral suffering when they act courageously by doing what they believe is morally right despite anticipated disturbing consequences. Sometimes, doing the right thing or acting as a virtuous person would act is difficult.

Some people view suffering as something to accept and to transform, if possible. Others react to situations with fear, bitterness, and anxiety. It is important to remember that wisdom and inner strength are often most increased during times of greatest difficulty.

> **CRITICAL THINKING QUESTION**
>
> Has there ever been a time that you have experienced the dilemma of having to make a choice that you know will impact the well-being of another individual? Have you ever experienced moral suffering?

Using a Team Approach

When trying to navigate ethically laden situations, patients and families may experience extreme anguish and suffering. Physicians, nurses, and other healthcare providers may explain to a patient or family that to continue the patient's treatment would be nonbeneficial and futile while patients or family members insist on continued treatment. When patients are weakened by disease and illness and families are reacting to the pain and suffering of their loved one, decisions regarding treatment may become sensitive and challenging for everyone concerned. Members of the healthcare team may question the decision-making capacity of the patient or family. The patient's or family's decision may conflict with the physician's or healthcare team's opinions regarding treatment. Nurses who care for patients and interact with families sometimes find themselves caught in the middle of these conflicts.

It is important to note that most problematic ethical decisions in health care are not be made unilaterally—not by physicians, nurses, or any other single person. Still, nurses are an integral part of the larger team of decision makers. Although nurses often make ethical decisions independently, many ethical dilemmas require nurses to participate interdependently with others in decision making. In analyzing healthcare ethics and decision making, nurses participate in extensive dialogue with others through committees, clinical team conferences, and other channels. Nurses are part of the larger team approach to ethical analysis. Commonly, the team is called an ethics consultation team or ethics committee.

Members of the team usually are physicians, nurses who represent their patients, an on-staff chaplain, nurses who regularly participate on the consultative team, a social worker, administrative personnel, possibly a legal representative, a representative for the patient in question or surrogate decision maker, and others drafted by the team. The number and membership of the ethics team vary among organizations and specific cases. When ethical disputes arise among any members of a patient's healthcare team, including disputes with patients and families, nurses often are the ones that seek an ethics consultation. It is within the right and duty of nurses to seek help and advice from the team if they encounter moral dilemmas or experience moral suffering.

In healthcare settings, moral reasoning to resolve an ethical dilemma is often a case-based, or bottom-up, inductive, casuistry approach. This approach begins with relevant facts about a particular case and moves toward a resolution through a structured analysis. A practical case-based ethical analysis approach that is used commonly by nurses and other healthcare professionals is the Four Topics Method or, often called in jargon, the 4-Box Approach (Table 4-1) (Jonsen, Siegler, & Winslade, 2006, p. 11). The Four Topics Method, developed by Albert Jonsen, Mark Siegler, and William Winslade, was published first in 1982 in their book *Clinical Ethics: A Practical Approach to Ethical Decisions in Clinical Medicine*, which is in its sixth edition.

> In healthcare settings, moral reasoning to resolve an ethical dilemma is often a case-based, or bottom-up, inductive, casuistry approach.

This case-based approach facilitates critical thinking about the issues and problems of a particular situation and facilitates construction of the case through information gathering in a structured format. Each problematic ethical case is analyzed according to four topics: medical indications, patient preferences, quality of life, and contextual features (Jonsen et al., 2006). Nurses and other healthcare professionals on the team gather information in an attempt to answer the questions in each of the four boxes.

The Four Topics Method promotes a dialogue between the patient, family, and members of the healthcare ethics team. Each patient's case is unique and should be considered as such, but the subject matter concerning the dilemma involves common threads among cases, such as withdrawing or withholding treatment and right to life. Applicability of the four fundamental bioethical principles—autonomy, beneficence, nonmaleficence, and justice—are considered along with data generated by using the Four Topics Method in analyzing a

TABLE 4-1 FOUR TOPICS METHOD FOR ANALYSIS IN CLINICAL ETHICS CASES

Medical Indications

The Principles of Beneficence and Nonmaleficence

1. What is the patient's medical problem? history? diagnosis? prognosis?
2. Is the problem acute? chronic? critical? emergent? reversible?
3. What are the goals of treatment?
4. What are the probabilities of success?
5. What are the plans in case of therapeutic failure?
6. In sum, how can this patient be benefited by medical and nursing care, and how can harm be avoided?

Patient Preferences

The Principle of Respect for Autonomy

1. Is the patient mentally capable and legally competent? Is there evidence of incapacity?
2. If competent, what is the patient stating about preferences for treatment?
3. Has the patient been informed of benefits and risks, understood this information, and given consent?
4. If incapacitated, who is the appropriate surrogate? Is the surrogate using appropriate standards for decision making?
5. Has the patient expressed prior preferences, e.g., advance directives?
6. Is the patient unwilling or unable to cooperate with medical treatment? If so, why?
7. In sum, is the patient's right to choose being respected to the extent possible in ethics and law?

Quality of Life

The Principles of Beneficence and Nonmaleficence and Respect for Autonomy

1. What are the prospects, with or without treatment, for a return to normal life?
2. What physical, mental, and social deficits is the patient likely to experience if treatment succeeds?
3. Are there biases that might prejudice the provider's evaluation of the patient's quality of life?
4. Is the patient's present or future condition such that his or her continued life might be judged undesirable?
5. Is there any plan and rationale to forgo treatment?
6. Are there plans for comfort and palliative care?

Contextual Features

The Principles of Loyalty and Fairness

1. Are there family issues that might influence treatment decisions?
2. Are there provider (physicians and nurses) issues that might influence treatment decisions?
3. Are there financial and economic factors?
4. Are there religious and cultural factors?
5. Are there limits on confidentiality?
6. Are there problems of allocations of resources?
7. How does the law affect treatment decisions?
8. Is clinical research or teaching involved?
9. Is there any conflict of interest on the part of the providers or the institution?

Source: Jonsen, A. R., Siegler, M., & Winslade, W. J. (2002). *Clinical ethics: A practical approach to ethical decisions in clinical medicine* (5th ed.). New York: McGraw-Hill. Reprinted with permission of The McGraw-Hill Companies.

patient's case. In Table 4-1, each box includes principles appropriate for each of the four topics. The additional principles of fairness and loyalty are included in the contextual features section.

Intense emotional conflicts between healthcare professionals and the patient and family may occur and hurt feelings can result. Nurses need to be sensitive and open to the needs of patients and families, particularly during these times. As information is passed back and forth between healthcare professionals and patients and families, an attitude of respect is indispensable in keeping the lines of communication open. Nurses play an essential role in the decision-making process in bioethical cases because of their traditional roles as patient advocate, caregiver, and educator. Nurses must attempt to maximize the values and needs of patients

CASE STUDY   MS. CRANFORD

You are a student nurse who is caring for Ms. Cranford. She is an 87-year-old mentally competent woman who has lived alone since her husband died 10 years ago. She was admitted to the hospital with chest pain, feeling faint, a pulse of 48, and a blood pressure of 98/56. The physician and nurses stabilized Ms. Cranford with medications and intravenous fluids but later informed Ms. Cranford and her only son that she would need a heart pacemaker to regulate her heartbeat. After the physician explained the procedure and risks involved, Ms. Cranford pondered the situation for a long while before discussing it with her son and the physician. Her medical history includes long-term adult-onset diabetes, chronic renal failure, and arterial insufficiency. She feels very tired. She decides that she does not want a pacemaker. Once Ms. Cranford tells her son her wishes, he is quite upset, and thus, he meets with the physician to discuss the options. The physician and Ms. Cranford's son revisited this issue with her in an attempt to persuade her to change her mind, but she continues to refuse the recommended treatment. She and her son argue. The physician tries to explain to Ms. Cranford that the pacemaker is for her benefit, in her "best inter-

est," and involves very minimal risks to her. She feels as if they are "ganging up" on her. Once the registered nurse becomes aware of the problem, you and the nurse visit with Ms. Cranford and her son to assess and evaluate the ethical issues involved with her case.

CASE STUDY QUESTIONS:

Imagine that you are a nurse on the ethics committee consulted about Ms. Cranford's case. Answer the following questions:

1. What are the central ethical issues and questions in this case?
2. What principles are in conflict in this case?
3. What did the physician mean by "best interest" for Ms. Cranford?
4. Use the Four Topics Method to discuss issues, to identify additional information that may be needed, and to analyze this case. What are your recommendations on behalf of the ethics committee?
5. What is the role of the nurses caring for Ms. Cranford in resolving this situation with the ethics team, her other healthcare providers, Ms. Cranford, and her son?

and families. A key component in preserving patient autonomy, respect, and dignity is for the nurse to have all of the essential information necessary for wise and skillful decisions.

Conclusion

With any type of ethical matters in health care, a nurse must ask "What is good in terms of how one wants to be?" and "What is good in terms of what one ought to do?" Becoming ethically savvy does not *just happen* in nursing. Nurses must consciously cultivate ethical habits and use theoretical knowledge about how to navigate ethical dilemmas. Moral suffering cannot be eliminated from nursing practice; however, the cultivation of wisdom and skill in decision making can help to alleviate some of its effects.

References

American Nurses Association. (2001). *Code of ethics with interpretive statements.* Washington, DC: Author.

Angeles, P. A. (1992). *The Harper Collins dictionary of philosophy* (2nd ed.). New York: Harper Perennial.

Beauchamp, T. L., & Childress, J. F. (1979). *Principles of biomedical ethics.* New York: Oxford University Press.

Beauchamp, T. L., & Childress, J. F. (2001). *Principles of biomedical ethics* (5th ed.). New York: Oxford University Press.

Bentham, J. (1988). *The principles of morals and legislation.* Loughton, Essex: Prometheus Books. (Original work published 1789)

Broadie, S. (2002). Commentary. In C. Rowe (Trans.), *Aristotle: Nicomachean ethics: Translation, introduction, and commentary.* New York: Oxford University Press.

Callahan, D. (1995). Bioethics. In W. T. Reich (Ed.), *Encyclopedia of bioethics: Revised edition* (Vol. 1, pp. 247–256). New York: Simon & Schuster Macmillan.

Chambliss, D. F. (1996). *Beyond caring: Hospitals, nurses, and the social organization of ethics.* Chicago: University of Chicago Press.

Daly, B. J. (2002). Moving forward: A new code of ethics. *Nursing Outlook, 50,* 70–99.

Dossey, B. M. (2000). *Florence Nightingale: Mystic, visionary, healer.* Springhouse, PA: Springhouse.

Fowler, M. D., & Benner, P. (2001). Implementing a new code of ethics for nurses: An interview with Marsha Fowler. *American Journal of Critical Care, 10*(6), 434–437.

Fry, S., & Veatch, R. M. (2000). *Case studies in nursing ethics* (2nd ed.). Boston: Jones and Bartlett.

Gilligan, C. (1993). *In a different voice: Psychological theory and women's development.* Cambridge, MA: Harvard University Press.

Grimshaw, J. (1993). The idea of a female ethic. In P. Singer (Ed.), *A companion to ethics* (pp. 491–499). Oxford, England: Blackwell.

International Council of Nurses. (2006). *The ICN code of ethics for nurses.* Geneva, Switzerland: Author. Retrieved December 2, 2007, from http://www.icn.ch/icncode.pdf

Johnstone, M. J. (1999). *Bioethics: A nursing perspective* (3rd ed.). Sydney, Australia: Harcourt Saunders.

Jonsen, A. (1998). *The birth of bioethics.* New York: Oxford University Press.

Jonsen, A. R., Siegler, M., & Winslade, W. J. (2002). *Clinical ethics: A practical approach to ethical decisions in clinical medicine* (5th ed.). New York: McGraw-Hill.

Jonsen, A. R., Siegler, M., & Winslade, W. J. (2006). *Clinical ethics: A practical approach to ethical decisions in clinical medicine* (6th ed.). New York: McGraw-Hill.

Kant, I. (2003). *Groundwork of the metaphysics of morals.* New York: Oxford University Press. (Original work published 1785)

Kelly, C. (2000). *Nurses' moral practice: Investing and discounting self.* Indianapolis, IN: Sigma Theta Tau International Center Nursing Press.

Kuhse, H., & Singer, P. (1998). What is bioethics? A historical introduction. In H. Kuhse & P. Singer (Eds.), *A companion to bioethics* (pp. 3–11). Oxford, England: Blackwell.

Mappes, T. A., & DeGrazia, D. (2001). *Biomedical ethics* (5th ed.). Boston: McGraw-Hill.

Mill, J. S. (2002). *Utilitarianism* (G. Sher, Trans.). Indianapolis, IN: Hackett Publishing. (Original work published 1863)

Munson, R. (2004). *Intervention and reflection: Basic issues in medical ethics* (7th ed.). Victoria, Australia: Thomson Wadsworth.

Pieper, J. (1966). *The four cardinal virtues.* Notre Dame, IN: University of Notre Dame Press.

Pullman, D. (1999). The ethics of autonomy and dignity in long-term care. *Canadian Journal on Aging, 18*(1), 26–46.

Thomas, L. (1993). Morality and psychological development. In P. Singer (Ed.), *A companion to ethics* (pp. 464–475). Oxford, England: Blackwell.

chapter 5

Social Context of Professional Nursing

Mary W. Stewart

LEARNING OBJECTIVES

After completing this chapter, the student should be able to:
1. Describe the social context of professional nursing.
2. Identify factors that influence the public's image of professional nursing.
3. List ways that nurses can promote an accurate image of professional nursing in the media.
4. Discuss the gender gap in nursing.
5. Recognize strategies to broaden the cultural and ethnic diversity in nursing.
6. Evaluate current barriers to health care in our society.
7. Analyze present trends in society that influence professional nursing.
8. Suggest research needs related to the future of nursing in our society.

Key Terms and Concepts

- Stereotype
- Multiculturalism
- Access to care
- Capitalistic society
- Nurse-managed centers
- Violence
- Mental health
- Global aging
- Nursing shortage
- Consumerism
- Complementary and alternative medicine
- Disaster preparedness

When you hear the word *nurse,* what image comes to mind? Ask yourself, "Why did that picture come into focus?" The answer to this question will tell you much about the social context of nursing. For many people, the image that first comes into view is one of a white female who is dressed in white and who is wearing a stiff cap. For those of us in nursing, we recognize that this traditional American view of nursing is rarely seen in the real world of professional nursing. Thus, how do we fill the gap? How do we want the public to perceive us? What influences the image of today's professional nurse?

105

In this chapter, we look at the social context of professional nursing. We explore the major influences that affect nursing in today's society. This journey toward a deeper understanding of nursing will challenge us to identify our individual responsibilities in educating our patients and the public about professional nursing. The end result will not necessarily be an immediate change in the picture that comes to mind when one says "nursing." However, we may begin to see nursing and those of us committed to nursing in new, more accurate ways.

Public Image of Nursing

The public values nursing. When asked to defend this support of nurses, people often respond with anecdotal stories of personal experiences with nurses. Popular stories include those of relatives or friends who are nurses. The fact that nurses serve society seems to have an automatically positive impact on society's value of nursing. However, a gulf divides the public's perception of nursing from the reality of nursing. The public will confess to holding nurses in high regard. Nevertheless, the public has few specific impressions of nursing, good or bad. Unfortunately in health care, nursing is the invisible majority (Sullivan, 2004).

We must first begin with the realization that "a nurse is a nurse" is not true. Unfortunately, many well-educated persons do not understand the varying educational programs available to become a registered nurse. Moreover, the difference in preparation and responsibility between licensed practical nurses, registered nurses, and advanced practice nurses (e.g., nurse practitioners) is vague.

What created this muddy view of nursing? As you are preparing to be a professional nurse, ask yourself, "How do I clarify and communicate the significance of professional nursing?" First, know what it is that professional nurses do and understand the multifaceted roles for which you are being educated. Second, be able to identify specifically the unique place that professional nurses have in the healthcare system. This comes about by not only knowing your own field, but also knowing about others' responsibilities and contributions in health care. Finally, and most importantly, tell your story. Suzanne Gordon, an award-winning journalist, dedicates much of her writing to telling the stories of nursing. Not a nurse herself, Gordon writes to empower nurses to find their voice and be heard. According to Buresh and Gordon (2000), although the public holds nurses in high regard, they know very little about what nurses actually do. Without articulating more clearly and loudly on our profession's behalf, we may be at a loss when trying to defend our place in the current healthcare system.

When asked about the nurse's failure to promote nursing effectively, we respond with excuses such as our lack of time. Professional nurses work in very demanding jobs. Often we are so consumed with the responsibilities of our work that we fail to notice what we are actually accomplishing. Moreover, we rarely take time to become aware of what our colleagues in nursing around us are doing. Although organizations exist to communicate and support these achievements, only a slim percentage of registered nurses are members of professional nursing associations.

Better insight into professional nursing must first come from within. Then, we have an obligation to communicate our necessary place to the public. Only at that point will we begin to see the public image of nursing change. We want to maintain the positive impression the public now holds of nursing, but nursing and the public deserve more than that. All of us should be convinced of the expertise professional nursing offers: mastery of complicated technologic skills; appreciation for the whole person; commitment to public health for all people; a keen knowledge of anatomy, physiology, biochemistry, pharmacology, and other disciplines; the ability to connect the dots in a fragmented healthcare system; and proficiency in communication. The list continues.

Social change takes place one person at a time. Reflecting on the changes in racial relationships, for example, we understand that improvements have not come solely because of the civil rights movement in the 1960s. Granted, that was a period of radical change for which we should all be indebted. Nonetheless, real change in race relationships in our society has come

> Social change takes place one person at a time.

from exposure and experience. Someone once said, "Ignorance is only removed by experience." Is it any different for our image as nurses?

Media's Influence

Clearly, the media plays a major part in how society views professional nursing. Historically, the nurse has been portrayed in the media in several ways. First, the nurse appears as a young, seductive female whose principal qualification is the length of her slender legs. Needless to say, this nurse is usually depicted as an airhead. The other popular view in the media is also female, but at the other end of the spectrum of physical attractiveness. She is round and rough. Often she is shown in a threatening way to patients, such as holding a syringe with a 3-inch needle in her hand. Neither of these views is accurate, and probably no one would argue with that. At the same time, we continue to draw a blank when asked to define the professional nurse.

In their book *From Silence to Voice: What Nurses Know and Must Communicate to the Public,* Buresh and Gordon (2000) asserted that nurses have to create a "voice of agency." They described this as nurses recognizing not only what they do as important, but also recognizing their own importance. A voice of agency says, "I'm here. I am doing something important" (p. 35). As nurses, we have been complacent with refuting the negative stereotypes portrayed in the media. Furthermore, we have been remiss in articulating our expertise to the media.

Buresh and Gordon (2000) wrote extensively about ways for us as nurses to communicate our essential message clearly. Nurses need to face the stereotypes present

CRITICAL THINKING QUESTION

How do you tell society what professional nurses do?

in our society and erase the lines that define us. To do this, we must first recognize within ourselves our value. When introducing ourselves in the professional role, we should do so with confidence and clarity, for example, "Good morning, Mr. Smith. I'm Susan Jones, your registered nurse." This introduction should be accompanied by a kind and self-assured handshake. Such day-to-day engagement is important. Still, we must tell the world what we do.

In *From Silence to Voice,* the authors identified the following actions to promote the real image of nursing:

- Educate the public in daily life.
- Describe the nurse's work.
- Make known the agency—independent thinker—of the registered nurse.
- Deal with the fear of angering the physician.
- Accept thanks.
- Be ready to take advantage of openings to promote nursing.
- Respond to queries with real-life stories from nursing.
- Tell the details.
- Avoid using nursing jargon.
- Be prepared ahead of time to tell your story.
- Do not suppress your enthusiasm.
- Reflect the nurse's clinical judgment and competency.
- Connect your work to pressing contemporary issues.
- Respect patient confidentiality.
- Deal with the fear of failure.

Finally, Buresh and Gordon provided a history and understanding of modern media and provided examples of how to interconnect with them. How to write a letter to the editor, present oneself on television, and converse with community groups are among the guidelines provided. This is an exciting, proactive work for nursing, and it comes at a time when healthcare costs demand that only the fundamental players are left standing.

Sigma Theta Tau International commissioned the 1997 Woodhull Study on Nursing and the Media, which reported the paucity of representation that nurses have in the media (Sigma Theta Tau International, 1998). Of approximately 20,000 articles from 16 major news publications, nurses were cited only 3% of the time. Among the healthcare industry publications, only 1% of the references were nurses. Although nurses are highly relevant participants in patients' stories, they were neglected in almost every case (Sigma Theta Tau International Web page). Key study recommendations from the Woodhull Study include the following:

- If the aim is to provide comprehensive coverage of health care, the media should include information by and about nurses.

- Nurses must not wait for the media to discover their contributions.
- *Health care* needs to be clearly identified as the umbrella term for specific disciplines, such as medicine and nursing.
- Nurses with doctoral degrees should be identified correctly as doctors, and those with medical doctorate (MD) degrees should be identified as physicians.
- Language needs to reflect the diverse options for health care by avoiding phrases such as, "Consult your doctor." Rather, media needs to state, "Consult your primary healthcare provider."

In recent years, we have seen more accurate portrayals of nurses supported in the media. Johnson & Johnson continues the *Campaign of Nursing's Future* to raise public awareness of professional nursing. This positive promotion has supported student and faculty recruitment into the profession. Further, Johnson & Johnson has recognized the valiant efforts of many nurses, including those who were intensely engaged in responding during national crises such as Hurricane Katrina. Nurses must continually evaluate the portrayal of nurses in the media. After all, if the image is inaccurate, we have a responsibility to correct it.

The Gender Gap

Women in Nursing and the Socialization of That Tradition

In Western culture, women have traditionally been socialized as the more passive of the sexes—to avoid conflict and yield to authority. The implications of this conventional thought are still seen in nursing practice today. Many nurses lack confidence in dealing with conflict and communicating with others in authority. For some, it is a matter of a short supply of energy. There are too many other commitments. For others, we see assertiveness as clashing with people's expectations of us. Isn't the reward of knowing we do a good job enough?

As female nurses assuming multiple roles, the career is often not at the top of our priorities. This may be attributed to the fact that the role of women in past society was primarily geared toward family responsibility, not a career. For women who chose nursing, many did so without the expectation of a long-term commitment to the profession. Rather, nursing was a "good job" when and if a woman needed to work. This centeredness on service by women continues in nursing today, albeit with less intensity than in the past.

The women's movement in the 1960s empowered intelligent career-seeking women to professions other than the traditional ones of teaching and nursing. After some years of competing for students, nursing saw a return of interest in the 1980s and 1990s. At this point, women chose nursing because nursing provided a natural complement to their gifts and not because it was one of a few options available to them (Chitty & Campbell, 2001). As the message of varied opportunities for women and men in nursing is shared, the social status of all of nursing is elevated to a higher level.

Men in Nursing

As we started the new millennium, men represented approximately 5.4% of the registered nurse population in the United States (Trossman, 2003). Although relatively small in number (146,902), this is a 226% increase in the number of male nurses from the previous 20 years (2003). Recruitment campaigns to attract men into nursing are frequently advertised. For example, the Oregon Center for Nursing (2003) created a poster of men in nursing using the slogan, "Are you man enough to be a nurse?" The Mississippi Hospital Association published an all-male calendar with monthly features of men in nursing, from nursing students to practicing professionals in a variety of roles. Needless to say, these actions are resulting in less of a stigma for men to enter the modern world of professional nursing.

The American Nurses Association (ANA) inducted the first man into its Hall of Fame in 2004 (American Nurses Association, 2007). Dr. Luther Christman was recognized for his 65-year career and contributions to the profession, including the founding of the American Assembly for Men in Nursing. In 2007, the ANA established the Luther Christman Award to recognize the contributions of men in nursing. Current literature keeps alive the discussion of men in nursing.

Although a popular topic, men have been in nursing for a long time. In the 11th, 12th, and 13th centuries, men played a major role in providing nursing care. Nursing became a predominantly female discipline late in the 1800s. Despite her many positive contributions to nursing, Nightingale did not encourage the participation of men in nursing. Rather, she defined nursing as female work. This **stereotype** has continued to today and is also evidenced in foreign reports (Lliffe, 2002).

Men are open to nursing as a career choice (Berlin, Stennett, & Bednash, 2004). In the fall of 2003, the percentage of men enrolled in undergraduate schools of nursing was 8.4%. Frequently, men choose the high-technology, fast-paced, intense environments to practice nursing. Emergency departments, intensive care units, and nurse anesthesiology are examples of areas to which men are often attracted (Gibbs & Waugaman, 2004). Some speculate that men make these choices because of the potential role strain if they were to choose other areas, such as obstetrics and pediatrics (Chitty & Campbell, 2001).

Some argue that men in nursing have an advantage over their female peers. It is not unusual for patients to assume that a male nurse is a physician or a medical student. Discrepancies in salaries exist (Kalist, 2002). Furthermore, men assume leadership roles in nursing at a much higher percentage than that reflected in the overall composition of men in nursing. As a result, women in nursing are challenged to learn from our male colleagues how to promote ourselves within the profession—regardless of gender.

What issues do men face in nursing? Because most nursing faculty are female, most nursing textbooks are written by females, and most leaders in nursing are female, men may have to learn new ways of thinking and understanding in order to find a comfortable place of belonging in the nursing profession. An example is given of a male nursing student who was having difficulty answering questions on a nursing examination. When the student shared a sample question with his wife (who was not a nurse), she answered the question correctly (Brady & Sherrod, 2003).

Because of gender bias, some patients may refuse to allow men in the nursing role to care for them (Cardillo, 2001). In labor and delivery, for example, patients and their partners may request a female nurse to be at the bedside during labor. In the least, the presence of a male nurse alone in the room is out of the ordinary. On the other hand, men in nursing are assumed to be physically stronger and willing to do the heavier tasks of nursing care, such as lifting and moving patients (Cardillo, 2001). Still, many men and women are learning to appreciate and enjoy the emerging culture in the profession (Meyers, 2003). The old biases are disappearing as patients and providers become more educated about the need for diversity.

> **CRITICAL THINKING QUESTIONS**
>
> What advantages do women have in nursing? What advantages do men have in the profession? What are the risks of being gender exclusive?

Cultural and Ethnic Diversity

In addition to gender diversity, we are also privileged as a profession to experience a diversity of race, age, and socioeconomic backgrounds. However, the presence of this **multiculturalism** force can lead to people feeling threatened, especially if the culture within the profession does not encourage mutual respect and acceptance (Waters, 2004).

Even though most registered nurses are Caucasian women, more minorities are being represented in the schools of nursing. The American Association of Colleges of Nursing reported that 12.2% of students enrolled in baccalaureate programs in the fall of 2003 were African-American, which represented a 0.9% increase and the largest minority population in nursing. American Indians or Alaskan Natives at 0.6% represented the lowest minority population and revealed no change in the same time frame. The Hispanic nursing population grew slightly from 5.1% to 5.4% (Berlin, Stennett, & Bednesh, 2003, 2004).

As the population becomes increasingly diverse, consumers of health care are more knowledgeable about the need for culturally competent care (Jacob & Carnegie, 2002). To provide such nursing care, we must encourage a nursing population that more accurately represents our communities. Partnerships between the healthcare agencies and other community agencies are vital to increased understanding.

The National Advisory Council on Nurse Education and Practice (NACNEP) was established to advise the secretary of the US Department of Health and Human Services and the US Congress on policy issues related to Title VIII programs administered by the Health Resources and Services Administration. NACNEP identified the need to increase racial and ethnic diversity of the RN workforce. In its third report, NACNEP recommended that the country "expand the resources available to develop models that will effectively recruit and graduate sufficient numbers of racial/ethnic students to reflect the nation's diverse population" (National Advisory Council on Nurse Education and Practice, 2003). More details about the council's advocacy of a national action agenda to address nursing workforce diversity are available at www.diversitynursing.com.

Dr. Madeleine Leininger, a nurse theorist and anthropologist, began the field of transcultural nursing. In her work, Dr. Leininger has advanced nursing's thinking to include people from all cultures and to understand the significance of cultural context (Leininger, 1991). Being culturally competent, that is, having the ability to interact appropriately with others through cultural understanding, is an expectation for people entering the nursing profession (Grant & Letzring, 2003). Keep in mind that there is a difference between learning *of* another culture and learning *from* another culture.

Efforts to Recruit and Retain Minorities in Nursing

In a recent literature review of ethnic diversity in the nurse workforce, Otto and Gurney (2006) explored two aspects: academic and career factors that influence diversity; and recruitment, retention, and other strategies to diversify the workforce. First, there is a paucity of scholarly research investigating ethnic diversity in nursing. However, some progress is being made. In a 2000 national survey, New York State reported a minority RN population similar to their overall minority population. Authors also reported that in one study, 56% of hospital units had a nursing team that represented at least three different ethnic groups (Otto & Gurney).

Kavanagh (2001) indicated that failure to recognize the issue of ethnic diversity ignores health issues and potential resources. Historically, people of ethnic minorities have not been afforded equal opportunities for education. As a result, the nursing population has yet to represent the population that we serve. The number of nurse educators and nurse researchers from minority groups is even less representative of the population. Jacob and Carnegie (2002) identified the following strategies to promote minorities in the nursing workforce:

- Raise the awareness level of diversity issues through educational offerings in the workplace and through organizational meetings.
- Seek experts on cross-cultural nursing issues from reputable sources, such as the Transcultural Nursing Society.
- Use mentoring programs where people are matched based on their cultural backgrounds.
- Use technology and media to connect with people of different cultures.

Additional implications include the increase in scholarly nursing research to demonstrate the value of a diverse workforce (Otto & Gurney, 2006). Analysis of recruitment and retention interventions is also necessary. Finally, professional nurses must become actively engaged in the political arena to influence the policy and legislation ensuring diversity in nursing (Otto & Gurney).

Access to Health Care

Populations at risk for poor health care include the vulnerable among us; some are easily spotted, whereas others are masked by propriety. In the richest country in the world, why do we have people who we label "at risk"? The answer is not simple and is in part related to our segregated healthcare system. Of all developed countries in the world, the United States is the only country that does not guarantee health care for all its citizens. Barriers to access include issues of economics, geography, and sociocultural differences.

> Of all developed countries in the world, the United States is the only country that does not guarantee health care for all its citizens.

Economic Barriers

Undoubtedly, poverty poses the greatest risk to health care. The United States has a long-standing reputation for providing the highest quality health care to persons in the highest socioeconomic strata; likewise, the lowest quality health care is

> **CRITICAL THINKING QUESTION**
>
> Who is entitled to health care?

provided to those at the other end of the socioeconomic continuum (Jacob & Carnegie, 2002). As the largest segment of the healthcare industry, registered nurses can have a positive impact on the needed change in this established system. Recognizing the stronghold that poverty currently has on the health care of citizens is a beginning to the much needed work in the fight for equality.

Although stereotypes communicate that poverty is limited to certain groups, we understand that poverty affects people of all cultures and ethnicities. We must recognize the impact that poverty has on healthcare practices. People who are forced to live day to day will have difficulty accepting the teaching surrounding primary care; they strive to meet the immediate needs and cannot think of anything else. "Universally, the greatest threat to positive health status is poverty" (Kavanagh, 2001, p. 215). Our most vulnerable could be saved if poverty was eradicated. There would be no more homeless people, no more uninsured, and no more choices between food and medicine. Until that time, nursing continues to face the challenge of meeting the needs of all the people.

Geographic Barriers

Those living in rural areas have unique concerns regarding **access to care**. As finances influence the closing of many rural hospitals, more communities find themselves struggling to find primary care providers who will work in those areas. State and national efforts have attempted to provide more service to these areas, but the demand is outweighing the supply.

Urban dwellers are not immune to geographical barriers. Large cities have economically depressed sections with fewer healthcare providers than the more affluent areas. Dependency on public transportation is another factor to be managed. Finally, most rural and many urban communities do not support a full range of healthcare services in one location. These variables impact patients' access to care and their continuation in prescribed treatment plans.

Sociocultural Barriers

We have already discussed the need for cultural and ethnic diversity in the nursing workforce. Moreover, healthcare settings are challenged to provide an environment where people of various sociocultural backgrounds are respected. For example, having translators on site or within easy contact is critical for ensuring safe care to non-English-speaking clients. Written materials should also be provided in appropriate languages. Specifically, consent forms for surgery and other procedures should be available in the client's language. To ignore the need for language-appropriate literature may lead to patient harm, as well as disrespect for the uniqueness of others.

One subculture that has garnered much attention in recent years is the military patient population. The Department of Defense operates and finances health care through TRICARE, a comprehensive healthcare coverage program for members of the uniformed services, their families, and survivors. With national resources decreasing and demands for health care of our military population on the rise, nurses play a pivotal role in influencing the direction of care for this special group.

Healthcare Delivery in the United States

Economic variables pervade our nation's value of health care. Individuals who are unable to secure a health insurance plan are at great risk for inadequate care. Further, insurance companies now dictate to care providers what is permissible by determining covered benefits. The confusing patterns of payment for health care are prohibitive and further increase the stress of individuals in poor health conditions. In addition to the complexity of healthcare payment options, the availability of charitable care in this country is shrinking.

Even though we live in a **capitalistic society**, nursing in the United States has been protected against the details of healthcare finance. Our roles have been focused on the patient, nothing more. Such days are no longer, and wishing for their return is futile. The changing economy has thrust all of us in health care to reconsider and restructure the very nature of our delivery systems. Hospitals have resisted a more decentralized approach to management, which has led to distrust and disloyalty to the organization. Crow (2002) encouraged the establishment of trust in the organizational culture—from the top executive to the shift supervisor—so social capital (shared values between employees and organizations) can be restored.

In addition to participating in new and creative management styles, nurses represent the intermediary for patients and the healthcare system. Part of the responsibility that comes with that role is being knowledgeable about healthcare finance and educating others about the current vocabulary in charges, reimbursement, and coverage. Moreover, nurses need to be involved in the policy-making processes that regulate the healthcare system. We are in an unprecedented time of change in our nation's health care. Professional nurses should be at the forefront, leading the charge to ensure adequate health care for all people.

Nurse-Managed Centers

Nurse-managed centers are increasing access to health care in a cost-effective way (Turkeltaub, 2004). Also called nursing clinics and nurse practice arrangements, these healthcare delivery options are meeting needs in communities across the country. Based on the philosophy of primary care and education, nurses are offering vital services at a lower cost.

In addition to providing care and cure, nurse-managed centers are enhancing relationships with the community. Faculty performing advanced practice and community nursing provide role models for the community while making clinical experiences available for students. In 2002, 18 grants to support nurse-managed centers were funded through the Health Resources and Services Administration's Bureau of Health Professions, Division of Nursing. As a result, 36 access points to care were provided for underserved populations. Service delivery options include school-based clinics, homeless shelters, correctional facilities, mobile health units, shelters, and public housing units. Federal support for these worthy programs is promising (Turkeltaub, 2004).

Trends

At any time in history, societal trends color the nursing profession. Major current movements include violence in the workplace; mental health needs; global aging; imbalance of supply and demand of nursing professionals; consumerism; complementary and alternative care; technologic changes; disaster preparedness; and nursing research. Discussion of these issues allows us to see more clearly the professional landscape and some of our challenges.

CRITICAL THINKING QUESTIONS

What barriers to health care do you see in your community? How are the underprivileged served in our current healthcare system? What actions should be taken to ensure universal access to health care?

Violence in the Workplace

The **violence** in our society is astounding. What is more alarming is our desensitization to it. As nurses, we can easily put a face on violence. We see the man in the emergency department with a gunshot wound to the chest. Only 30 minutes before, he was leaving work for a weekend with family when someone decided that they needed his car more than this man needed his life. We see violence at the women's shelter when we rotate through that clinical site in community health nursing. Why and how does it happen? We are puzzled—not just because we are nurses. We are also members of our communities where violence is far too common.

The sexual assault nurse examiner (SANE) is an example of how nursing is working aggressively to deal with one of the major types of violence (Littel, 2001). To be a SANE, a registered nurse must have advanced education and preparation in forensic examination of sexual assault victims. The Office for Victims of Crime of the US Department of Justice has led the development of SANE programs across the country and provides materials and resources to encourage new programs. As a result of the SANE programs, victims of sexual assault consistently receive attention and compassion without delay (Littel).

Nurses must become politically involved in preventing violence. We have to support legislation that proactively addresses violence and lobby for funding that provides nursing research into violence prevention and treatment. In every potential case, nurses have to use keen assessment skills to identify people at risk and to promote reporting, treatment, and rehabilitation. The national initiative to increase health for all US citizens, *Healthy People 2010,* outlines objectives for violence and abuse prevention (Table 5-1).

Mental Health Needs

As professional nurses experience the stresses that come with today's healthcare environment, we are obliged to assess our own **mental health** needs. Consider the registered nurse who works for 20 years with the same agency. During this time, he learns the practices of his department and agency. In fact, he becomes highly specialized in his area of nursing expertise. Economic changes require workforce reductions, and he becomes a victim. With the high demand of professional nurses, one would think securing employment an easy task. However, due to his specialization, he is forced to take a job outside his area to maintain an income. In addition to the stress of losing a position after a two-decade investment, he finds himself being challenged with some of the fundamental aspects of nursing care. Yet, they are not fundamental to him, and there is no one to help him. People try, but after all, they are very busy fulfilling their own roles. He becomes depressed, unfilled, and wondering what his future holds.

Following the national crises in the last several years, we have witnessed an increase in the mental health needs of our society. Professional nurses are not immune to this reality. Historically, mental health concerns have taken a backseat to other concerns, such as cancer and heart disease. True, these conditions require our resources, but so do the less glamorous conditions that affect emotional, spiritual, and mental health. In a following chapter, the writers examine care of professional self and address key concepts pertinent to this discussion.

Global Aging

The Year of the Older Person—this is what the United Nations called the year 1999 to recognize and reaffirm **global aging**—the fact that our global population is aging

TABLE 5-1 *HEALTHY PEOPLE 2010* VIOLENCE AND ABUSE PREVENTION OBJECTIVES

Objective to Reduce	Target by 2010	Baseline Data (1998)
Homicides	3 per 100,000	6.5 per 100,000
Maltreatment of children 17 years and younger	10.3 per 1000	12.9 per 1000
Fatalities caused by maltreatment, 17 years and younger	1.4 per 100,000	1.6 per 100,000
Rate of physical assault by current or former intimate partners	3.3 per 1000	4.4 per 1000
Annual rate of rape or attempted rape, persons aged 12 years and older	0.7 per 1000	0.8 per 1000
Sexual assault other than rape, persons aged 12 years and older	0.4 per 1000	0.6 per 1000
Physical assaults, persons aged 12 years and older	13.6 per 1000	31.1 per 1000
Physical fighting among adolescents in grades 9 through 12	32%	35%*
Weapon carrying by adolescents on school property in grades 8 through 12	4.9%	6.9%*

*Baseline data from 1999.
Source. Centers for Disease Control and Prevention (2000).

at an unprecedented rate (US Census Bureau, 2001). After World War II, fertility increased, and death rates at all ages decreased. Not only are people in developed countries living longer and healthier but so are those in the developing world. In the 1990s, developed countries had equal numbers of young (people 15 years and younger) and old (people 55 years and older) at approximately 22% of the population in each category. On the other hand, 35% of the people in developing countries were children compared with 10% who were older. Still, absolute numbers of older persons are large and growing. In the year 2000, more than half of the world's older people (59% or 249 million people) lived in developing nations. That projection is expected to increase to 71% (686 million) by the year 2030 (US Census Bureau).

For the first time in our history, people 65 years and older are expected to match closely in number those 18 years and younger in the next 30 years (Table 5-2). In the United States, a decrease in fertility, an increase in urbanization, better education,

TABLE 5-2   PROJECTED POPULATION AND PERCENTAGE OF POPULATION CHANGE IN THE UNITED STATES BY AGE, 2000–2050, IN THOUSANDS

	2000	2010	2020	2030	2040	2050	Percentage Population Change by Age (2000–2050)
Total	282,125	308,936	335,805	363,584	391,946	419,854	48.8%
0–4 years	19,218	21,426	22,932	24,272	26,299	28,080	46.1%
5–19 years	61,331	61,810	65,955	70,832	75,326	81,067	32.2%
20–44 years	104,075	104,444	108,632	114,747	121,659	130,897	25.8%
45–64 years	62,440	81,012	83,653	82,280	88,611	93,104	49.1%
65–84 years	30,794	34,120	47,363	61,850	64,640	65,844	113.8%
85+ years	4,267	6,123	7,269	9,603	15,409	20,861	388.9%

Source: US Census Bureau (2004).

improved health care, and the aging of the baby boomers are all contributors to this social phenomenon. The impact this will have on our healthcare system is daunting.

We must have clear health policy at a national level if we are to be prepared to care for our aging. Approaches from the past are inadequate. Because this is a new challenge for us, the correct actions are not clearly defined. Still, the responsibility is ours as a society, and nursing professionals should have a major role to play in ensuring that quality health care is available and provided.

In the last several years, schools of nursing have incorporated a greater number of gerontology courses and concepts into the curriculum. Clinical experiences in the adult health settings are heavily saturated with older persons. Still, we lack an organized plan to make certain that healthcare needs will be met—not just for the aging, but also for those who will come after them. Recent legislation in federal and local governments has called for improvements in medication coverage, insurance reimbursements, and reform in malpractice law. Thus far, these attempts have been inadequate to provide the comprehensive care that will be vital if we are to make the right to health care real for everyone.

Nursing Supply and Demand

Few topics regarding nurses have garnered the level of publicity that the current **nursing shortage** has attracted in recent years. As our general population ages, so does our nursing population. As a result, the number of nurses and nurse faculty is shrinking (Peterson, 2001). The major concern is related to what was discussed in the previous section—who will care for the old? As people age and experience health problems, their needs are often more complex and acute, thereby demanding an even greater skilled nursing force.

With a downturn in the nation's economy, healthcare systems tried to cut costs to stay in business. Unfortunately, nursing care was not exempt from the cutbacks. In the mid-1990s, nurses were asked to do more with less, and that expectation continues. Patients are sicker, and the nurse to patient ratio is often unbearable. Nurse burnout is too common (Weinberg, 2003). As a result, nurses leave the profession (Bingham, 2002). For female nurses, 4.1% left the profession in 2000 compared with 2.7% in 1992. Male nurses left at a rate of 7.5% in 2000, up from 2% in 1992 (Nelson, 2002).

In September 2002, the nursing shortage in the United States was labeled a national security concern (Nelson, 2002). Although the historical picture of nursing supply and demand has fluctuated, other variables influence the current shortage. In 2000, 9% of nurses were less than 30 years old. Additionally, more than 330,000 registered nurses are expected to retire by 2008. When you combine the number of older people requiring care with the number of nurses expected to retire, we expect the projected nursing vacancy rate to reach 800,000 by 2008. By 2020, the national nursing shortage is predicted to reach a 20% deficit (Nelson).

The majority of registered nurses work in hospitals; therefore, the onus is on those facilities to find better ways of recruiting and retaining professional staff. Cooper (2003) presented some strategies for nursing managers, staff, and faculty to negotiate through this crisis:

- To retain older nurses, reconstruct the patient care environment to make it more ergonomically sensitive, supportive, and tailored to the physical limitations of an aging workforce.
- Provide for and encourage educational pursuits.
- Evaluate and modify work schedules to complement circadian rhythms.
- Provide auxiliary staff around the clock.
- Attend to special needs of the nighttime workers; for example, provide fresh foods and healthy snacks.
- Provide a "resting room" for sleep breaks, especially if employees have a distance to drive home.

Still on the supply side of the equation, nursing faculty are also aging. Assistant and associate professors are an average of 52.1 and 48.5 years old, respectively (Cooper, 2003). The shortage of doctoral-prepared faculty is even more severe. On average, nurses receiving new doctorates are 45 years old (Cooper). Who will teach our future nurses?

Wieck (2003) pointed out that people are not choosing nursing as a profession. The younger generation is not attracted to the nursing career option. Some of the reasons for that may be related to issues currently being discussed in the literature—inflexible work environments, low compensation, poor recognition, high stress, and so on. Another possibility is the tendency for nursing education to resist change to meet the expectations of college-degree-seeking students. Nursing education programs must be aware of what this new generation desires in relationship to a learning experience and be prepared to reconfigure and create anew ways of instruction: offering courses online; providing personal, frequent feedback; and focusing on outcomes and not just the process are some of the suggestions in the literature (Wieck). The emerging workforce cannot be convinced to enter nursing for the same reasons that once attracted people to the profession. If we are to draw from the rich pool of young people, we have to find out what they need and find ways to provide it.

Consumerism

Since the American Hospital Association's development of "A Patient's Bill of Rights" in 1973, consumers have assumed more control of their healthcare experiences; this shift is called **consumerism**. The 1992 version of that document has recently been replaced by the brochure, "The Patient Care Partnership: Understanding Expectations, Rights, and Responsibilities" (American Hospital Association, 2003). A summary of that document is presented in Box 5-1. Gone are the days when patients blindly follow the instructions that their physicians give to them. In part, this is cause for celebration in the nursing arena. Professional nursing has long sought to empower patients to take responsibility for their own health. Although pockets of medical paternalism continue, the general shift is to hold healthcare providers to a higher standard than ever before.

BOX 5-1   THE PATIENT CARE PARTNERSHIP

What to expect during your hospital stay:

1. High-quality patient care
2. A clean and safe environment
3. Involvement in your care
   a. Discussing your medical condition and information about medically appropriate treatment choices
   b. Discussing your treatment plan
   c. Getting information from you
   d. Understanding your healthcare goals and values
   e. Understanding who should make decisions when you cannot
4. Protection of your privacy
5. Preparing you and your family for when you leave the hospital
6. Help with your bill and filing insurance claims

O'Neil and the Pew Health Profession Commission (1998) provided another example of attempts to respond to the changing needs of the American healthcare system. From 1989 to 1999, with a grant from the Pew Charitable Trusts, a commission was established to focus on the healthcare workforce. To improve health care of the American people, professionals in the healthcare delivery system need guidelines to respond to trends and developments. In 1998, the Commission presented their report *Twenty-One Competencies for the Twenty-First Century*. These competencies are presented in Box 5-2.

Bulger (2002) stated that four major points must be kept in mind when considering the healthcare system of the future. First, the influence of technology and science will have a major impact. Although research and experimentation have brought the United States to be a global leader in informatics, robotics, and genetics, we are cautioned to pause and consider the full potential of such a revolution. Second, multiprofessional collaboration will determine the efficiency and effectiveness with

---

BOX 5-2 TWENTY-ONE COMPETENCIES FOR THE TWENTY-FIRST CENTURY

1. Embrace a personal ethic of social responsibility and service.
2. Exhibit ethical behavior in all professional activities.
3. Provide evidence-based, clinically competent care.
4. Incorporate the multiple determinants of health in clinical care.
5. Apply knowledge of the new sciences.
6. Demonstrate critical thinking, reflection, and problem-solving skills.
7. Understand the role of primary care.
8. Rigorously practice preventive health care.
9. Integrate population-based care and services into practice.
10. Improve access to health care for those with unmet health needs.
11. Practice relationship-centered care with individuals and families.
12. Provide culturally sensitive care to a diverse society.
13. Partner with communities in healthcare decisions.
14. Use communication and information technology effectively and appropriately.
15. Work in interdisciplinary teams.
16. Ensure care that balances individual, professional, system, and societal needs.
17. Practice leadership.
18. Take responsibility for quality of care and health outcomes at all levels.
19. Contribute to continuous improvement of the healthcare system.
20. Advocate for public policy that promotes and protects the health of the public.
21. Continue to learn and help others learn.

Source: O'Neil and the Pew Health Professions Commission (1998).

which we respond to the demands in health care. Third, we must educate ourselves as healthcare providers and the public as consumers of health care. Finally, as health professionals, we are dependent on the research being conducted, which guides our actions and practice. In the end, nursing professionals have a heavy responsibility to be actively engaged in shaping and determining the future healthcare system.

Complementary and Alternative Approaches

As the consumer's perspective grows in influence, and individuals take on a greater investment in their healthcare decisions, they explore approaches to health care that may actually contrast with Western traditions. Different terminology has been used synonymously to define this growing field, such as *complementary care practices* and *alternative medicine.* According to the National Center for Complementary and Alternative Medicine (2002), "Complementary and alternative medicine is a group of diverse medical and healthcare systems, practices, and products that are not presently considered to be part of conventional medicine." Complementary medicine refers to an approach that *combines* conventional medicine with less conventional options, whereas alternative medicine is an approach used *instead* of conventional medicine. Major types of **complementary and alternative medicine** include:

- Alternative medical systems (built on complete systems of practice such as homeopathic medicine or naturopathic medicine)
- Mind-body interventions (techniques designed to enhance the mind's capacity to affect bodily function such as meditation, prayer, music, and support groups)
- Biologically based therapies (use of substances found in nature such as herbs, foods, and vitamins)
- Manipulative and body-based methods (based on manipulation or movement of one or more parts of the body such as chiropractic manipulation or massage)
- Energy therapies (involves the use of energy fields through either biofield therapies such as therapeutic touch, qi gong, or Reiki; or bioelectromagnetic-based therapies such as magnetic therapy)

Alternative and complementary therapies impact the selection of traditional choices for treatment, and ignoring that they exist is not an option. People persist in the use of alternative and complementary therapies for obvious reasons: (1) the therapies have been found valuable, and (2) Western medicine has limited options. A duty of the professional nurse is an accurate assessment of the patient's needs and circumstances. Therefore, it is imperative that nurses be educated on treatment choices the patient has selected. Nurses should provide a safe, trusting atmosphere where patients feel free to discuss their healthcare routines and preferences. Additionally, nursing educational programs should incorporate more information about the research in this growing field.

Technological Changes

Although technology influences in professional nursing are presented in detail later in this text, the mention of those changes here is warranted. Undeniably, technologic advances have impacted professional nursing practice in ways never imagined. The dream of connecting with patients in their homes via remote video and satellite is now commonplace. Digital, point-of-care documentation systems are the upcoming standard for patient records. Moreover, the equipment used in treatment plans changes at an exponential rate.

Although technology has presented new challenges—higher costs, greater educational demands, threats to bedside care—nurses can respond proactively. Ways of caring through technology exist. One example is the adoption of electronic patient records, which provide clearer communication between members of the multidisciplinary team. Also, documentation can be recorded in real time, thereby allowing the nurse to spend time with the patient. Additionally, patient safety is not compromised with poor handwriting and delayed orders (Meadows, 2003). Another example is the use of telehealth approaches to improve healthcare service in rural and underserved communities (Buckwalter, Davis, Wakefield, Kienzle, & Murray, 2002).

Information technology has given patients and care providers an enormous resource for gaining knowledge about diseases, medications, treatment options, and support groups. A basic part of any nursing plan of care should include reputable resources for the patient that can be accessed through the Internet. In today's healthcare environment, people are searching for answers to their healthcare questions. Who better to guide them to good information than a professional registered nurse?

Disaster Preparedness

Prior to the turn of this century, **disaster preparedness** was not a major topic of discussion in programs of nursing. Further, the key roles that professional nurses now play in preparing and responding to disasters were unexplored until recent history. The World Trade Center attack in 2001 and the shock of Hurricane Katrina in 2005 have opened eyes to our vulnerability and our strength. As a result, disaster management has become common language in our schools, agencies, and communities.

Disaster management has become common language in our schools, agencies, and communities.

Disaster management, plans designating response during an emergency, is coordinated by local, state, and federal groups. Firefighters, police officers, and healthcare professionals are part of response teams. Disaster training is also available to other volunteers. We have learned that caring for large groups affected by disaster requires an organized, thoughtful, unbiased approach by our leaders. Professional nurses carry the burden of being knowledgeable about such potential disasters as Avian influenza, educating the public about the risks, and responding when persons are affected.

Research regarding the future of nursing must center on efforts aimed at creating practice environments that increase nurse satisfaction and improve productivity.

Research Needs

Addressing the context of professional nursing in today's world gives rise to important research questions. Key are the changes in patient acuity and the effect on nurse staffing (Robert Wood Johnson Foundation, 2007). Models of nurse staffing, including fixed minimum ratios and pay-for-performance, are being tested. Although not independently, staffing ratios offer promise to improve nursing work environments. Research regarding the future of nursing must center on efforts aimed at creating practice environments that increase nurse satisfaction and improve productivity. Specific areas identified by the Robert Wood Johnson Foundation (2007) include increasing nurses' authority, increasing trust between nurses and management, reorganizing nurses' work, and prohibiting mandatory overtime.

Conclusion

Now, when you hear the word *nursing*, what image comes to mind? If the picture is blurry or confused by the expanding social context presented in this chapter—good! The cloudiness indicates that the tradition is questioned. We have looked at some of the social phenomena that help define nursing. Because those experiences change constantly, what we envision now will also be transformed. Nevertheless, we have to question the image and explore the factors that influence it. We are challenged to do this on a regular basis. Only then can we evolve in meaningful ways to better meet the nursing needs of our society.

Web Resources

American Assembly for Men in Nursing: http://www.aamn.org
American Association of Colleges of Nursing: http://www.aach.nche.edu
American Hospital Association: http://www.aha.org
American Nurses Association: http://www.nursingworld.org
Campaign for Nursing's Future: http://www.discovernursing.com
Diversity Nursing: http://www.diversitynursing.com
Healthy People 2010: http://www.healthypeople.gov
Minority Nurse: http://www.minoritynurse.com
National Association of Hispanic Nurses: http://www.thehispanicnurses.org
National Black Nurses Association: http://www.nbna.org
National Center for Complementary and Alternative Medicine: http://www.nccam.nih.gov
National League for Nursing: http://www.nln.org
National Student Nurses Association: http://www.nsna.org
Office for Victims of Crime, US Department of Justice: http://www.ojp.usdoj.gov/ovc
Pew Health Professions Commission: http://futurehealth.ucsf.edu/pewcomm.html
Sexual Assault Nurse Examiners: http://www.sane-sart.com

Transcultural Nursing Society: http://www.tcns.org

TRICARE: http://www.tricare.mil

US Bureau of the Census: http://www.census.gov

US Department of Labor: http://www.stats.bls.gov

References

American Hospital Association. (2003). *The patient care partnership: Understanding expectations, rights and responsibilities.* Retrieved April 24, 2008, from http://www.aha.org/aha/issues/Communicating-With-Patients/pt-care-partnership.html

American Nurses Association. (2007). American Nurses Association recognizes the contributions of men in nursing with the (ANA) Luther Christman Award. *Wyoming Nurse, 20*(2), 13.

Berlin, L. E., Stennett, J., & Bednash, G. D. (2003). *2002–2003 Enrollment and graduations in baccalaureate and graduate programs in nursing.* Washington, DC: American Association of Colleges of Nursing.

Berlin, L. E., Stennett, J., & Bednash, G. D. (2004). *2003–2004 Enrollment and graduations in baccalaureate and graduate programs in nursing.* Washington, DC: American Association of Colleges of Nursing.

Bingham, R. (2002). Leaving nursing [Electronic version]. *Health Affairs, 21,* 211–218.

Brady, M. S., & Sherrod, D. R. (2003). Retaining men in nursing programs designed for women [Electronic version]. *Journal of Nursing Education, 42,* 159–163.

Buckwalter, K. C., Davis, L. L., Wakefield, B. J., Kienzle, M. G., & Murray, M. A. (2002). Telehealth for elders and their caregivers in rural communities. *Family and Community Health, 25*(3), 31–40.

Bulger, R. J. (2002). What will health care look like in the future? In E. J. Sullivan (Ed.), *Creating nursing's future: Issues, opportunities and challenges* (pp. 14–31). St. Louis, MO: Mosby.

Buresh, B., & Gordon, S. (2000). *From silence to voice: What nurses know and must communicate to the public.* New York: Cornell University Press.

Cardillo, D. W. (2001). *Your first year as a nurse: Making the transition from total novice to successful professional.* Roseville, CA: Prima.

Centers for Disease Control. (2000). *Healthy People 2010.* Retrieved April 24, 2008, from http://www.healthypeople.gov/Document/tableofcontents.htm#partb

Chitty, K., & Campbell, C. (2001). The social context of nursing. In K. K. Chitty (Ed.), *Professional nursing: Concepts and challenges* (pp. 64–100). Philadelphia: W. B. Saunders.

Cooper, E. E. (2003). Pieces of the shortage puzzle: Aging and shift work [Electronic version]. *Nursing Economics, 21*(2), 75–80.

Crow, G. (2002). The relationship between trust, social capital, and organizational success [Electronic version]. *Nursing Administration Quarterly, 26*(3), 1–12.

Gibbs, D. M., & Waugaman, W. R. (2004). Diversity behind the mask: Ethnicity, gender, and past career experience in a nurse anesthesiology program [Electronic version]. *Journal of Multicultural Nursing & Health, 10,* 77–82.

Grant, L. F., & Letzring, T. D. (2003). Status of cultural competence in nursing education: A literature review [Electronic version]. *Journal of Multicultural Nursing & Health, 9*(2), 6–13.

Jacob, S. R., & Carnegie, M. E. (2002). Cultural competency and social issues in nursing and health care. In B. Cherry (Ed.), *Contemporary nursing: Issues, trends, & management* (pp. 239–262). St. Louis, MO: Mosby.

Kalist, D. E. (2002). The gender earnings gap in the RN labor market [Electronic version]. *Nursing Economics, 20,* 155–163.

Kavanagh, K. H. (2001). Social and cultural dimensions of health and health care. In J. L. Creasia & B. Parker (Eds.), *Conceptual foundations: The bridge to professional nursing practice* (pp. 294–314). St. Louis, MO: Mosby.

Leininger, M. M. (1991). *Culture care diversity & universality.* New York: National League for Nursing Press.

Littel, K. (2001). *Sexual assault nurse examiner (SANE) programs: Improving the community response to sexual assault victims.* Retrieved April 25, 2008, from http://www.ojp.usdoj.gov/ovc/publications/bulletins/sane_4_2001/welcome.html

Lliffe, J. (2002). Time to address nursing's gender imbalance [Electronic version]. *Australian Nursing Journal, 9*(1), 1.

Meadows, G. (2003). Improving the patient experience with information technology [Electronic version]. *Nursing Economics, 21,* 300–302.

Meyers, S. (2003). Real men chose nursing [Electronic version]. *Hospitals & Health Networks, 77*(6), 72–74.

National Advisory Council on Nurse Education and Practice. (2003). *Third report to the secretary of Health and Human Services and Congress.* Retrieved April 25, 2008, from http://bhpr.hrsa.gov/nursing/NACNEP/reports/third/default.htm

National Center for Complementary and Alternative Medicine. (2002). *What is complementary and alternative medicine (CAM)?* Retrieved April 25, 2008, from http://nccam.nih.gov/health/whatiscam

Nelson, R. (2002). US nursing shortage a "national security concern" [Electronic version]. *Lancet, 360,* 855–857.

O'Neil, E. H., & the Pew Health Professions Commission. (1998). *Twenty-one competencies for the twenty-first century.* San Francisco: Pew Health Professions Commission.

Oregon Center for Nursing. (2003). *Are you man enough . . . to be a nurse?* Retrieved March 21, 2008, from http://www.oregoncenterfornursing.org/documents/Poster%20order%20forms.pdf

Otto, L. A., & Gurney, C. (2006). Ethnic diversity in the nurse workforce: A literature review. *Journal of the New York State Nurses Association, Fall/Winter,* 16–21.

Peterson, C. (2001). Issues update. In short supply: Around the world, the need for nurses grows. *American Journal of Nursing, 101*(9), 61–64.

Robert Wood Johnson Foundation. (2007). *Charting nursing's future: Reports on policies that can transform patient care.* Princeton, NJ: Author.

Sigma Theta Tau International. (1998). *The Woodhull study on nursing and the media: Health care's invisible partner.* Indianapolis, IN: STTI Center Nursing Press.

Sullivan, E. J. (2004). *Becoming influential: A guide for nurses.* Upper Saddle River, NJ: Prentice Hall.

Trossman, S. (2003). Caring knows no gender: Break the stereotype and boost the number of men in nursing. *American Journal of Nursing, 103,* 65–68.

Turkeltaub, M. (2004). Nurse-managed centers: Increasing access to health care [Electronic version]. *Journal of Nursing Education, 43*(2), 53–54.

United States Census Bureau. (2001). *An aging world: 2001.* Retrieved April 25, 2008, from http://www.census.gov/prod/2001pubs/p95-01-1.pdf

United States Census Bureau. (2004). *U.S. interim projections by age, sex, race, and Hispanic origin.* Retrieved April 10, 2004, from http://www.census.gov/ipc/www/usinterimproj

Waters, V. L. (2004). Cultivate corporate culture and diversity [Electronic version]. *Nursing Management, 35,* 36–40.

Weinberg, D. B. (2003). *Code green.* Ithaca, NY: Cornell University Press.

Wieck, K. L. (2003). Faculty for the millennium: Changes needed to attract the emerging workforce into nursing. *Journal of Nursing Education, 42,* 151–159.

Education and Socialization to the Professional Nursing Role

Patricia Becker Hentz and Melanie Gilmore

LEARNING OBJECTIVES

After completing this chapter, the student should be able to:

1. Describe how the history of nursing has affected the socialization of nurses.
2. Discuss professionalism and nursing.
3. Describe socialization to professional nursing.
4. Describe how nursing education affects the socialization of nurses.
5. Identify cognitive stages related to professional socialization.
6. Discuss social influences on professional socialization and role development.
7. Describe the stages of skill and knowledge acquisition as defined by Benner.
8. Identify factors that facilitate professional role development.

Key Terms and Concepts

- Socialization
- Professional values
- Novice
- Advanced beginner
- Competent
- Proficient
- Expert
- Core values

Professional **socialization** involves a process by which a person acquires the knowledge, skills, and sense of identity that are characteristic of a profession. According to Cohen (1981), it involves the internalization of the values and norms of that profession. Professional socialization has four goals: (1) to learn the technology of the profession—the facts, skills, and theory—(2) to learn to internalize the professional culture, (3) to find a personally and professionally acceptable version of the role, and (4) to integrate this professional role into all of the other life roles.

127

A profession is generally distinguished from other kinds of vocations and occupations by (1) its requirement of prolonged, specialized training to acquire a body of knowledge specific to the work to be performed, and (2) the commitment of the individual toward service. The professional standards of education and practice for the profession are determined by the profession rather than outsiders (Blais, Hayes, Kozier, & Erb, 2002, p. 10). Nursing as a learned profession continues to evolve into a profession with a distinct body of knowledge, specialized practice, standards of practice, and social contract.

Professional Nursing Values

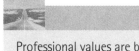

Professional values are beliefs or ideals that guide interactions with patients, colleagues, other professionals, and the public.

Educational preparation for nursing should facilitate the development of **professional values** and value-based behaviors. The development of professional values begins with professional education in nursing and continues along a continuum throughout the years of nursing practice (Shank & Weis, 2001). Professional values are beliefs or ideals that guide interactions with patients, colleagues, other professionals, and the public. Watson (1981) identified values critical to the profession of nursing. The values of (1) commitment to public service, (2) autonomy, (3) commitment to lifelong learning and education, and (4) a belief in the dignity and worth of each person epitomize the caring, professional nurse. Nurses, guided by these values, demonstrate ethical behaviors in the provision of safe, competent health care (American Association of Colleges of Nursing [AACN], 1998).

Nursing is a helping profession directed toward health promotion and disease prevention of individuals, families, and communities. Caring is a concept central to the profession of nursing. Inherent in this value is a strong commitment to public service. The role of the nurse is focused on assessing and promoting the health and well-being of all humans. Registered nurses remain in nursing to promote, advocate, and strive to protect the health and safety of patients, families, and communities (American Nurses Association [ANA], 2004).

Autonomy is the right to self-determination as a profession. The role of the professional nurse is to honor and assist individuals and families to make informed decisions about health care and provide information so that they can make informed choices. The professional nurse respects patients' rights to make decisions about their health care.

Commitment to lifelong learning and education is necessary in the dynamic healthcare arena that surrounds nursing practice in this century. Nurses need continuous education to maintain a safe level of practice and expand their level of competence as professionals. With new technologies and the rapid expansion of medical and nursing knowledge, the nurse must continuously seek to expand the body of professional knowledge. Professional nursing involves a commitment to be resourceful, to respond to the dynamic challenges of delivering health care, to incorporate technology into their art and caring, and to remain visionaries as the future unfolds (ANA, 2004).

Human dignity is respect for the inherent worth and uniqueness of individuals and communities. It is the basic belief in human life and the worth of a person regardless of nationality, race, creed, color, age, sex, politics, or social class (Blais et al., 2004, p. 15). "The essence of caring in nursing is respect for human dignity" (Fahrenwald et al., 2005, p. 47).

> **CRITICAL THINKING QUESTIONS**
>
> As a nursing student, do you share the values of commitment to public service, autonomy, commitment to lifelong learning and education, and the belief in the dignity and worth of each person? Do nurses with whom you have interacted demonstrate these values?

Socialization of Nurses: A Historical View

Early nursing education, an apprenticeship model or training as it was called, reflected the values and beliefs of Florence Nightingale, which emphasized character development over skills. The finished products (the Nightingale nurse was simply the ideal *lady*) were transplanted from the home to the hospital and were absolved of reproductive responsibilities. To the doctor, she brought the wifely virtue of absolute obedience. To the patient, she brought the selfless devotion of a mother (Ehrenreich & English, 1973, p. 36). In addition to service and obedience, training in the hospital school reflected military and religious models with an emphasis on duty, obligation, and order. Loyalty to the physician and trustworthiness were key values. The image of a nurse was "to be a 'gentle woman' with all the virtues and qualities that defined idealized middle- and upper-class womanhood in Victorian America" (Reverby, 1987, p. 49).

Obedience, loyalty, and character development remained central in the socialization of women in the 1900s. Isabel Hampton Robb's text *Nursing Ethics: For Hospital and Private Use* echoed this sentiment, as reflected in the following: "Above all, let her remember to do what she is told to do, and no more; the sooner she learns this lesson, the easier her work will be for her, and the less likely will she be to fall under severe criticism" (Jameton, 1984, p. 37).

The shadows of obedience and loyalty to the physician as core values for nursing practice were dominant throughout a major portion of the 1900s. "Until the 1950s, virtually every school required that the student nurse live in the hospital's residence, so the hospital was school, workplace, and home combined. Separated from her family and community, the young woman took her place in a world of female authority, where she underwent a rigorous apprenticeship into nursing, learning her craft in the classrooms and on the ward" (Melosh, 1982, p. 37). In the 1950s, loyalty to the physician was presented as the nurse's first duty. McAllister asserted that "by virtue of her profession, as well as her implied contract, the nurse owes the physician not only efficient care of patients but also such evidence of loyalty as will strengthen the patient's confidence in him" (Davis & Aroskar, 1978, p. 33). The nurse's loyalty to the physician was also reflected in the International Code for Nurses (1965 version) that stated, "The nurse is under the obligation to carry out the physician's orders intelligently and loyally." There was a cultural shift in the 1970s, as reflected in the 1973 revision of the International Code for Nurses, which read, "The nurse sustains a cooperative relationship with coworkers in nursing and other fields" (p. 3).

With the move from diploma programs to baccalaureate and associate degree nursing schools, the question arose how new nurses would be socialized into the real world of nursing in a different educational environment. During this time there was an emerging shift from obedience to a more self-directed practice; however, the transition was slow. Stein (1967) described the power struggle that nurses were facing in their practice. Evident was a work environment that did not promote nurses' autonomy.

Isabel Maitland Stewart was an early advocate of nursing education. She developed the first course dealing specifically with the teaching of nursing at Teacher's College (Donahue, 1983). She differentiated training from education. Training was aimed at fixed habits and skills by a process of repetition, relied on authority and coercion, and fostered dependency. Discipline, obedience, and conformity were outcomes of training. Training was not seen as a process that inspired confidence and self-esteem. Education, on the other hand, according to Stewart, promoted self-discipline, responsibility, accountability, and self-mastery. Autonomy and freedom were expected outcomes. Like Dewey (1938), Stewart envisioned education as a process that was liberating—one that actively engaged the learner in the process. Learners were free to explore and were active in the learning culture. Stewart emphasized the science, skill, and spirit of nursing as interrelated and as essentials for nursing. She was a strong proponent of theory. She believed that practice without intelligent understanding of its purpose is not only wasteful but also dangerous.

Unlike other professions, the registered nurse may be educationally prepared for competent entry into practice via three educational routes (diploma, associate, and baccalaureate). However, since 1965, the American Nurses Association has affirmed the baccalaureate degree in nursing as the preferred educational preparation to entry into nursing practice (ANA, 2004). Educational preparation at the baccalaureate level provides a broader education to better address the complexities of society and the profession.

Socialization Process

There are two types of sociologic conditions involved in the professional socialization process: structural and cultural (Cohen, 1981). Structural conditions refer to the rules that determine the roles for individuals. Hospital policies, doctors' orders, and job descriptions reflect structural conditions. "Cultural conditions are the idea systems prevalent in a society as expressed in words, symbols, and ceremonies.

These words, symbols, and ceremonies are referred to as the cultural climate" (Cohen, 1981, p. 31). In Melosh's (1982) text, the physician's hand symbolizes the nurses' position in the medical hierarchy and identifies the role of the nurse in executing the physician's work. It also can be seen to symbolize nurses' work as hands-on and skill based. In addition, the physician's hand could also symbolize the nurse as an extension of the physician and nurses' ongoing struggle for professional autonomy. Structural and cultural conditions are interrelated. In authoritarian cultures there are more structured rules. In such systems, conformity rather than individual autonomy is the norm. As words are reflective of a culture, clearly the idea of nursing training is very different from the idea of nursing education.

Professional Socialization

There are several models in the literature that describe professional socialization, a few of which will be discussed later in this chapter. Regardless of the model embraced, socialization into the nursing profession must include the new competencies for this century. O'Neil and the Pew Commission on Nursing Socialization (1998) referred to societal changes as well as changes in healthcare financing and reform when it identified the competencies. Among the competencies identified were:

- Embracing a personal ethic of responsibility and service
- Exhibiting ethical behavior in all professional activities
- Contributing to the continuous improvement of the healthcare system
- Continuing to learn and help others

Model of Professional Socialization: Cognitive Development

Cohen (1981) adapted the cognitive stages of development from Piaget to describe the cognitive development of the student from neophyte to competent and confident professional. This model of professional socialization describes the stages of development within the individual but does not prescribe the time for each stage. Cohen proposed that each of these stages must be experienced for the student to feel comfortable in one's professional role. In stage 1, Unilateral Dependence, the individual places complete reliance on external controls and searches for the one right answer (Cohen, 1981, p. 16). As the student gains foundational knowledge and skill, there begins the process of questioning the authority. During stage 2, Negative/Independence, the student begins to pull away from external controls and is characterized by cognitive rebellion. Historically, this has been a difficult stage for nurses because of its traditions of obedience and conformity. Authoritarianism in nursing education had made it too risky to be openly defiant. However, similar to the development of independence of adolescents, exerting one's self is an essential process for the development of the competent, authentic professional. Stage 3, Dependence/Mutuality, marks the beginning of empathy and commitment to others (Cohen, 1981, p. 18). In this stage, the student moves from a position of opposition toward a more realistic evaluative stance, critically thinking about the theory and its application. Applying knowledge to practice, the student tests information and facts and begins to make judgments. In this stage, the student is actively engaged in the learning, thinking through problems. "Students have a knowledge base upon which to anchor critical thought and can relate new material to their previous knowledge base" (Cohen, 1981, p. 18). For this stage to emerge, the learning environment must support and value risk taking. The role of the teacher is that of coach, mentor, and senior learner.

Stage 4, Interdependence, is when neither mutuality nor autonomy is dominant. Learning from others and the ability to independently solve problems are evident. This is the stage of the professional lifelong learner who demonstrates reflection in practice and is responsible for continued learning. Professional socialization toward the stage of interdependence requires a supportive educational climate that values autonomy, independent thinking, and authenticity. The historical roots of nursing, with emphasis on obedience and service, have certainly undermined this professional development as described by Cohen's stages. Shadows of these traditions in nursing education may still be evident in many nursing programs.

Model of Professional Socialization: Social Influence

Kelman (1967) discussed how the social influences have affected the professionalization process. In contrast to Cohen's stages of internal processes, these are the external forces that affect the individual. Kelman described three stages: compliance, identification, and internalization. The first stage, compliance, occurs when an individual accepts the influence from another in order to gain acceptance and positive responses. Students take their cues on how to think and act from role models reflecting a stage of dependence. The second stage, identification, occurs as the student adopts attitudes and behaviors of a role model because the student becomes aware that the behaviors will enable him or her to perform the professional role (Cohen, 1981). This stage reflects dependence and mutuality, as described by Cohen. Students test the aspects of the role and gain experience in the professional role with faculty guidance and support.

To progress toward independence, the students need to experience a culture of trusting tolerance. It is critical that the student's self-esteem is maintained in the process in order to progress to the third stage, internalization. In this stage, professional norms and values are incorporated into the student's self-concept. Key in this stage is that the motivation for behavior is intrinsically rewarding and independent of external sources. At this stage, the individual moves from a position of dependence to one of interdependence within a profession.

Model of Professional Socialization: From Novice to Expert

Benner (1984) described the development of professional clinical practice of nurses. Benner's model identifies the stages of novice, advanced beginner, competent, proficient, and expert that are based on the nurse's experience in practice. Understanding this progression of knowledge and skills, educational programs have developed supportive curricula using a continuum of experiences to enhance skill and knowledge development. Healthcare environments have also incorporated this model to facilitate the nurse's professional practice by assessing the nurse's stage of development. This model is not limited to the student experience or to that of the new graduate nurse. Experienced nurses too can benefit from experiences designed to move toward expert.

Benner's model identifies the stages of novice, advanced beginner, competent, proficient, and expert that are based on the nurse's experience in practice.

The first stage, **novice**, is characterized by a lack of knowledge and experience. In this stage, the facts, rules, and guidelines for practice are the focus. Rules for practice are context free, and the student task is to acquire the knowledge and skills. The stage of novice is not related to the age of the student but rather to the knowledge and skill in the area of study. For example, learning how to give injections would be presented with the procedural guidelines, and the novice would then practice the skill. At this stage, much of the student's energy and attention is aimed at remembering the rules.

In the next stage, **advanced beginner**, the student is able to formulate principles that dictate action (Benner, 1984). For example, the advanced beginner would grasp the rationale behind why different medications require different injection techniques. However, advanced beginners still lack the experience to know how to prioritize in more complex situations and may feel at a loss in terms of what they can safely leave out. There is emphasis on the rules, and there is not the experience to adjust or adapt the rules to the situation. Both the advanced beginner and the novice stage require guidance. These stages parallel Cohen's professional development stage of dependence.

Benner's stage 3, **competent**, is characterized by the ability to analyze problems and prioritize. The nurse has a solid grasp of the rules and principles. Although the movement from one stage to the next does not have distinct boundaries, the nurse at this stage has had experience in a variety of clinical situations and is able to draw on prior knowledge and experience. There is the ability to plan as well as to alter plans as necessary. Students who have the opportunity to have extended internships in a specialty area during their education may graduate entering this stage. Cohen's stage, dependence/mutuality, corresponds to this stage. Given the complexity of nursing practice and the range of clinical experiences, many new graduates may be described as advanced beginners.

Stage 4, **proficient**, refers to the professional who is able to grasp the situation contextually and as a whole. They have a solid grasp of the norms as well as solid experiences that shed light on the variations from the norm. Incorporated into practice is the ability to test knowledge against situations that might not fit and to solve problems with alternative approaches. In this stage, the professional is testing the rules and theories and looking at cases that may lead to developing alternative rules and theories. One might say that this is the stage when the professional begins to "break the rules" as he or she sees that the rules do not always apply.

Benner's final stage, **expert**, has moved beyond a fixed set of rules. There is an internalized understanding grounded in a wealth of experience as well as depth of knowledge. The expert is always learning and always questioning using subjective and objective knowing. Benner (1984) proposed that not all nurses are able to obtain this stage.

Reality Shock

Professional socialization requires that the student learn the technology of the profession, learn to internalize the professional culture, find a personally and professionally acceptable version of the role, and integrate this professional role into all the other life roles (Cohen, 1981). In the 1974 book *Reality Shock,* Kramer presented the disillusionment of new graduates entering the clinical world. The authoritarian culture, traditions of subservience and obedience, and the lack of recognition and professional autonomy left nurses feeling conflicted. The culture of the classroom and the culture of clinical practice were seen as worlds apart. New graduates cited disparity between the values espoused by educational establishments and those in the clinical area (Philpin, 1999). Technical aspects of nursing were emphasized in clinical practice with very little time to talk with patients. In essence, students experienced a sense of role confusion with difficulty finding a personally and professionally acceptable version of the role. Similarly, Campbell, Larrivee, Field, Day, and Reutter (1994) cited that nursing students equated a good day of practice with good patient care that was based primarily on good relationships. Good relationships included patient–student nurse relationships and student–instructor relationships. Making a difference along with good relationships were core values for nurses personally and professionally.

Wilson and Startup's (1991) research also identified the dichotomy between the values of school and those in the ward. Students experienced "anxiety dealing with the conflicting expectations of conformity" (p. 1481). Reality shock occurs when the perceived role (how one believes he or she should perform in a role) comes into conflict with the performed role. Many new graduates experience this role conflict between what they know to do and how to do it, but they experience circumstances that do not allow them to perform the role in that way (Blais et al., 2005, p. 21).

> **CRITICAL THINKING QUESTIONS**
>
> What do you think are the barriers to professional socialization? Do you think different environments might foster or hinder professional socialization? Do you think that personal characteristics of nurses might influence professional socialization?

Facilitating Reflective Professional Practice

In 1998 the American Association of Colleges of Nursing (AACN, 1998) developed five **core values** to facilitate the development of professional nursing values.

The core values embraced by the AACN are human dignity, integrity, autonomy, altruism, and social justice. Chenevert (1994) discussed a path for developing a sense of self that values self and others. Her model on assertiveness depicts a process of developing one's voice—moving from position of low self-esteem and high anxiety toward the development of high esteem for self and toward others and a sense of personal power. As presented earlier, learners who experienced a caring culture felt supported in their personal and professional development. The following highlight some of the characteristics for the professional nurse:

The core values embraced by the AACN are human dignity, integrity, autonomy, altruism, and social justice.

- High esteem for self and others
- Ability to view conflict as potentially positive
- Ability to be open to the perspectives of others, valuing open dialogue
- Willingness to take risks personally and professionally with a strong sense of integrity and accountability
- Feeling empowered to advocate for self and others
- High tolerance of ambiguity
- Views power as that of power with others rather than power over others
- Confidence in practice and self-directed
- Values collaboration and interdependence
- Exhibits a strong sense of internal locus of control, experiencing practice as intrinsically rewarding
- Practices caring for self and others
- Values self-reflection
- Theory informs practice and practice is used to inform theory

Experiences with caring role models and mentors in the educational environment as well as in clinical practice were identified as critical for professional role development. Students voiced that the most positive factor in their ability to gain confidence and progress professionally was a caring, competent clinical teacher. As a role model, the most effective clinical teacher was one who enjoyed teaching and demonstrated excellent clinical skills and sound clinical judgment (Campbell et al., 1994, p. 1125). Concerns for each individual's achievement are addressed within a context of cooperation and confirmation. When expectations are not met, it is the teacher's responsibility to respond with compassion and understanding to assist the student to achieve (Chinn, 2008).

Caring cultures that were supportive of student growth as individuals and professionals had a positive impact on professional development. Such environments encouraged self-exploration and self-care (Campbell et al., 1994, p. 1125). The student–teacher relationship based on a philosophy of caring resembles the nurse–client relationship and fosters honest and open communication. Students involved in these types of relationships experience therapeutic approaches firsthand and are more able to internalize the behaviors and values into their practice. Thus, professional socialization, self-actualization, self-fulfillment, and self-concept are enhanced by caring interpersonal relationships (Clayton & Murray, 1989, p. 48).

Based on Bandura's social learning, the impact that role models have on students is significant in regard to professional socialization. Caring as the core value in nursing practice and nursing education is operationalized as:

> a total way of being, of relating, of acting; a quality investment and engagement in the other—person, idea, project or self as "other"—in which one expresses the self fully, and through which one touches most intimately and authentically what it means to be human. (Roach, 1991, p. 131)

Professional socialization of nurses toward a profession that fully embraces caring for self and others reflects the internalization of what Roach refers to as "the five C's: compassion, competence, confidence, conscience, and commitment" (Roach, 1991, p. 132), representing a framework for human response from which professional caring is expressed.

Caring as a core value of nursing represents the essence of the history of nursing and the foundation for the future (Watson, 1988). Caring is presented as a moral ideal of nursing with concern for preservation of humanity, dignity, and fullness of self (Watson, 1989, p. 75). This moral imperative relates to the education of nurses as well as the practice of nursing. How indeed can the profession expect to have graduates empowered as professionals if the education is not one that demonstrates caring and encourages students in an environment that is not driven by fear and anxiety? Education cannot be grounded in the ultimate fear "someone could die" but rather with knowledge that experienced nurses will make a difference for the patient.

Lauterbach and Hentz-Becker (1996), in their article "Caring for self: Becoming a self-reflective nurse," presented caring for self as a personal and professional mandate. "For nurses as persons, it has the potential to become a route for self-empowerment, self-fulfillment, and advocacy" (p. 98). The goal in the socialization of nurses today and for the future is to achieve caring with autonomy. Educational programs must depart from the training model toward a schema that fosters caring and critical thinking professionals. An education should depart from control and conformity to one that fosters authenticity, responsibility, growth, and reflective practice.

Conclusions: Reflective Professional Practice

Nursing education should be humanistic and caring, with caring experts as role models who will contribute to the socialization of future generations of nurses and help them become caring experts in nursing practice. Regarding role development and socialization, it is important to remember that we learn what we live (Becker-Hentz, 2004).

CLASSROOM ACTIVITY

Incorporate actual quotes from the nurses who were interviewed as provided in Benner's book *From Novice to Expert* (1984) in class to illustrate the differences between each of the stages: novice, advanced beginner, competent, proficient, and expert. This activity is simple but enlightening to students.

References

American Association of Colleges of Nursing. (1998). *Essentials of baccalaureate education.* Washington, DC: Author.

American Nurses Association (ANA). 2004. *Scope and standards of practice.* Washington, DC: Author.

Becker-Hentz, P. (2004). *Understanding relationships: Learning what we live.* Unpublished manuscript.

Benner, P. (1984). *From novice to expert.* Menlo-Park, CA: Addison-Wesley.

Blais, K. K., Hayes, J. S., Kozier, B., & Erb, G. (2002). Socialization to professional nursing roles. In K. K. Blais, J. S. Hayes, B. Kozier, & G. Erb (Eds.), *Professional nursing practice: Concepts and perspectives* (4th ed.). Upper Saddle River, NJ: Prentice Hall.

Campbell, I. E., Larrivee, L., Field, P. A., Day, R. A., & Reutter, L. (1994). Learning to nurse in the clinical setting. *Journal of Advanced Nursing, 20,* 1125–1131.

Chenevert, M. (1994). *STAT: Special techniques in assertiveness training.* St. Louis, MO: Mosby.

Chinn, P. L. (2008). Philosophical foundations for excellence in teaching. In B. Moyer (Ed.), *Nursing education: Foundations for practice excellence.* Philadelphia: F. A. Davis.

Clayton, G. M., & Murray, J. P. (1989). Faculty-student relationships: Catalytic connection. In National League for Nursing (Eds.), *Curriculum revolution: Reconceptualizing nursing education* (pp. 43–53). New York: National League for Nursing Press.

Cohen, H. A. (1981). *The nurse's quest for a professional identity.* Menlo-Park, CA: Addison-Wesley.

Davis, A. J., & Aroskar, M. A. (1978). *Ethical dilemmas in nursing practice.* Stamford, CT: Appleton & Lange.

Dewey, J. (1938). *Experience and education.* New York: Collier Books.

Donahue, M. P. (1983). Isabel Maitland Stewart's philosophy of education. *Nursing Research, 32*(3), 140–146.

Ehrenreich, B., & English, D. (1973). *Witches, midwives and nurses: A history of women healers.* New York: The Feminist Press.

Fahrenwald, N. L., Bassett. S. D., Tschetter, L., Carson, P. P., White, L., & Winterboer, V. J. (2005). Teaching core nursing values. *Journal of Professional Nursing, 21*(1), 46–51.

Jameton, A. (1984). *Nursing practice: The ethical issues.* Englewood Cliffs, NJ: Prentice Hall.

Kelman, H. (1967). *Three processes of social influence. Current perspectives in social psychiatry.* New York: Oxford University Press.

Kramer, M. (1974). *Reality shock, why nurses leave nursing.* St. Louis, MO: Mosby.

Lauterbach, S. S., & Hentz-Becker, P. (1996). Caring for self: Becoming a self-reflective nurse. *Holistic Nursing Practice, 10*(2), 57–68.

Melosh, B. (1982). *"The physician's hand": Work culture and conflict in American nursing.* Philadelphia: Temple University Press.

O'Neil, E. N., and the Pew Health Professions Commission. (1998). *Recruiting health professional practice for a new century.* San Francisco: Pew Health Professions Committee.

Philpin, S. M. (1999). The impact of Project 2000 educational reforms on the occupational socialization of nurses: An exploratory study. *Journal of Advanced Nursing, 29*(6), 1326–1333.

Reverby, S. M. (1987). *Ordered to care: The dilemma of American nursing, 1850–1945.* New York: Cambridge University Press.

Roach, M. S. (1991). Creating communities of caring. In National League for Nursing (Eds.), *Curriculum revolution: Community building and activism* (pp. 123–138). New York: National League for Nursing Press.

Shank, M. J., & Weis, D. (2001). Service and education share responsibility for nurses' value development. *Journal for Nurses in Staff Development, 17*(5), 226–231.

Stein, L. I. (1967). The doctor-nurse game. *Archives of General Psychiatry, 16,* 699–703.

Watson, J. (1981). Socialization of the nursing student in a professional nursing education program. *Nursing Papers, 13,* 19–24.

Watson, J. (1988). *Nursing: Human science and human care.* New York: National League for Nursing Press.

Watson, J. (1989). *Toward a caring curriculum: A new pedagogy for nursing.* New York: National League for Nursing Press.

Wilson, A., & Startup, R. (1991). Nurse socialization: Issues and problems. *Journal of Advanced Nursing, 16,* 1478–1486.

chapter 7

Career Management and Care of the Professional Self

Luann M. Daggett

LEARNING OBJECTIVES

After completing this chapter, the student should be able to:

1. Describe the difference between an occupation and a career.
2. Articulate the importance of assuming a proactive role in managing your nursing career.
3. Set career goals and formulate objectives designed to meet the goals.
4. Describe specific strategies for increasing personal visibility within an organization.
5. Explain methods for obtaining feedback on personal performance.
6. Describe the effects of work-related stress on health and career longevity.
7. Articulate the importance of life management for optimal personal and professional health.

Key Terms and Concepts

- Career management
- Journaling
- Core values
- Mission statement
- Success
- Objectives
- 5-year plan
- Public speaking
- Networking
- Mentoring
- Feedback
- Lifelong learning
- Burnout
- Self-care
- Life management

Sharon is a 23-year-old registered nurse who graduated from an associate's degree nursing program 3 years ago. Since graduation, she has worked at a large university-based hospital in a major metropolitan area. Her first assignment was in an oncology unit where she worked as a staff nurse for a year before transferring to the cardiovascular recovery unit. Sharon is an outstanding staff nurse, providing excellent care to her patients and working well as a member of the healthcare team. Her performance appraisals have been positive. Although Sharon would like to return to school for her baccalaureate

139

degree, working rotating shifts with varying schedules has prevented her from taking classes.

Recently, there was an opening on her unit for an assistant nurse manager. Sharon hoped to be considered for the position and was disappointed when another nurse whom she considered less qualified got the position. Discussing the decision with her supervisor, Sharon asked why she had not been given the job. To her surprise, the supervisor replied, "Why, Sharon, I had no idea you were interested!" Sharon left the meeting feeling hurt, angry, frustrated, and devalued. She could not understand why all of her hard work had gone unnoticed (and unrewarded) by her supervisor. Although inconvenient, Sharon is thinking about changing jobs and moving to a new hospital in a different part of the city.

Sharon's story, unfortunately, is typical of the way many nurses approach their jobs. Career management is not a concept that is familiar to them. For many, nursing is still viewed as a calling or vocation rather than as a career that needs managing. Despite the increasing number of men entering nursing in the past few years, nursing is still a female-dominated profession, and women see career management as self-promotion. They are uncomfortable calling attention to their accomplishments, asking for recognition, or negotiating raises and promotions. As a result, many nurses do not receive the positive feedback, recognition, and career advancement opportunities that they deserve. Feeling chronically undervalued and unappreciated, nurses become burned out, change jobs, or leave the profession altogether.

Occupation vs. Career

Nursing as a career is as much a philosophical approach as it is a professional choice. The difference is whether one considers nursing an occupation or a career. Occupation is defined as (1) an activity that keeps a person busy or (2) one's job or employment (Oxford University Press, 1996). In comparison, a career is a course of professional life or employment that affords the individual opportunities for personal advancement, progress, or achievement (Miller, 2003). Some people view nursing as a job or an occupation, whereas others take the approach that nursing is a profession requiring a lifelong commitment. Table 7-1 compares attitudes toward nursing as either an occupation or a career. If you choose to view nursing as a professional career, then you will behave differently than if you consider it as merely a job that is most likely temporary or a means to an end.

A career is not something that is automatically conferred along with a college degree; it is a life choice that must be actively planned and pursued. A degree and a nursing license may be the ticket that gets you started on the journey, but without a destination, an itinerary, and a map, you will not travel very far. Like any important journey, a career requires research and planning; otherwise, you risk missing opportunities and critical milestones along the way. One should always assess the current location before planning future directions. Just as you track progress with a map

TABLE 7-1	COMPARISON OF ATTITUDES: OCCUPATION VS. CAREER	
	Occupation	Career
Longevity	Temporary, a means to an end	Lifelong vocation
Educational Preparation	Minimal training that is required, usually associate degree	University professional degree program based on a foundation of core liberal arts
Continuing Education	Only what is required for the job or to get a raise/promotion	Lifelong learning, continuous efforts to gain new knowledge, skills, and abilities
Level of Commitment	Short-term, as long as job meets personal needs	Long-term commitment to organization and profession
Expectations	Reasonable work for reasonable pay; responsibility ends with shift	Will assume additional responsibilities, volunteer for organizational activities and community-based events

while on a road trip, you should have a plan for managing your career, lest you find yourself wandering in the wilderness without making any true progress toward your career goals. **Career management** can be defined as a planned logical progression of one's professional life that includes clearly defined goals and objectives and a plan for achievement. Joel (2003) advised building a nursing career cautiously and deliberately, laying each brick in a predetermined pattern. This requires careful consideration of what it is you like to do, what you are good at, where you would eventually like to be professionally, and what skills and education you will need to get there.

> **CRITICAL THINKING QUESTIONS**
>
> Do you view nursing as a career or a job? What are your goals related to nursing?

Common Myths and Misconceptions

Table 7-2 lists a number of common myths and misconceptions that many nurses hold. The attitude that one's supervisor is responsible for taking care of you is a common example of an employee's flawed thinking. Good works do not speak for themselves—mistakes speak for themselves, and they speak loudly and clearly. Quality patient care is an expectation of the nurse's job and generally goes unnoticed until either a mistake is made or a complaint is received. Your supervisor has many role responsibilities—looking out for your career is not one of them.

Your supervisor has many role responsibilities—looking out for your career is not one of them.

Many nurses believe that because of the nursing shortage they will be guaranteed a job. In fact, a large number of students enter nursing programs think that they will always have job security. Although graduates of nursing programs generally have

TABLE 7-2 COMMON MYTHS AND MISCONCEPTIONS
• If I work hard, I will be rewarded.
• Good works speak for themselves.
• It is my boss's job to recommend me for special assignments or promotion.
• As a registered nurse, I will always have a job.
• My hospital will look out for me.

highly marketable skills, nursing positions are as susceptible to economic fluctuations as those in any other field. The nursing shortage does not mean job security; a nursing shortage usually leads to a proliferation of unlicensed assistive personnel that actually erodes the role of professional nurses. The notion that hospitals and healthcare agencies look out for the concerns of nurses is unrealistic. Whether operated for profit or not, healthcare facilities are businesses that are concerned with providing services to customers for a fee. If production costs exceed profits, adjustments must be made or the business will fold. Nursing care is expensive to provide, and thus, it is often targeted for cost reduction. Healthcare agencies operate in their own best interests, which may not coincide with the interests of the nursing staff.

It is our responsibility to manage our own careers. Your boss has other things to do than to follow your career. It is your responsibility to get the level of recognition that you need and to seek opportunities that will advance your own career. Passive, obedient behavior does not get you far in the real world and neither does sitting back waiting for others to look out for you. In the real world, you cannot afford to wait your turn for good things to happen—you have to make them happen.

Setting Personal Goals

The first step in career management is to know where you want to go professionally. Unless you have a clear understanding of the final destination, it is impossible to select the best route to follow to get there. If you set out on a trip without knowing your final destination, how can you possibly choose the best road to take to get there? This is probably the most difficult part of career management. A reasonable approach would be to consider which aspects of nursing are most appealing to you. Do you like the interaction of direct patient care, or do you prefer to direct others in providing care? Are you more comfortable in an acute care setting, or do you favor the stability of long-term care or rehabilitation settings? Do you like to teach others? Are you more at ease leading or following? Because professional activities always take place within the context of personal needs and responsibilities, it is important to consider what those might be as well.

For many of us, goal setting and visualizing a desired future are difficult tasks. At some point in our early education, we made the decision to become a nurse and set our sights on preparing for entrance into a nursing program. Then we focused on surviving the rigorous course of study and graduating. After graduation came the challenge of finding and adjusting to our first nursing position. Long-range goals were not something we gave much thought to until reaching a point where being a staff nurse was no longer exciting or challenging. At this point, many nurses decide to return to school to seek an advanced degree in nursing with little thought as to what exactly they wish to study or what they ultimately plan to do with an additional degree. They choose programs that are convenient or assessable rather than searching for the right educational program to meet specific learning needs. Often they decide to apply to school because friends or colleagues are doing so, and they do not want to feel left behind.

The decision to return to school or make a major career change should never be made hastily; rather, it should occur after a period of careful introspection and discernment. Consideration should be given to issues such as:

- Personal values
- Professional values
- Family issues and responsibilities
- Lifestyle choices
- Economic factors
- Community and recreational involvement

Educational programs are demanding and costly—financially, psychologically, and socially. Returning to school requires commitment, not just from the individual who will be studying, but also from family members, friends, employers, and other people in one's social network. Likewise, job or career changes are stressful and have long-term effects on finances, personal happiness, and interpersonal relationships. These decisions should never be made casually or impetuously.

Journaling Techniques, Writing Objectives

Various exercises and books on values clarification are available in bookstores or on the Internet; however, one of the most effective means of introspection is journaling. **Journaling** is the process by which one sits down quietly on a daily or regular basis to think and record one's thoughts and ideas in a notebook. There are many suggested techniques for journaling; one useful method is to record three things—events, ideas, or thoughts—that were important to you that day. These may include things that happened at work or in your personal life. As you record your thoughts, be sure to include any particular insights that occur to you. It is important that you do this on a daily basis or at least five to six times a week. At the end of the week, review your journal entries, looking for themes or patterns in your writing. Be sure to write these observations. Once a month look back through your journal to assess the issues, ideas, or events that were important to you that month. Record your insights.

As you write, the emphasis should be on recording your thoughts as they occur to you. Grammar, spelling, sentence structure, and handwriting are not important. This journal is for your eyes only, and substance is more important than form. Some people are more comfortable writing fragments of sentences or making lists of their ideas, whereas others prefer the catharsis of writing pages of text. Either style is effective, whichever works best for you. The important thing is regularity. One's daily activities are like the fine stitches of a tapestry; examined close-up they are interesting but limited. By stepping back and looking at the details of one's life over a period of time, you see a more complete picture and gain a sense of the core values that give depth and meaning to life. **Core values** are those values that are most important to us, the values that define who we are as human beings. There must be congruence between what it is you value and what it is you do before satisfaction can be derived from one's work.

CRITICAL THINKING QUESTIONS

What are your core values? Do you see congruence between what you value and your career?

Once you have an appreciation of what is truly important to you, Covey (1989) recommended developing a personal mission statement that includes all of your life roles and the values that you attach to or express in those roles. A **mission statement** is a clear, concise statement of who you are and what you are about in life. It can be a powerful tool for helping you find meaning and give direction to your life. Until one understands what is truly important and essential to one's happiness in both the professional and personal arenas, it is impossible to plan a future or manage a career effectively. Understanding your values and life mission allows you to discern which professional activities provide you with a sense of accomplishment and reward. As you feel the need to grow professionally, it is important that you set goals and make choices based on core values instead of circumstance or whim. **Success** in life can be defined as doing what you want, where you want, and with the people you want to do it with. This implies balance within the various arenas of your life—professional, personal, social, and spiritual.

When you have decided on a direction for your professional career, it is essential that you be able to visualize clearly the outcome you desire. Covey (1989) believed that visualizing something organizes one's ability to accomplish it; one must begin with the end in mind. The more precisely you are able to visualize exactly what it is you desire, the more clearly you will be able to distinguish the steps it will take for you to achieve your goal. **Objectives** are specific measures that you will take in achievement of your goal. Writing objectives provides you with a plan on how you are going to get from where you are to your desired future. Objectives should be specific and measurable, serving as milestones that mark your progress. Objectives must include a time frame for their accomplishment. Table 7-3 shows an example of a goal and its concomitant objectives for a nurse who wants to become a family nurse practitioner. It is clear from this example that one could realistically attain this goal by following the objectives in this plan. The more detailed and specific your objectives, the easier it will be to follow the steps required to reach your goal. The difference between

---

TABLE 7-3   CAREER GOAL: FAMILY NURSE PRACTITIONER

Goal: To become a certified Family Nurse Practitioner

Objectives:

- Contact university for program information and application materials.
- Schedule the Graduate Record Examination.
- Purchase the Graduate Record Examination study guide and review one chapter per week.
- Contact three professional sources for reference letters.
- Complete health information forms and schedule physical examination.
- Submit application materials before the fall deadline.
- Apply for financial aid.
- Make appointment with academic advisor to plan program of study.
- Register for classes.

---

people who are successful in life and those who only dream of success is the ability to visualize their dreams and complete the steps that connect their present with their future.

Although it is highly desirable to know one's ultimate professional goals, for many of us, it may be unrealistic to look that far into the future. That does not mean your career should proceed without plan; rather, your plans may be more short term. Developing short-range goals such as where one would like to be in 5 years might be a more reasonable approach for you. Defining a **5-year plan** enables you to set clear objectives and follow specific steps on how to meet those objectives while allowing for flexibility in adjusting to changing life circumstances.

Career Management Strategies

Assessing your current position is a good place to begin managing your career. Are you engaged in work that is socially significant, challenging, rewarding, and fulfilling? Do you generally look forward to going to work and enjoy the time that you spend there? Do you like and respect the people with whom you work? Are the salary and benefits you receive for your work reasonable and sufficient to accommodate your lifestyle? Are there opportunities for advancement within your organization? If you cannot respond positively to these questions, you have two choices: Either stay where you are and work to improve the situation, or look for another position. Only you can make this decision; however, if your job situation is not working for you, it is up to you to do something about it.

Once you have decided that a job change is the right move for you, it is important that you set about finding a position that will meet your personal and professional needs. Knowing what you are looking for is vital to your success. A careful analysis of your old job—what you liked and disliked about the job and your role in creating and sustaining the situation—will help you avoid similar pitfalls in your next position. This is where journaling can be very useful in clearly defining your expectations.

If possible, never leave a job until you have a firm commitment from a new employer. Finding the perfect job is labor intensive and time consuming. Trying to do so when you are unemployed and facing financial hardship is almost impossible. The old adage "good jobs are hard to find" is very true. Many people hunt for prospective jobs in newspapers or visit Internet career Web sites. This strategy may be the best option if you are unfamiliar with the local job market or are relocating to a new area. Keep in mind, however, that most organizations first post position openings in house to allow their employees opportunities for advancement or lateral transfers. Because it may be difficult for outsiders to know about these openings, you might consider beginning your job search within your present organization. Along with contacting the human resources department for a listing of current job openings, it is important for you to begin networking and talking to people within your organization who might be able to help you advance your career goals. Your unit supervisor, other managers, or your nursing service administrator are all potential sources for leads. Even if there is not a current opening in the area you seek, expressing your interest to influential people will put you in mind if something becomes available.

If your job search takes you to unfamiliar territory, modern job hunting can be facilitated by technology. Most healthcare agencies have Web sites that post current position openings along with a description of the facility, the services it offers, and its mission statement and philosophy. You might also consider posting your résumé with an online health careers database where prospective employers can search for qualified employees. Because there is no control over who has access to your information, use caution in listing personal information in an online résumé. Alternatively, you might want to contact colleagues in a geographical locale by joining local chapters of a professional organization or registering for newsgroups or chat rooms to make professional contacts. Regardless of whether you choose to look internally or externally for job opportunities, creating a positive first impression of you and your work is exceedingly important.

First Impressions

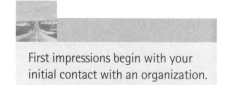

First impressions begin with your initial contact with an organization.

First impressions—whether it is by telephone, letter of inquiry, résumé, e-mail, or personal interview—begin with your initial contact with an organization. A favorable first impression creates a halo effect that lasts a long time. Likewise, it is very difficult to alter an initial negative impression, and the more negative the impression, the harder it is to change. You want to present yourself in such a way that people take you seriously and listen to what you have to offer. If your first contact is a written communication, either a letter of inquiry, résumé, or a job application form, be sure your writing conveys a true representation of who you are. Letters should always be typed and written clearly and concisely and be free of spelling, punctuation, and grammatical errors. Likewise, application forms should be typed or printed clearly using black ink. The information must be complete, accurate, and free of errors. If your written communication is sloppy or grammatically incorrect, the reviewer will assume that you are careless or uneducated. This is not the impression you want to convey to a prospective employer. Table 7-4 offers some useful hints for résumé preparation.

If your first contact with an organization is a personal interview, you must prepare yourself for the interview and present yourself as a serious prospect. Dress professionally. For men this means a coat and tie and for women a business suit or dress. Regardless of your personal style, the goal is to look like you will belong in this organization; thus, be sure to dress appropriately. Arrive at least 5 minutes before your scheduled appointment time. Do your homework by learning as much as you can about the organization, including its philosophy and mission statement. Keep in mind that you will be interviewing the organizational representatives as much as they will be interviewing you; thus, come prepared with questions. During the interview, you will want to learn as much as possible about the job expectations and convey information about what you have to offer to the organization. Be prepared to discuss your strengths and limitations. It is customary not to inquire about salary or benefits until a job offer has been made. Employers typically interview several prospects before deciding on an individual, and salary is based on education and experience. There is usually a salary range for a given position, and thus, be prepared to negotiate if the initial offer is unacceptable. Even if the employer is unwilling to increase the quoted salary, you will at least learn whether you were offered the maximum allocated to the position for someone with your experience and background.

The better the job, the more competition you will have in applying for it; thus, find positive ways to separate yourself from other applicants. Preparation and a professional appearance are a good start, but you may need to do more to stand out from the crowd. Discuss not only your present qualifications, but share your plans for future professional growth or aspirations. The more you align yourself with the mission and goals of the organization, the more acceptable you will be to an employer. Follow an interview immediately with a written letter thanking the interviewer for his or her time and consideration of your application. This crucial step is often overlooked by applicants and may tip the balance in your favor.

Before concluding the interview, ask about the time frame for decision making about the position. If you know when the employer expects to choose a candidate and you have not been notified of your selection, you can follow up with a telephone call at the appropriate time. Even if you are not selected for this position, maintain your positive first impression by thanking the employer for interviewing you and

TABLE 7-4   HINTS FOR RÉSUMÉ PREPARATION

Résumé Essentials

Begin with a self-assessment including the following:

- Skills
- Abilities
- Education
- Work experience
- Extracurricular activities

Content of Your Résumé

- Include contact information: Name, address, telephone, e-mail address, Web site address.
  - Avoid nicknames.
  - Use a permanent address and telephone number (include area code).
  - Record a neutral greeting on your answering machine.
  - Give your e-mail address; choose one that sounds professional.
  - Only include your Web page if it reflects your professional ambitions.
- Objective or summary: Tells employers the sort of work you hope to find.
  - Be specific about the type of job you want.
  - Tailor your objective to each employer/job you want; no generic objectives
- Education: New graduates without work experience should list education information first.
  - List your most recent educational information first.
  - Include your degree, major, institution attended, and minor/concentration.
  - Add your grade point average if it is higher than 3.0.
  - Mention any academic honors (scholarships/grants, awards, Dean's List, honor societies, etc.).
- Work experience: Give a brief overview of work that has taught you skills.
  - Use action verbs to describe your job duties.
  - List in reverse chronological order (last job, first).
  - Include title of position, name of organization, location (city, state), dates of employment, work responsibilities, skills, and achievements.
- Other information
  - Key or special skills or competencies
  - Leadership experience in volunteer organizations
  - Participation in sports

(continues)

TABLE 7-4   HINTS FOR RÉSUMÉ PREPARATION (continued)

- References
    - Ask people if they are willing to serve as references before giving their names to a prospective employer.
    - Do not list names and addresses of your references on your résumé. Note "references furnished on request" at bottom of your résumé and give later if requested.

Résumé Checkup

- Proofread for spelling and grammatical errors.
- Print on $8\frac{1}{2} \times 11$-inch white or off-white quality bond paper.
- Print on one side only using 10- to 14-point font; avoid decorative typefaces.
- Do not fold or staple; mail in large envelope.

Source: Reprinted and adapted from JobWeb (www.jobweb.com), with permission of the National Association of Colleges and Employers, copyright holder.

---

asking to have your application kept on file so that you might be considered for future positions.

As stated previously, the interview is also a time for you to find out more about the organization. The American Association of Colleges of Nursing (AACN) has identified eight key characteristics or hallmarks that each nurse should consider when screening potential employers (AACN, 2002). To assess the practice environment of the organization AACN suggests that the nurse ask questions during the interview that relate to the following eight key organizational characteristics:

1. Does the potential employer manifest a philosophy of clinical care emphasizing quality, safety, interdisciplinary collaboration, continuity of care, and professional accountability?
2. Does the potential employer recognize the value of nurses' expertise on clinical care quality and patient outcomes?
3. Does the potential employer promote executive-level nursing leadership?
4. Does the potential employer empower nurses' participation in clinical decision making and organization of clinical care systems?
5. Does the potential employer demonstrate professional development support for nurses?
6. Does the potential employer maintain clinical advancement programs based on education, certification, and advanced preparation?
7. Does the potential employer create collaborative relationships among members of the healthcare team?
8. Does the potential employer utilize technological advances in clinical care and information systems?

Other information about the organization that may be of interest to the potential nurse employee during the interview is the RN vacancy and turnover rate, patient satisfaction scores, educational mix of nursing staff, average tenure of nursing staff, employee satisfaction scores, percentage of travel nurses utilized, key human resource policies, whether the nurses are unionized (if so, a copy of the contract), and the most recent JCAHO (Joint Commission on the Accreditation of Healthcare Organizations) report on the organization (AACN, 2002). The full white paper and summary brochure are available online.

> **CRITICAL THINKING QUESTION**
>
> What kind of first impression do you make when searching for a new position?

Knowing the characteristics of the practice environment before you accept a position will assist you in making the best decision possible. Making an informed decision about where to practice nursing, whether you are a new graduate or an experienced nurse, will contribute to your long-term success and job satisfaction as a nurse.

Maximizing Your Visibility

If you wish to advance your career in a given institution, you must be seen as a committed member of that organization.

Developing and managing a career is very different from merely showing up and doing your job. A career involves a commitment not just to the work of an employee but to the well-being of the entire organization. This means that your efforts extend beyond the care of your patients on your assigned nursing unit to assume responsibilities beyond those for which you were hired. Administering high-quality patient care is an important part of the nurse's role; however, this is only one aspect of the professional nursing role. If you wish to advance your career in a given institution, you must be seen as a committed member of that organization. To do this, you must be visible within the organization.

Remember the myth that good works speak for themselves. Nurses who show up on time, do their jobs well, and go home rarely come to the attention of influential people within the organization unless a problem occurs. Then the nurses receive a lot of negative attention. Nurses and other employees who work the night shift are rarely if ever seen by hospital administrators and risk being invisible within the organization unless they purposely engage in activities that take place during normal business hours. Thus, how does one increase his or her visibility in a positive way?

Most hospitals and healthcare agencies provide some degree of self-governance within the organizational structure. Committees composed of physicians, nurses, and administrators assume important functions of governance such as ethics committees, research protocol review committees, patient care review committees (quality assurance), and others. Volunteering to serve on self-governance committees not only contributes to nurses' professional autonomy but also affords opportunities for you to be seen in a different light by people who can be helpful to you in your career. Similarly, most healthcare institutions are committed to supporting health-related community activities such as blood drives, fundraising walks, and health fairs. These also provide opportunities for nurses to contribute to their community while getting to know people in other areas of their organization.

As a professional nurse, you represent your organization both in and out of the workplace. Volunteering to be a spokesperson for the organization can increase your visibility dramatically. **Public speaking** is a daunting task for many nurses who are otherwise fearless in their other professional activities. Most nurses would rather work double shifts, manage disasters, or care for multiple acutely ill unstable patients simultaneously than stand up in front of a group and deliver a speech. Unfortunately, it is hard to be a spokesperson for an organization without engaging in some public speaking. The higher in an organization you rise, the more you are going to be called on to speak in public. If you are comfortable speaking in front of others, it will be much easier for you to establish your authority and credibility with a group. The good news is that it is not only possible to become a skilled speaker but to enjoy that aspect of your professional nursing role. The bad news is that the only way to become comfortable being a public speaker is to speak in public.

If you are inexperienced or uncomfortable speaking before a group, start slowly. Begin by speaking out in a staff meeting or volunteering to do an in-service presentation for the staff on your nursing unit. Agree to chair a hospital committee, accept a leadership position in your professional nursing organization, or travel to local schools or colleges to recruit nurses for your institution. Soon you will be making presentations to community organizations, church groups, or schools. Developing this important skill will increase your poise and self-confidence, ensuring that your ideas will be heard.

Writing letters is a powerful tool to support others while increasing your own visibility within the organization. Writing letters to individuals who have done a good job or gone out of their way to help you, thanking them for their efforts, not only supports your colleagues but also ensures that you will receive similar high levels of cooperation in the future. By directing the letter to the supervisor while sending a copy to the individual, a powerful message is sent that has the secondary benefit of marking you as a team player. This strategy may seem manipulative and self-serving; however, members of an organization have an obligation to support each other. We must reframe our thinking to understand that by advancing the careers of our colleagues and ourselves we are in fact strengthening the organization.

Likewise, it is important to get letters of support for ourselves. Think of all of the times patients and family members have complimented you on the care they have received from you. Although it is always nice to know that your efforts are appreciated, would it not be nice if your supervisors were able to hear those comments? The next time you receive a verbal compliment, ask the person to put it in writing. Good work counts when someone sees it or knows about it. Try saying, "Thank you. I really appreciate you telling me that. I wish my boss could hear it. Would you mind putting that in writing?" Most people will respond positively and wonder why they had not thought to do it themselves.

Letters document your skills and validate your abilities. Save these letters and use them to get new jobs or promotions. Letters may be presented as samples of your work. Never leave a job without getting at least three letters of reference from supervisors and colleagues. If you are not immediately moving to another position, have the references addressed "To Whom It May Concern." Often, if there is a gap in your employment, when you go to apply for a new position, the people who knew you before and who could attest to your work have retired or moved to other institutions themselves. These letters of reference are just as valid as those written currently by specific individuals.

Networking

The more people who know you and who know the quality of your work and what you have to offer, the more doors will be open to you and greater opportunities will come your way.

The more people who know you and who know the quality of your work and what you have to offer, the more doors will be open to you and greater opportunities will come your way. **Networking** is the process by which you get to know people within your organization and within your profession. Networking is important because it allows people to know one another on a personal level, forging relationships that enhance communication and increase productivity. Networking creates a sense of belonging among members of an organization or professional group.

One of the best ways to network with other nurses is to join or become more active in your professional organization. By attending meetings, working on a committee, contributing to the newsletter, or speaking at an organizational function, you increase your professional contacts and enhance your reputation in your field. Attend regional or national conventions, join a panel discussion, or make a presentation. Be sure to send a copy of your speech to your supervisor and nursing service administrator so that they will know that you are representing your organization well.

If you tend to shy away from meetings because you are uncomfortable in social situations where you may not know people, keep in mind that others probably feel the same way. Assume that you are going to be welcomed and accepted. Take on the role of welcoming other people and putting them at ease. Come prepared with small talk—topics that you can share comfortably with others. Keep abreast of developments in your field, controversial legislative proposals, news items, or amusing anecdotes. If you arrive at the meeting with ideas to share, it will be much easier to strike up conversations with relative strangers. Occasionally you may find that it is difficult to detach yourself from someone with whom you have started a conversation. If this is a concern, stand by the door and greet people as they arrive. Speak to them briefly before directing them to others or the refreshments. You will find you get to meet a lot of people for a short time and you will not have to worry about disengaging. Table 7-5 offers further hints on getting the most out of meetings. If you are still uncomfortable, give yourself an assignment: stay for 1 hour, and speak to five people; then you can leave. You may find that you remain for the entire meeting and enjoy doing so. After one or two meetings, you'll arrive to a meeting of friends and colleagues rather than strangers. The informal conversations that take place at professional meetings may be more valuable to you and your career than the formal business of the group.

Mentoring

Just as we are responsible for developing and managing our own careers, we are obliged to encourage others to develop professionally as well. Too often nurses compete to maintain the status quo rather than supporting the advancement of colleagues. Nurses who choose to further their careers by returning to school for advanced degrees or seeking promotions are somehow perceived as a threat and are frequently discouraged or even sabotaged in subtle ways by their colleagues. There is a scarcity mentality in which another's progress is perceived as a loss in one's own status. This phenomenon has a detrimental effect on the profession as a whole.

Experienced nurses can usually recall other nurses who served as role models or mentors providing leadership and guidance to them as they began their nursing careers or faced professional challenges. The relationships between new and experienced nurses take many forms and vary from friend and informal advisor

---

TABLE 7-5   GETTING THE MOST OUT OF MEETINGS

- Attend three meetings before deciding about a group; once to overcome your fear, once to learn about it, and once to decide if you like it.
- Introduce yourself by giving your first and last name and telling something about yourself to get the conversation going.
- Say your first and last name as you meet people. Even people that know you well or have met you before can have temporary amnesia for names.
- Wear your name tag on the right side so people can see it when you shake hands.
- Wear comfortable shoes and clothing; you may be standing for a while.
- Plan your conversation ahead of time. Come prepared with small talk.
- Keep your business cards handy; use them to leave a tangible reminder of who you are.
- Relax and try to enjoy yourself. If you are uncomfortable, find someone who looks nervous and try to set them at ease.

to that of a formal contractual mentor. **Mentoring** has been defined as a developmental, empowering, and nurturing relationship that extends over time and in which mutual sharing, learning, and growth occur in an atmosphere of respect, collegiality, and affirmation (Vance & Olson, 1998). Ideally, all graduate nurses should be assigned mentors who work closely with them during the difficult transition between the student and staff nurse roles. A true mentor, however, is someone who is willing to maintain a long-term relationship, advising and guiding an individual as needed throughout the professional career.

Unfortunately, few organizations are able to provide formal mentors for all new employees. Mentorship, however, is such an important component of successful career management that individuals should actively seek out formal or informal mentors to guide and support them. Mentoring relationships can develop through networking as you meet and interact with colleagues who you respect and admire. When selecting a mentor, it is important to seek someone with whom it is easy to communicate and who has the time and interest to work with you to discuss various professional issues. A mentor is not just someone who offers advice, but someone who will challenge your ideas and encourage you to strive for excellence.

Evaluating Your Performance

What do people really think of you and your work? Aside from asking a trusted colleague how he or she rates your performance professionally, you may either rely on the formal process of the performance appraisal done annually by your supervisor, or you can actively solicit feedback from others. Most people are creatures of habit and will continue behaviors that seem to have been effective in the past until someone informs them otherwise. It is difficult for us to directly observe the effects of our words or actions on another person. We must rely on the social mirror in which we see ourselves reflected through the responses of others. **Feedback** is information that we receive from others about the impact of our behavior on them; it allows us to view ourselves from another's perspective. Soliciting feedback from peers is one way to gain direct information on how people perceive our words, actions, and abilities. Feedback differs from advice in that it describes the effect of another's behavior on us. It does not include advice on changing that behavior; rather, it is up to the individual soliciting feedback to decide if change is warranted (Riley, 2004).

Feedback may be difficult to hear, especially if it is unexpectedly negative. Be sure that you truly want to hear the information you are asking another to give. If you only want to receive positive feedback, forget about asking people to be honest with you. It is risky asking others to jeopardize a relationship by divulging opinions that may not be welcomed. Riley (2004) recommended the following steps be taken when you solicit feedback:

- Get focused: Ensure that you are not distracted by other issues and can give your full attention to the information you are receiving.

- Allocate sufficient time: Schedule enough time so that you can listen and reflect on the information without being rushed.
- Understand the feedback: Seek clarification or ask for repetition of information that is unclear.
- Ask for guidance: If the feedback indicates the need for a change in behavior, ask for advice or directions for change.
- Show appreciation: The person giving feedback has taken a big risk and made an effort to provide you with useful information. Thank him or her for the effort.
- Think about the feedback: Evaluate your behavior in light of this new information. Reflect on the implications and consider changes.

Asking for and receiving feedback, especially if it is negative, is a courageous act. Regardless of whether you choose to act on the information, it is important to know how others perceive you.

CRITICAL THINKING QUESTIONS

Do you have the courage to ask for honest feedback? Do you have the courage to give honest feedback to a friend or colleague? How do you respond to negative feedback?

The process of performance appraisal is a more formalized means of obtaining feedback on your professional activities. Performance appraisals are formal evaluations of employees by a superior, usually a manager or supervisor of some kind, comparing the employee's behavior with a set of standards (Tappan, 2001). When done correctly, the performance appraisal process can be a highly effective tool for motivating employees to continue high-level performance and to strive for even greater accomplishments. Too often, however, the process is perfunctory or, at worst, punitive, serving rather to discourage rather than reward employees. Optimally, a good manager will collect data for the employees' annual reviews throughout the reviewing period, which is usually 1 year. Collecting anecdotal notes on incidents of positive performance as well as negative episodes will help to present a balanced picture of an individual's performance. Annual reviews are too often based on an employee's performance during the week or weeks immediately preceding the review, thus creating an artificial halo or horns effect (Table 7-6). To counter this possibility, it is important for you to take a proactive role in the process by providing your supervisor with accurate information about your performance and accomplishments throughout the reporting period.

Most organizations have a set time in the year when performance appraisals are conducted. Commonly, this takes place early in the calendar year and reflects employee performance during the previous 12-month period. Newer employees may be evaluated more frequently. Keeping in mind the fact that your supervisor has more important things to do than to track your career, you can assist in this process by providing your supervisor with information that you believe should be included in your performance appraisal such as:

- Continuing education courses, workshops, seminars, or formal programs of study attended

TABLE 7-6   HALO VS. HORNS EFFECT

Halo Effect: Overrating an employee's total performance based on a single positive event.

- Strong social skills and a pleasant personality masking poor performance
- Rating based on past positive performance rather than current observations
- History of mediocrity punctuated by a single recent stellar performance
- Friendship or shared interests with the manager

Horns Effect: Underrating an employee's total performance based on a single negative event.

- Positive performance interrupted by a serious error committed recently
- Consistent good work but disagrees with manager
- Associating with substandard peers
- Poor physical appearance in dress, manners, or hygiene

- Special projects completed, such as preparing teaching materials, in-service educational programs, or developing patient care policies
- Special assignments carried out in other areas of the organization
- Awards, letters of commendation, or recognition received for your professional activities
- Examples of instances when you performed above and beyond what was expected or required
- Plans for further education and/or professional development activities in the next year

Most managers will appreciate this type of assistance and welcome having the information at their disposal as they fill out the appraisal forms. If you have made serious errors or committed a recent professional faux pas, this may still show up on your evaluation; however, you are more likely to receive a balanced review.

Once the performance appraisal evaluation form has been completed, most organizations require a conference between the employee and supervisor to discuss the review. If your unit manager does not already do this, request a meeting at a time that is convenient for both of you when you can be relatively free from interruptions. For many of us, these meetings conjure up painful memories of being called to the principal's office in school to be reprimanded for some infraction of the rules—not a pleasant association. Keep in mind, however, that the purpose of the meeting is to discuss the review ratings, identify strengths and limitations, and brainstorm activities that will contribute to your professional growth. Motivation is the goal. Your role in the meeting is to listen carefully to what is being said, whether or not you agree with the findings. If the review is positive, the discussion will be easy for both sides. If the review is disappointing, it is important that you remain neutral and not react negatively, making a difficult situation worse.

Coping with Adversity

No one likes to hear negative things about their performance, especially if the comments are unexpected or unwarranted. Responding to a negative performance appraisal with anger or defensiveness is not going to advance your career. Whether or not you agree with the appraisal, the report reflects your supervisor's perceptions of your performance, which may or may not be accurate. Either way, you have a problem. Remember, your role in this meeting is to listen to feedback. Your career is at stake here; thus, you do not have the luxury of getting angry and storming out of the meeting. If you become emotional or feel that you may lose control, ask for time to reflect on the report and schedule another meeting to continue the discussion.

Be careful what you sign and know what your signature implies. Does it mean that you concur with the performance appraisal or only that you have received the report? If your supervisor insists that you sign the report, it is appropriate that you write in what your signature indicates (e.g., "signature reflects receipt of report only, not concurrence with findings" or "see attached response"). It is strongly recommended that you take time to distance yourself and gain perspective about a negative performance appraisal before responding either in person or in writing. You might want to validate the findings with your mentor or trusted colleagues.

If you believe the findings are inaccurate, you will need to explore how your supervisor reached those conclusions. This can only be accomplished by having a frank discussion with him or her about your performance and how it varies from the expectations. This discussion should afford you an equal opportunity to describe your point of view. If you are concerned about the emotional level of the meeting, you may request that a disinterested third party attend to mediate. You can do a great deal to diffuse a potentially hostile meeting by acknowledging your role in creating the situation: "Given the information you have, I can see where you might draw that conclusion," or "I see where you might think that." This does not mean that you agree with your supervisor's statements but allows for the possibility that the supervisor's impressions may be accurate given limited or erroneous information. If the appraisal is inaccurate, you should present specific facts that contradict the findings and request that the ratings be changed. It is hoped the outcome of the interview will be that you each have a greater appreciation for the other's perspective and expectations.

If your supervisor disagrees or is unwilling to change the ratings, you should then attach a typewritten page of comments to the report stating factually the events from your point of view. Be sure to keep copies of all documents for your personal records. At the end of the meeting, if you are still dissatisfied or believe that you have been treated unfairly, you will need to seek redress by following the chain of command in your organization. Consult your employee handbook or policy manual for information on how to appeal an erroneous performance appraisal. As much as it might give temporary relief, if would be a grave mistake to go outside the chain of command and storm the nursing administrator's or CEO's office. At some point, you will have to decide how far the matter is worth pursuing. If you are unable to resolve your differences with the supervisor, it may be time to look for another position either within the organization or at a different agency.

Given the numbers and types of decisions that nurses are required to make daily, it is practically inevitable that mistakes will be made in the clinical area. Fortunately, most errors can be corrected without patients experiencing adverse effects. Whenever a mistake is made, however, it is important that the nurse notify the patient and family if appropriate, the supervisor, the physician, and any other members of the healthcare team who may be concerned. Every organization has a procedure for documenting errors or events that may cause a risk of injury or possible litigation. The manner in which mistakes are handled on a unit is indicative of the relationships among the individuals working there. Errors are generally symptoms of more important problems that must be addressed. Although errors are obviously undesirable, they create opportunities for learning as well as developing policies and procedures for preventing their occurrence in the future. As a professional, you should always be honest and take responsibility for your actions. When an error is made, admit that you did something wrong, apologize, and do whatever is necessary to either correct the error or mitigate the consequences. Take steps to ensure that similar mistakes are prevented. Making excuses or blaming others only makes an adverse situation worse. Hospital administrators and managers would much prefer honest employees who make mistakes and take steps to correct the situation than individuals who lie or attempt to cover up errors that might lead to costly litigation later.

Commitment to the Profession

Nursing is more than just a job; it is a profession and requires serious commitments from its members.

Nursing is more than just a job; it is a profession and requires serious commitments from its members. One of the characteristics of a profession is a commitment to **lifelong learning**. Undergraduate nursing programs, regardless of whether they are diploma, associate degree, or baccalaureate degree programs, are designed to prepare individuals to function in entry-level nursing positions under the supervision of more experienced nurses. Successful completion of the NCLEX-RN examination and qualifying for state licensure imply that you have met the minimal requirements to practice safely as a registered nurse. Many nurses have said that their real education began not in school, but on their first job. Nursing is one of the most rapidly developing professional disciplines. It is impossible for any educational program to provide nurses with all of the information that they will need to know to practice over the course of a lifetime. The best that education can do is to provide the basics while teaching students how to learn and how to access information. It is up to the individual to continue to develop professionally by acquiring new skills and knowledge.

As members of a professional discipline, we have an obligation to support our profession. Our responsibilities do not end at the close of our shift; we are responsible for keeping abreast of developments in the field and ensuring that the care our patients receive is the highest quality and most current treatment available. It is also important for nurses to have a voice in health care and related issues. The public considers nurses to be the most trusted of all healthcare providers, yet few people are able to describe exactly what it is that nurses do. The media more often portrays nurses as sex objects than as competent clinical practitioners. The media rarely views nurses as experts in health-related issues. It is vital that we articulate our role and educate elected officials and the public about the valuable contribution that nurses make. Nurses should take every opportunity to promote their profession.

One important way to do this is by joining professional organizations. Whatever your clinical interests, there is a professional organization that supports them. By joining an organization, you have access to journals, continuing education offerings, professional meetings, and a network of other nurses who share your interests. The American Nurses Association along with its state chapters is the recognized voice of nursing in the United States, although only 10% of registered nurses are members. This means that the vast majority of nurses are not heard or consulted when public policies concerning healthcare issues are discussed. Organizations such as the National League for Nursing and the American Association of Colleges of Nursing have an important role in setting educational standards and ensuring that those standards are met. These organizations depend on the contributions of members who volunteer their time, energy, and support to advance the goals of nursing.

> **CRITICAL THINKING QUESTIONS**
>
> Do you plan to be a part of a professional organization after graduation? Why or why not? What do you anticipate will be your level of involvement?

Commitment to Ourselves

As nurses, we have the privilege of interacting with people during the most significant moments of their lives—birth, death, and times of illness and injury. In the course of our work we routinely engage in activities that impact the lives of others at times when they are most vulnerable and in need of caring professionals. Our work matters, our actions count. As a result, the public views nurses very positively. We have the reputation of being honest, caring, reliable, concerned, and approachable. Although we enjoy the status of being members of this prestigious profession, there is a downside to it.

Nurses, unfortunately, are particularly vulnerable to stress and burnout. Nursing is publicly perceived to be not just a profession, but a vocation to which members pledge lifelong commitment. There is an assumption that nurses should be readily available at all times to listen to problems and discuss health issues even when they are not on the job. Nurses are caring and approachable; therefore, people often seek out nurses for advice and treatment where they would never presume to impose on a physician outside of a working situation. Family members frequently assume that nurses will step forward and volunteer to care for sick or elderly relatives simply because they are nurses, regardless of their professional career responsibilities—and we respond as expected. Men and women who are attracted to the nursing profession tend to be "people pleasers" who are generous with their time and resources. They often having trouble saying "no" to requests for assistance. Being needed makes us feel valued and important. Although there is nothing inherently wrong with this trait, it does open us up to abuse and disregard for our personal needs.

Stress in the Work Environment

Nursing is demanding work. Nurses work long hours in high-stress environments caring for clients whose conditions are often unstable. The decisions nurses make have serious implications for the health and lives of their patients. Our clients are sick and family members are stressed by the hospitalization, so nurses regularly interact with people who are not at their best. Hospitals are fast-paced, intense work environments where situations change rapidly and nurses must respond quickly and accurately to a multitude of competing demands. The nursing shortage further complicates the situation in that many units are chronically understaffed. There is often a rapid turnover of staff members and a lack of experienced nurses. Many hospitals have implemented 12-hours shifts for nurses, and although this scheduling offers certain advantages, it creates a lifestyle that leaves little time for personal self-care activities. A 12-hour shift easily stretches to 14 or more hours when considering report time, paperwork, and commuting. The work is physically and mentally taxing and, at the end of the day, nurses arrive home with little time or energy left to care for their families, let alone themselves.

Nurses in general are a resilient group capable of dealing with work-related stress and thriving in the demanding healthcare environment. Unfortunately, it is easy for our professional lives to overrun our personal lives with the result that we lack a positive balance between work, home, and personal interests. Maintaining this pace for prolonged periods can have untoward effects on one's health, relationships, and overall quality of life. The effects of stress are multiple and varied and may affect the following:

- Feelings, including anxiety, irritability, fear, anger, and moodiness
- Thoughts, including self-criticism, difficulty concentrating and making decisions, forgetfulness or mental disorganization, preoccupation with the future, repetitive thoughts, and fear of failure
- Behaviors, including crying, acting impulsively, nervous laughter, snapping at friends, teeth grinding or jaw clenching, smoking, alcohol or drug abuse
- Physical sensations, including headaches, tight muscles, cold or sweaty hands, back or neck problems, difficulty sleeping, stomach aches, colds

and infections, fatigue, rapid breathing or pounding heart, or trembling (Sikorsky & Malaney, 2007).

The means by which we deal with stress becomes very important. All too often, nurses use coping methods that are detrimental to their overall well-being. Lack of exercise and poor nutrition increase the deleterious effects of stress. Addictive behaviors such as smoking, overeating, self-medication, and substance abuse can develop. Some nurses are attracted to needy people and enter into toxic relationships. The results of these negative behaviors can lead to physical illness, increased risk of injuries, and burnout.

Burnout—An Occupational Hazard

Burnout occurs when nurses can no longer cope with the stresses and strains of professional nursing and choose to leave the profession to seek employment elsewhere. Symptoms of burnout include physical, psychological, and emotional exhaustion; lack of enthusiasm and decreased interest in work-related activities; and depression, negativism, and anger. Nurses experiencing burnout withdraw emotionally from both clients and coworkers. There may be an increase in physical symptoms that results in absenteeism. Nurses who continuously give of themselves

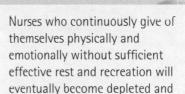

Nurses who continuously give of themselves physically and emotionally without sufficient effective rest and recreation will eventually become depleted and develop burnout.

physically and emotionally without sufficient effective rest and recreation will eventually become depleted and develop burnout. Savvy employers recognize this danger and implement measures and programs designed to identify nurses at risk and intervene to prevent burnout from occurring. All too often, however, this workplace crisis is overlooked until nurses resign in frustration. Ultimately, we as nurses are responsible for our own physical and mental health. It is imperative that nurses understand the effects of workplace stress and the symptoms of burnout in order to prevent this occupational hazard.

Stress Management and Self-Care

To survive and thrive in the profession, nurses must be as attentive to their own needs as they are to the needs of their clients. **Self-care** means acknowledging and meeting your own physical, psychological, social, and spiritual needs. It means caring for yourself *before* you care for others, not after you have tended to everyone else. In an emergency, airline attendants always advise individuals traveling with young children to place the oxygen masks over their own faces before placing them on the children. We cannot help others if we are starved and depleted ourselves.

Individuals are happiest and function at their best when there is balance in their lives. Meeting one's physical needs is a good place to begin. Nurses understand the importance of nutrition on wound healing and illness recovery in their clients; therefore, they must similarly nourish their own bodies with healthy, balanced, nutritious meals for optimal performance. Problems with overweight and obesity should be addressed through programs of sound nutrition and planned exercise. One of the cruel ironies of nursing is that, although the work is physically demanding, it is not particularly good exercise. Nurses must make time in their busy schedules for aerobic activities such as walking, jogging, swimming, tennis, spinning, bicycling, or dancing in addition to basic weight training to strengthen muscles and build stamina. Habits such as smoking, consuming alcohol, and taking nonprescription medications must be avoided.

Rest is as important as diet and exercise in dealing with stress. Most people require a minimum of 8 hours of sleep at night. Nurses who rotate shifts or work nights often have problems sleeping during the day and fail to get adequate rest. Sleep aids may offer temporary relief; however, most sleep-inducing medications cause dependency and may have side effects. Melatonin is a naturally occurring hormone that induces sleep and may be purchased over the counter in drugstores or health food stores. To date, melatonin has not been shown to have negative side effects when taken as directed for short-term relief of sleeplessness. The most effective sleep aid, however, is good nutrition, physical exercise, and an environment conducive to rest and relaxation.

Whether one considers nursing a vocation, an occupation, or a career, it remains only one aspect of an individual's life and must not become all-consuming.

Psychological, social, and spiritual needs are as important to one's well-being as the physical needs. Unfortunately, these are often sacrificed when time and energy are at a premium. Whether one considers nursing a vocation, an occupation, or a career, it remains only one aspect of an individual's life and must not become all-consuming. Time away from the job is as important as time spent on the job. Socializing with people we love and who contribute positively to our lives is crucial; however, not all relationships with friends or family members are healthy. When you regularly leave social encounters feeling worse than before, it is time to re-evaluate that relationship. By all means, address interpersonal issues and resolve conflict whenever possible; seek counseling if necessary, but if the relationship remains toxic, you must limit your exposure to that person. We are social beings who rely on each other for validation, stress relief, and sheer enjoyment of life. Without positive social relationships, we lose perspective and problems can rapidly become overwhelming.

Human beings naturally strive to find meaning in their existence. All of us have spiritual needs, but for nurses who deal with life and death on a daily basis, spirituality becomes particularly important as we struggle to come to terms with these issues. Belief in a higher being, in a planned universe, and in a rich afterlife helps provide context for the joys and tragedies we witness regularly. Regardless of one's personal spiritual beliefs, participation in prayer, religious services, and fellowship with others sharing your beliefs are important to maintain balance and perspective.

Time Management—Life Management

For most of us, the greatest challenge and key to life balance is time management. Each of us has 24 hours a day, 168 hours per week, or 8760 hours per year to manage. If a third of your daily allotment is spent sleeping and another third working, that leaves only eight hours to attend to all of the other activities of daily living— shopping, meal preparation, dining, housekeeping, laundry, errands, childcare, carpooling, commuting, and so on. Precious little time remains at the end of the day for quiet reflection, recreation, reading, relaxing, or relationships; yet, these are the activities that are vital to restoring our physical and mental health. The more activities we cram into our day, the more the stress builds. It is impossible to do it all! Yes, we can have it all—career, friends, family relationships, children, home— we just might not be able to have it all at the same time or manage it all by ourselves.

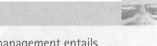

Many people approach the challenge of time management by attempting to become more organized, employing to-do lists, daily planners, or personal assistive devices to gain control over multiple demands for time and attention. These strategies may help you organize your activities, but they cannot add hours to the day. An alternative approach to time management is **life management**. Life management entails determining what is truly important to you and making positive choices about how, where, and with whom you spend your precious hours. Life management means letting go of the minutia that clutters our lives and saps our strength. It involves simplifying our environments, our commitments, and our relationships in order to eliminate the physical and psychological baggage that weighs us down.

> Life management entails determining what is truly important to you and making positive choices about how, where, and with whom you spend your precious hours.

The popular press abounds with books written by life coaches and time management specialists with suggestions on how to identify your values, formulate personal mission statements, and set priorities that allow you to incorporate the relationships and activities that nourish and enrich your life into your schedule. Take advantage of whatever tools are available to you to learn to put into place the people and systems that assist you to accomplish that which is truly important.

> **CRITICAL THINKING QUESTION**
>
> Think about what it is that is truly important to you. Do the choices you make about how, where, and with whom you spend your time reflect what is important to you?

Conclusion

As nurses our professional lives are both challenging and rewarding. Simply by introducing yourself as a nurse, you are invited into the lives of others in a way that rarely happens in other disciplines. People entrust you with the most intimate details of their lives and literally place their lives and the lives of their loved ones in your hands. On a daily basis, you have the opportunity to make a difference in the life of another human being. Few professions offer this level of interaction. This is, at the same time, a rare privilege and an awesome responsibility. As members of a widely respected profession, we must keep in mind the responsibility that we bear and strive to uphold continuously the standards of excellence that our profession holds.

One crucial aspect of this responsibility lies in caring for ourselves both personally and professionally. We must attend to our own needs first so that we will be able to address the needs of our clients and of our profession. This chapter has discussed the importance of career management, life management, and personal self-care. As individuals make the decision to enter the nursing profession, they also choose whether nursing, for them, will be an occupation or a career. The future of nursing depends on members caring for themselves and choosing to approach nursing as a lifelong profession. We hope that you will choose wisely.

CLASSROOM ACTIVITY: NURSING SCHOOL SURVIVAL GAME

Before class the instructor will prepare the board game. Spaces on the board will reflect self-care activities and give instructions for moving forward or backward depending upon if the activity reflected in the space promotes self-care or is detrimental. Divide students into small groups to play the Nursing School Survival Game. Students roll the dice to determine how many spaces to move. As they move around the board they will progress from nursing school admission to second semester, third semester, fourth semester, and then graduation.

As the groups land on different spaces take time to discuss the self-care activity and why it will help them to be successful in nursing school. Activities might include things such as buying a planner to get organized, reading assignments before class, finding a study group, regular exercise, eating nutritious meals, and specific stress management techniques. This game is a good one to use at the beginning of the first semester to help students get to know one another as well as discuss ways in which students can begin using self-care strategies from the very beginning of their nursing school career.

Spaces on the board may alternately reflect categories if verbal questions will be asked during the game. If this approach is used, the group will answer questions about self-care categories in order to progress around the board. Another approach to this game that is fun is to have different colored pieces of paper labeled as categories of self-care questions on the floor creating a game board effect and letting the students (either alone or in groups) move around the "game board" as they answer questions related to self-care.

References

American Association of Colleges of Nursing. (2002). *White paper on the professional practice setting.* Retrieved March 21, 2008, from www.aacn.nche.edu/Publications/positions/hallmarks.htm

Covey, S. R. (1989). *The 7 habits of highly effective people.* New York: Simon & Schuster.

Joel, L. A. (2003). Career management. In L. A. Joel (Ed.), *Kelly's dimensions of professional nursing* (9th ed.). New York: McGraw-Hill.

Miller, T. W. (2003). Work versus career. In T. W. Miller (Ed.), *Building and managing a career in nursing*. Indianapolis, IN: Sigma Theta Tau.

Oxford University Press. (1996). *The Oxford English dictionary*. New York: Oxford University Press.

Riley, J. B. (2004). Feedback. In J. B. Riley (Ed.), *Communication in nursing* (5th ed.). St. Louis, MO: Mosby.

Sikorski, E., & Malaney, K. (2007). Personal and financial health. *Vermont Nurse Connection, 10*(3), 9.

Tappan, R. M. (2001). Individual evaluation procedures. In R. Tappen & C. Lynn (Eds.), *Nursing leadership and management concepts and practice* (4th ed.). Philadelphia: F. A. Davis.

Vance, C., & Olson, R. (1998). *The mentor connection in nursing*. New York: Springer.

Unit II

Professional Nursing Practice and the Management of Patient Care

chapter 8

The Healthcare Delivery System and the Role of the Professional Nurse

Sharon Vincent

LEARNING OBJECTIVES

After completing this chapter, the student should be able to:

1. Describe how health care is delivered and how the system is changing.
2. Compare and contrast nursing delivery models of patient care.
3. Define the case management model of care.
4. Analyze the role of the nurse in health promotion.
5. Describe the advocacy role of the professional nurse.
6. Explain how effective delegation can benefit both the client and the healthcare delivery system.
7. Identify the need for consultation and collaboration with other healthcare providers.
8. Describe the importance of continuity of care and collaboration between healthcare providers in other departments or facilities.
9. Discuss the need for referral of a client to other departments or community resources.

Key Terms and Concepts

- Healthcare delivery system
- Models of patient care
- Functional nursing
- Team nursing
- Total patient care
- Primary nursing care
- Case management
- Critical pathway
- Case manager
- Collaborative critical path
- Role of the professional nurse
- Caregiver
- Holistic care
- Advocate
- Manager
- Delegation
- Collaborative practice
- Interdisciplinary healthcare team
- Consultations
- Continuity of care
- Collaboration
- Comanagement
- Referral
- Performance improvement

Perhaps you are wondering why hospitals or clinics are called healthcare delivery systems and not just hospitals or clinics, or why nurses are referred to as professional nurses? In this chapter, we will explore what the healthcare delivery system means to us. Also, we will discuss some of the various roles we play as nurses that define what it means to be a professional nurse. Various models of nursing care delivery will be explored so that the graduate nurse possesses a greater understanding of the healthcare delivery environment. The method used to assign staff nurses and technicians might seem like a distant concept at this moment, but as a baccalaureate entry-level nurse, you could be making assignments soon after graduation.

All nurses today are managers. Registered nurses manage the care of a specific group of patients, do some of the care themselves, direct others to provide care, and collaborate with other healthcare providers. Nurses must know how to delegate, supervise, evaluate, motivate, and communicate with other disciplines, other nurses, and unlicensed personnel. They must also lead teams. In the management of care, each nurse directs the nursing care within a delivery setting to protect the clients, significant others, and healthcare personnel. The professional nurse utilizes critical thinking skills to assess clients and to evaluate the expertise of nursing staff when making assignments. The nurse's role encompasses collaboration in the continuity of care from admission to discharge and rehabilitation. This chapter will clearly define some of the concepts that are needed for the entry-level nurse to maintain safe and competent entry-level nursing practice.

Healthcare Delivery System

The **healthcare delivery system** has changed profoundly over the past several decades for several reasons. Population shifts (demographic changes), cultural diversity, the patterns of diseases, advances in technology, and economic changes have all impacted the practice of nursing. Population changes are affecting the need for the delivery of health care. Health care is needed now more than in the past. The population is increasing, and the composition of that population is changing. Birth rates are decreasing, and the life span is increasing due to improved health care. For example, people older than 85 years of age make up one of the fastest-growing segments of the population; the number was 34 times larger in 1999 than in 1900 (Smeltzer, Bare, Hinkl, & Cheever, 2007). More senior citizens are a factor, many of whom are women. A significant portion of the population resides in urban areas, with a steady migration of ethnic minorities. Homeless persons, including homeless families, are on the rise. Cultural diversity increases as people from different nationalities enter the country.

It is important for the professional nurse to possess an appreciation for the diverse needs of people from varied cultural backgrounds. With increased immigration, it is projected that by 2030, racial and ethnic minority groups will constitute 40% of the population of the United States (Smeltzer et al., 2007). Nursing care must be sensitive to cultural differences. For example, the nurse might provide special foods that are significant or provide for the arrangement of religious observances. Many hospitals provide a cultural guide for healthcare providers of the foods, spiritual practices, and life, death, and illness practices for diverse cultural groups. Being culturally aware within the healthcare delivery system helps the nurse avoid imposing personal value systems when the patient has a different point of view.

In the last 50 years, evolving patterns of diseases have brought significant changes to the healthcare delivery system. Diseases such as tuberculosis, acquired immuno-deficiency syndrome (AIDS), and sexually transmitted infections are increasing. Because of the widespread inappropriate usages of antibiotics, an increasing number of infectious agents are becoming resistant to antibiotic therapy. Obesity is now a major health challenge as well as its comorbidities—hypertension, coronary heart disease, diabetes mellitus, and cancer. Also, the improvement in techniques for trauma and acute care means that more people are living decades longer with chronic conditions. Technology has boosted surgical and diagnostic service areas so that patients can receive sophisticated treatment on an outpatient basis. Communication techniques provide a means to train and deliver health care to remote countries and islands by satellite. For example, the military on a small island functions with a limited number of healthcare providers. Attending physicians monitor surgical procedures and train military personnel via Web-based satellite signal; this is an example of telemedicine healthcare delivery.

In the past, the healthcare delivery system was mainly hospital based with an acute care focus. Currently, many clients stay in the hospital for a short time, just 23 hours. Other facets of current healthcare delivery include hospital testing and precertification, telecommunications, home health, mobile vans, and mall clinics. Historically as healthcare costs became alarmingly high, cost-containment mandated by Congress initiated the beginning of diagnosis-related groups (DRGs), a plan to cut costs related to Medicare reimbursement. Care became focused on cost and profit, and the quality of nursing care declined. Nurses experienced work-related stress, burnout, and many left the nursing arena as hospitals operated with fewer resources. Because of cost constraints and a shortage of available nurses, cross-training became a common practice. For example, one nurse may be cross-trained in the operating room and the postanesthesia care unit and is thus able to work in either unit with specialized skills (Blais, Hayes, Kozier, & Erb, 2006). Nurses in those areas are trained to fill two departments or more, since fewer nurses are being hired due to cost constraints.

Nurses are challenged more than ever to provide quality care with fewer resources. With the two major issues of cost-containment and access to care at the forefront of healthcare delivery, many people have limited or no access to health care. Reducing personnel has been a major challenge with the restructuring of resources—fewer patients are covered by insurance and many have lower percentages of coverage, copayment problems, or no insurance coverage at all. The uninsured segment of the population is increasing. About 40 million Americans are estimated to be uninsured at a time, and 60 million Americans are without health insurance for a portion of the year (Blais et al., 2006). Many more are underinsured and limited from receiving health care.

Current healthcare delivery systems utilize interdisciplinary teams, collaboration techniques, and case management, whereas the physician used to direct all patient care with everyone else following the physician's lead. The professional nurse is currently career focused, with an interest in continuing credentials for specialty training or professional organization memberships, whereas nurses previously were simply job-focused employees. The care of clients has shifted from care of the sick to health promotion and prevention programs, continuity of care, and complementary health alternatives. The focus on billing with cost containment has shifted to a focus on accountability of caregivers, continuous quality improvement (CQI), and care maps or critical pathways (Blais et al., 2006).

Representing a step in the shift from a centralized biomedical model of caring, community nursing centers are a creative healthcare delivery model with a more holistic nursing model of caring. The focus of attention of the traditional biomedical model of illness over the past century has been on discovering the pathology, or the cure to one problem, rather than understanding the illness and its various components (Wade & Halligan, 2004). Community centers located in churches, mobile units, shelters, and schools are set up to meet the underserved populations by providing a range of services to the public that are not normally available. The needs of the patient become the focus, instead of a medical diagnosis for pathology and a single cure. These centers offer education and preventive measures for topics of interest to the local community. A nurse or group of caregivers might go to community centers to assess and teach health promotion and prevention strategies for cancer or hypertension. This represents a shift from seeking a single cure to the promotion of health, wellness, and well-being (Blais et al., 2006).

The healthcare delivery system is continuously changing and evolving. Within the healthcare delivery system there are several models of patient care delivery.

> **CRITICAL THINKING QUESTION**
>
> Positive health promotion is a process of enabling people to improve and increase control of their maximum health potential. Think of positive health promotion behaviors that you have demonstrated since beginning nursing school. What have you noticed since using these behaviors in your daily routine?

Models of Patient Care

Nurses are leaders and managers within various **models of patient care** delivery. The methods might differ significantly from one organization to another. The purpose of a nursing care delivery system is to provide a framework for nurses to deliver care to a specific group of patients. The delivery of care implements the nursing process and includes assessing and triaging clients so that the order of care may be prioritized, a care plan formulated, and client responses to nursing interventions evaluated in collaboration with other health team members (Wendt, Kenny, & Anderson, 2007).

The purpose of a nursing care delivery system is to provide a framework for nurses to deliver care to a specific group of patients.

The methods and models of nursing care have evolved over the years and have included functional nursing (task nursing), team nursing, total patient care or the case method, primary nursing, and case management. The most common models of nursing care delivery are discussed in this chapter. The continual evaluation of nursing models of care has been prompted by changes in nursing staff availability, reduction in hospital revenue and reimbursement, changes in acuity levels (critical illness levels), shorter stays in the hospital, consumer demands for quality care and lesser charges, and demands by healthcare workers for improvements.

Functional Nursing

Most hospitals use a combination of models of care to meet the needs on specific care units. Functional nursing (task nursing) was utilized as early as the 1940s when there was a national nursing shortage due to many registered nurses (RNs) serving in World War II. With fewer numbers of registered nurses in the hospitals, the use of licensed practical nurses (LPNs/VNs) and unlicensed assistive personnel (UAPs) increased widely. In the **functional nursing** system client needs are divided into tasks, and each task is assigned to RNs, LPNs, or UAPs. This system is advantageous because each assigned caregiver becomes highly efficient in performing the assigned tasks. However, disadvantages become apparent when the caregivers are assigned new or different tasks. Also the consideration of a holistic view of the client is nearly nonexistent. Communication regarding each task may become too time consuming. Because care becomes fragmented, the functional method of nursing care is not used very often in today's health care.

Team Nursing

The **team nursing** model of care is used in the United States most frequently in hospitals and in long-term and extended-care facilities. This arrangement evolved after the functional nursing of the 1940s. With this approach, the nursing staff is divided into teams, and total patient care is provided to a group of patients. The assigned patients might also be grouped according to their diagnoses. For example, a team might consist of an RN, LPN, and two UAPs. The RN is the team leader, is responsible for making assignments, and has overall responsibility for patient care by team members. The team works together, performing activities they are best trained to do. The team communicates client care needs and possible changes in the care plan to the team leader. The team acts as a whole with a holistic perspective of the personal needs of each client. The team leader takes the lead to resolve problems that the team encounters, updates care plans, and communicates with physicians and other healthcare personnel. Often the team leader makes rounds with physicians. The nursing reports communicated at the beginning of each shift are a key feature of team nursing.

There are several advantages to team nursing. One is that UAPs can carry out some of the functions that do not require a registered nurse's expertise. Team nursing also allows for tasks that require several persons to be carried out with an assigned team readily available. Several disadvantages may surface with multiple care providers on a team, however. If communication skills are not consistent, a holistic view of the patient may be fragmented. Also, resentment may be experienced by UAPs and LPNs if they view the RN as a person focused totally on paperwork and documentation, with less focus on the physical or real needs of the client. For a team leader to be effective, delegation, communication, and problem-solving skills are essential.

Total Patient Care

As early as the 1920s, the first model of patient care delivery was **total patient care** (Sullivan & Decker, 2005). In this model, the RN has the responsibility for all aspects of care of the patient(s). The RN works directly with the client, other nursing staff, and physician in implementing a plan of care. The objective of total patient care is to have one nurse provide all care to the same patient(s) for the entire shift. Currently this model is practiced in areas such as critical care units or postanesthesia recovery units, where a high level of expertise is required. This system's advantages provide holistic, continuous care, continuity of communication from clients to other healthcare team members, and total accountability for that shift. The disadvantage is that some of the tasks could be performed by lesser skilled persons, which would be more cost-effective.

Primary Care

The **primary nursing care** model of delivery was developed in the 1960s after team nursing first became popular and was designed to put the nurse back at the bedside (Sullivan & Decker, 2005). Primary nursing allows the nurse to provide care to a small number of clients for their entire stay. The nurse provides and is accountable for care, communicates with clients and their families and other healthcare providers, and performs discharge planning. The actual care is given by the primary RN or associate nurses (other RNs). So with the primary nursing care system, several nurses provide care to the same patient. Primary nursing has appeared to advance professional nursing for several reasons. It is a knowledge-based model, it gives staff nurses some decision-making opportunity and authority, and it improves continuity of care. This contributes to nurse, client, and physician satisfaction.

Disadvantages exist in primary nursing. Excellent communication between associate nurses and primary nurses does not always occur. Also, the primary nurse sometimes has difficulty holding the associate nurse accountable for care as prescribed. Sometimes the associate nurses are not willing to take direction from the primary RN. One reason many hospitals dropped this system was because they thought it required all RNs, and since this was not cost-effective, they adopted other models of care.

Case Management

A current nursing model of nursing care delivery is **case management**, which relies on clinical pathways to evaluate care. The **critical pathway** refers to expected outcomes and interventions that the collaborative practice team establishes (Sullivan & Decker, 2005). The professional nurse is responsible for initiating and updating the plan of care, care map, or clinical pathway used to consistently guide and evaluate client care. The clinical pathway provides a time frame for expected outcomes of care and involves an interdisciplinary team of caregivers.

Nursing case management focuses on managing a group (caseload) of clients and the members of the healthcare team caring for those clients. The **case manager** organizes patient care by major diagnoses or DRGs and focuses on specific time frames to achieve predetermined patient outcomes and contain costs. The case manager makes referrals to other healthcare providers and manages the quality of care. Important characteristics of the role of nursing case managers are collaboration, identification of patient outcomes with time frames, and the use of performance improvement (PI) and quality assurance (QA) analysis. The case manager does not usually provide direct patient care, but supervises the provision of care by UAPs and licensed personnel.

A case manager's role in an acute care setting involves the management of a caseload of 10–15 patients. They follow the patients' progress from admission through discharge and solve problems of variances from the expected outcomes. A variance would be, for example, that a total hip surgery patient did not get discharged on day 6 (expected outcome by time frame) as planned; instead, that person was hospitalized for 10 days. The case manager intervenes and communicates with the team to analyze the critical path and determine why the patient was not discharged. Usually case managers have considerable nursing experience and an advanced degree.

When a group of clients is case managed, a team is selected with clinical experts from the disciplines needed, such as nursing, medicine, or physical therapy. The key features of a case management team are support by administration and physicians, a qualified case manager, collaboration of the teams, a quality assurance system in place, and critical pathways. All members of the team must agree on the critical pathways that are established and accept responsibility and accountability for interventions and patient outcomes. Case management contributes to the reduction of complications that arise during hospitalization. Specific measurable patient outcomes with time frames for the group of clients are determined.

The groups selected are high-volume, high-cost, and high-risk cases. One such example is the total hip replacement client population in orthopedics. The numbers of hip replacement surgeries performed are higher than many other procedures; they cost more and include higher risks such as pulmonary emboli and surgical site infections. The total cost to the client and related departments is higher, so careful monitoring is necessary. Other high-risk clients are those in critical condition, in ICU more than 2 days, or on a ventilator. Baseline data are collected on these groups and analyzed such as length of stay, cost of care, and complications.

The critical path quickly orients the staff to the outcomes that should be achieved for that day. Nursing diagnoses identify the outcomes needed. If these are not achieved, the case manager is notified and the situation analyzed. An example of a **collaborative critical path** for a patient having a total hip replacement is described here. Segments of a critical path for a total hip client on days 1 and 3 postoperatively might include:

- **Day 1, Operating Room and Postoperative Care**
  Activity: Bed rest, turn/cough/deep breath q 2 hrs
  NSG: VS q h × 4, then q 4 hrs, circulation/neuro checks q h × 4, then q 4 hrs, Hemovac: check q hr × 4, then q 4 hrs, I & O
  Medications: Antibiotics, pain control
  Nutrition: NPO to clear liquids as tolerated
  Teaching: Pain control, assist devices, incentive spirometry, mobility plan, D/C plan, home health evaluation
- **Day 3 Postoperatively**
  Activity: Continue mobility plan, turn/cough/deep breath q 2 hrs, skin protocols
  NSG: VS q 8 hrs, D/C assessment, D/C hemovac, ck drainage, I & O q 8 hrs, D/C Foley, continue elastic hose
  Medications: Antibiotics, p.o. pain control, continue stool softeners, IV to heplock, continue Coumadin.
  Nutrition: Diet as tolerated, repeat teaching as needed
  D/C plans: Review transfer orders, D/C needs

Normally a total hip client would be expected to be discharged on the 6th day after surgery. The critical path continues all 6 days, with potential nursing diagnoses attached, such as pain control deficit, or impaired mobility. The critical path is also given to the family, so they know what to expect during an uncomplicated total hip surgery hospitalization. Case management is one role of professional nursing, but we will further define some of the many roles that nurses may assume.

Role of the Professional Nurse

The role of the professional nurse has expanded in response to changing populations and the philosophical shift toward health promotion rather than illness cure.

The **role of the professional nurse** is one of the most exciting areas to discuss for entry-level nurses. The role of the professional nurse has expanded in response to changing populations and the philosophical shift toward health promotion rather than illness cure. The list could be exhaustive, but roles of nurses include caregiver, advocate, educator, leader, manager, and researcher.

We will examine the most important aspects of the entry-level nurse role and also define basic concepts of management of care. Entry-level nurses will immediately manage their patients' care. Nurses practice health promotion (also referred to as primary prevention or illness prevention) through education of clients and their families.

Caregiver

The role of the nurse as **caregiver** has changed tremendously during the past century. The role as a dependent person to the physician who only provided personal care has evolved to that of the educated nurse who is an autonomous and informed professional. As a caregiver, the nurse practices nursing as a science. The nurse provides interventions to meet physical, psychosocial, spiritual, and environmental needs of clients and families using the nursing process and critical thinking skills. **Holistic care** is a philosophical approach that emphasizes the uniqueness of the individual, in which interacting wholes are more important than the sum of each part. That is, the whole person is greater than merely each component part of the client—their biophysical, psychological, social, and spiritual parts. The science (knowledge base) of nursing becomes the art of nursing through caring, where the nurse is concerned for the client. The nurse and client are connected. The nurse as a caregiver is skilled and empathetic, knowledgeable and caring.

Advocate

As the nurse–client relationship develops, the nurse needs professional knowledge to assist the clients in their decision making. The nurse fills the role of **advocate** in the healthcare delivery, intervening in crises of AIDS, homelessness, drug and alcohol abuse, teenage pregnancy, child and spouse abuse, and increasing healthcare costs. A client advocate is a person who pleads the cause for clients' rights. The purpose of this role is to respect client decisions and boost client autonomy. Client advocacy includes a therapeutic nurse–client relationship to secure self-determination, protection of patients' rights, and acting as an intermediary between patients and their significant others and healthcare providers (Blais et al., 2006). A client advocate is mainly concerned with empowering the client through the nurse–patient relationship. The nurse represents the interests of the client who has needs that are unmet and are likely to remain unmet without the nurse's special intervention. The professional nurse speaks for the client as if the client's interests were the nurse's own.

There are numerous situations where the nurse may speak up for the patient. Examples are pain control, the clients' refusal of treatment, or issues of resuscitation status. Challenges face the nurse as client advocate. To be an effective client advocate, the nurse must do the following:

- Be assertive.
- Recognize the client's values as more important than the healthcare providers'.
- Ensure adequate information so that clients and families can make decisions.

- Be aware that conflicts may arise that require consultation or negotiation between healthcare providers.
- Be able to work with unfamiliar agencies.

Nurses need to assist clients in the clarification of their values as they relate to a particular health problem or end-of-life issue. The nurse and the client are equally responsible for the outcomes of care, but the nurse is responsible for assisting the client to use their strengths to obtain the highest level of health possible.

Manager

In exploring the concept of management in practice, all nurses are **managers**. They direct the work of professionals and nonprofessionals in order to achieve expected outcomes of care. All nurses need to learn management and leadership skills to be efficient and effective in their respective fields. In the healthcare setting, a manager is an individual who is employed by an organization and is responsible and accountable for the goals of that organization (Sullivan & Decker, 2005). In practice, nurses are expected to manage the care of each patient assigned to them for that shift. So, imagine you've just received a report on your patients. Where do you begin? Assessments and medicines are due. Patients need to go to surgery and radiology. Breakfast trays are ready to pass out. Treatments are waiting. Charting is needed. So much to do, and so little time! How can you get everything done, provide quality care, and still be standing? Well, delegation is a terrific concept!

It is easy to say *delegate,* but delegation is a difficult leadership role for nurses to learn and one that is not readily learned during nursing education. Both experienced nurses and entry-level nurses struggle to continuously develop delegation skills. Nurse managers must continually develop delegation skills to survive. Nurses must also learn to delegate without the threat of litigation. With cost containment, it is necessary now more than ever to delegate effectively. **Delegation** is defined as the process by which responsibility and authority for performing a certain task are transferred to another individual. This individual accepts that authority and responsibility (Sullivan & Decker, 2005). When accepting responsibility, a nurse has the obligation to intervene and accomplish a task. Nurses become accountable when they accept ownership for the results, or the lack results, depending on the situation. When delegating, responsibility can be transferred to another individual whereas both individuals are accountable. Accountability is a shared concept. It is the quality or state of being accountable, especially the obligation or willingness to accept responsibility or to account for one's actions. To delegate, the person doing the delegating must be the one who is responsible for the task.

It is important to understand the acceptance of delegation. It is important that one knows exactly what is being asked of them. One must realistically decide if they have the skills and abilities for the task being assigned and if they have the time to do it. If they lack appropriate skills, then they must inform the person delegating that they do not have the skills. It does not mean that they cannot perform the function. The next step is to see if the person delegating has the time and willingness to train and assist in accomplishing the task. If they cannot do this, the assignment must be refused. When delegation is accepted, responsibility is accepted for outcome benefits and also for liabilities. The delegator has the option to delegate parts of a task, but one also has the option to negotiate for the parts of the task that can be accomplished. New skills may be obtained in the process. After agreeing on the responsibilities to assume, the time frame and other expectations must be clarified. One must communicate with the delegator effectively throughout the completion of the task. If a task is declined the delegator should be thanked, and the nurse should indicate a desire to help him or her in the future.

It is important to examine the liability issues of delegation. The National Council of State Boards of Nursing suggested five "rights of delegation":

- Right task
- Right circumstances
- Right person
- Right direction and communication
- Right supervision (Sullivan & Decker, 2005)

It is important to utilize these five "rights of delegation." According to the American Nurses Association (2001) *Code of Ethics for Nurses,* the nurse is responsible for using informed judgment and basing the decision to delegate on the person's competencies and qualifications. If the nurse fails to do this, it is considered negligence. So, the delegating nurse must follow the steps of delegation when defining the task. The nurse must assess the need for delegation based on client needs. Secondly, the nurse determines which personnel should perform the task as well as their education, skills, and experience in performing the delegated task. The procedure should be communicated with clear instructions and guidelines. The nurse must also delegate to accomplish the goals of care, not to dump undesirable tasks on someone else. After tasks have been delegated, the nurse must evaluate the tasks to ensure correct completion of each activity. Delegation is definitely a skill that can be learned and requires practice. Successful nurses learn the process of delegation. Nurses accomplish more by delegating than if they try and do everything themselves.

To summarize the concept of delegation, it is a contractual agreement in which authority and responsibility for a task are transferred by the delegating person who is accountable for the task to another person. Delegation necessitates proficiency in determining the task and level of responsibility, determining who has the skills that are required, communicating expectations clearly to assigned personnel, and monitoring the performance of assigned tasks. Tasks to be delegated are routine tasks that are not highly technical or controversial. In that situation, numerous problems could arise that the delegating nurse would have to solve in spite of delegating. Delegation that is ineffective is usually the result of inappropriate transference of authority or responsibility to another individual. When nurses carefully select a qualified person as a delegate and provide supervision, liability is minimized. All nurses and managers must learn to delegate in order to be successful.

Collaborative Practice

The purpose of collaboration is to achieve high-quality client care and client satisfaction. A collaborative framework with an interdisciplinary team can also limit costs as well as improve quality of care.

One of the many roles of the professional nurse is **collaborative practice**. The purpose of collaboration is to achieve high-quality client care and client satisfaction. A collaborative framework with an interdisciplinary team can also limit costs as well as improve quality of care. Other goals of collaboration include the following:

- Enhance continuity across the continuum of care, from wellness and prevention, through acute episodes of illness, to discharge or transfer and rehabilitation.
- Improve client and significant others' satisfaction with care.
- Provide research-based, high-quality, cost-effective care that is driven by expected outcomes.
- Promote mutual respect and communication between clients and members of the healthcare team.
- Provide opportunities to solve issues and problems.

Collaborative practice in caregiving can include nurse–physician interaction, nurse–nurse interaction, or the interaction of interdisciplinary teams or committees (Blais et al., 2006). Collaborative teams provide extensive care by providing a full range of expertise through each of the team members, and thus contributing to outcomes. Nurse–physician collaboration is essential to maximize quality patient care and requires knowledge sharing with joint responsibility for patient care. On some occasions, collaboration between nurses and physicians may involve fleeting encounters in patient areas. In this situation, there is no second chance to collaborate effectively on a committee, but the volume of these professional encounters may be increasing. This is due partly because physicians spend less time in each hospital unit than before, and many nurses work part-time. The challenge is to make the most of all interactions in order to utilize the best knowledge and abilities of all healthcare team members and produce positive client outcomes (Lindeke & Seickert, 2005). Bottom-line attention is given to compassionate and humanitarian patient care, and interdisciplinary collaboration can keep this central in spite of economic pressures. Motivated teams must work together to thrive by being optimistic and positive, thus inspiring hope in others when change is unsettling.

We have already examined how a critical pathway is implemented by collaboration with input from various departments. The **interdisciplinary healthcare team** can be especially effective in outpatient services. Here, the physician or nurse practitioner sees the client, and **consultations** are put into practice as needed. The teams deal with client-related problems and help the patient's progress through the clinic and hospital efficiently. Professional nurses practice consultations on a day-to-day basis. The primary nurse's role is to assess the need for consultations and identify expected outcomes of consultation, along with the need for revising care as client needs change. Nurse–nurse consulting might be between a staff nurse and an enterostomal therapist for the care of the client's excoriated ostomy site secondary to radiation and chemotherapy. This type of consultation is documented in the patient record by obtaining a physician's order for an enterostomal therapist consult, then the enterostomal nurse intervenes and documents the care rendered. The primary nurse provides for **continuity of care** with the initiation of appropriate interventions and assessment for collaboration, changing the current plan of care with continuous evaluation of outcomes.

The ability to collaborate is particularly important for staff nurses as well as nurses pursuing advanced practice roles. Collaboration is one of the key skills required in nursing. The advent of group practice, managed care, and practice standards has driven the need for collaboration and consultation. On a continuum, **collaboration** at the lowest level begins with communication between all involved disciplines and the client, with everyone asking similar questions (Blais et al., 2006). Each professional has separate interventions with a separate plan of care, and decision making is independent. Coordination and consultation represent a middle-range level of care, where the professionals seek to make best use of the effectiveness of resources. **Comanagement** and **referral** represent the highest level of collaboration, in which providers are responsible and accountable for their own aspects of care, and then patients are directed to other providers when the problem is beyond their expertise. The main levels of the continuum of collaboration are represented in Figure 8-1.

Successful consultation becomes apparent when each person making a contribution is recognized so that a unified plan can be put into practice. Nurses collaborate with clients, peers, and other persons in the healthcare delivery system. Specifically, the nurse's role as a collaborator with the client includes acknowledging and supporting the client in healthcare decisions, encouraging client autonomy, helping clients set goals for care, and providing client consultation in a collaborative

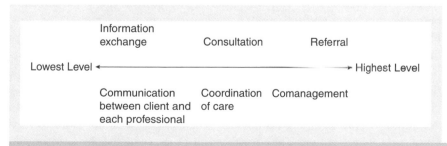

Figure 8-1
Levels of the Continuum of Collaboration

fashion. With other healthcare professionals, the nurse's role is to recognize the contribution of each member of the interdisciplinary team's expertise, listening, sharing responsibilities in exploring options and setting goals, and participating in collaborative interdisciplinary research to increase knowledge of a particular clinical problem. A nurse may also collaborate within professional organizations by serving on committees at the local, state, national, or international level to create solutions for professional and healthcare concerns.

Key elements needed for collaboration of the interdisciplinary healthcare team include effective communication skills, mutual respect and trust, giving and receiving feedback, decision making, and conflict resolution. Each professional group must center on common ground: the client's needs. A person-centered approach is essential, with formal training in consultation skills often nearly nonexistent (Brown, 2005). Mutual respect takes place in the team when individuals show honor or give credit to one another. When one is confident in the actions of another, trust occurs.

Mutual trust and respect must be verbalized by professionals, even though their actions may reflect a lack of respect or trust. Hospital delivery systems have not always fostered mutual caring and respect, so nurses must strive to promote positive relationships and practice in spite of past negative attitudes. When professionals work closely together on a team, giving and receiving timely and relevant feedback are some of the most difficult challenges. Feedback may be affected by each person's perceptions, roles, confidence, beliefs, and environment. Positive feedback is characterized by warm, caring, and respectful communication. Practicing basic communication with an opportunity to practice listening and giving and receiving feedback can enhance professional communication. Giving and receiving feedback helps the professional collaborative team develop an understanding and effective working relationship.

Another key element of collaboration by the interdisciplinary team involves responsibility for the expected outcome. To achieve a solution, team decision making must begin with a clear definition of the problem and be directed at the objectives of the specific effort. By focusing on the client's priority needs first, organization of interventions can be planned accordingly. The discipline best able to address the client's needs is given priority in planning and is responsible for providing its interventions in a timely manner. Take for example a terminal oncology patient requiring care postabdominal surgery following a bowel obstruction caused by an invasive tumor. Cancer has affected the spine, causing neurologic deficits of the extremities. The patient has an implanted port for chemotherapy, parenteral nutrition, and requires multiple antibiotic infusions. Several decubiti have developed. The primary nurse ensures total patient care by communicating with the client and significant others. The nurse then collaborates with the physician for pain

> **CRITICAL THINKING QUESTION**
>
> One of the most difficult challenges in promoting collaboration among professionals is giving and receiving feedback. What is your experience in giving and receiving timely and helpful feedback with a team? Think of an example of receiving both negative and positive feedback. Compare the effect of the negative and positive feedback. Compare the experience.

control and postoperative care. The nurse ensures expert intravenous lines for chemotherapy and multiple antibiotic infusions, collaborating with peers if necessary. The nurse consults via physician orders with the enterostomal therapist for wound care of the decubitus and consults with the dietician for hyperalimentation (total parenteral nutrition) needs. The nurse collaborates with physical therapy for resumption of activity for neurologic deficits. Each member of the interdisciplinary team contributes his or her own expertise to common goals of care. Nurses are often able to help the team identify priorities and focus on areas that require further referral or attention.

Role conflict may occur when individuals are working together and the expectations are incompatible. Conflicts may affect interdisciplinary collaboration. To reduce role conflict, team members can conduct interdisciplinary conferences, take part in interdisciplinary educational programs, and most important, recognize and accept personal responsibility for teamwork. Sometimes the failure of professionals to collaborate is due to lacking the skills necessary for effective teamwork. Nursing in the past has been interested in valuing "nursing" as a unique entity and concentrating on nursing research and nursing practice. The attention is now shifting to interdisciplinary collaboration and the recognition of different points of view. This requires the ability to articulate one's own theories as well as have the ability to mutually give and take to determine the best approach to specific problems. Sometimes organizational structure affects role conflict. Delivery systems that maintain a hierarchy of authority do not support interdisciplinary collaboration. In those situations where a traditional authority figure is strong, the promotion of collaboration by the organization between physicians and nurses can be effective. The relationship among participants must be one of trust and respect. The nurse's role in continuous quality improvement and performance improvement (PI) is especially true in hospitals that promote a culture of patient safety and view quality-related activities as priority "safety checks." Assuring high-quality patient safety cannot be overstated. Quality care results from caregivers doing the right thing the right way the first time.

Collaboration and evidence-based practice are key elements of successful quality programs, or **performance improvement** programs (Caramanica, Cousino, & Petersen, 2003). In the 1980s, hospitals and agencies implemented ongoing quality assurance programs (QAP). Quality assurance programs were required for reimbursement of services and for accreditation by the Joint Commission on Accreditation of Healthcare Organizations (JCAHO). In 1992 the revised JCAHO standards identified continuous quality improvement as a mechanism of health care. This differed from previous quality programs by purposely identifying the causes of problems or systems that needed improvement in health care. In 2002, JCAHO standard amendments further specified that patients have the right to age-specific and considerate health care that preserves dignity and respects cultural, psychosocial, and spiritual values (Smeltzer et al., 2007).

poor and less educated. Every client is a referral candidate. If the family believes that no help is necessary but the nurse believes otherwise, the nurse may suggest an evaluation visit by an agency once the client is at home. If a referral is made to a home care agency, it must proceed with a physician-approved treatment plan, which is a legal requirement. If physical therapy or other services are needed, the nurse or social worker arranges for these visits. The nurse is responsible for maintaining continuity of care between and among healthcare agencies. This includes providing and receiving reports on assigned clients and using appropriate documents to record and communicate client information such as medical records or transfer forms. Accurate transcription of primary healthcare provider orders is also necessary. The nursing process utilized in home care settings is the same as that practiced in any other healthcare setting.

Home care nursing is a specialty area that requires advanced knowledge and high-level assessment skills, critical thinking, and decision-making skills where other healthcare professionals are not available to validate conclusions and decisions about care. Because of this, the scope of medical-surgical nursing encompasses not only the acute care setting within the hospital but also the acute care setting as it expands into the community.

Collaborative practice should be a primary goal for nursing. This goal promotes shared participation, responsibility, and accountability in a healthcare environment that is striving to meet the complex healthcare needs of the public. Nurses with a significant practice that empowers others are those that value collaboration and develop the ability to associate effectively and positively with other healthcare personnel (Ponte et al., 2007). An influential professional nurse works well with others, is fair, and has perspectives that are sought out by other healthcare personnel. Leading and participating on interdisciplinary teams and partnering with others are essential to sound nursing practice.

Conclusion

This chapter has provided an introduction to the concepts necessary to understanding what a healthcare delivery system is and the role of the professional nurse. Various models of nursing care delivery were explored with methods of staff assignments. All nurses are managers of the care of a specific group of patients and collaborate with other healthcare providers in the delivery of client-centered and safety-focused care. Nurses must possess the skills of critical thinking, delegation, supervision, evaluation, motivation, and communication to work with other disciplines of care. This chapter has defined some of the concepts that are necessary for the entry-level nurse to maintain safe and competent entry-level nursing practice.

CLASSROOM ACTIVITY

You are planning the discharge of an 82-year-old man who has several chronic medical conditions. Divide the class into small groups of students to discuss how the case manager would intervene for the client and family, providing continuity of care from ICU to home. Have a spokesperson for each group briefly present their plan.

References

American Nurses Association. (2001). *Code of ethics for nurses with interpretive statements.* Washington, DC: Author.

Blais, K. K., Hayes, J. S., Kozier, B., & Erb, G. (2006). *Professional nursing practice concepts and perspectives* (5th ed.). Upper Saddle River, NJ: Pearson Prentice Hall.

Brown, F. (2005). *Nurse consultations: A person-centered approach.* Retrieved November 26, 2007, from http://findarticles.com/p/articles/mi_m0MDP/is_2_7/ai_n15679294

Caramanica, L., Cousino, J. A., & Petersen, S. (2003). Four elements of a successful quality program, alignment, collaboration, evidence-based practice, and excellence. *Nursing Administration Quarterly, 27*(4), 336–343.

LeMone, P., & Burke, K. (2007). *Medical-surgical nursing critical thinking in client care* (4th ed.). Upper Saddle River, NJ: Pearson Prentice Hall.

Lindeke, L. L., & Seickert, A. M. (2005). *Nurse-physician workplace collaboration.* Retrieved November 21, 2007, from http://www.nursingworld.org/ojin

Ponte, P. R., Glazer, G., Dann, E., McCollum, K., Gross, A., & Tyrrell, R. et al. (2007). The power of professional nursing practice: An essential element of patient and family centered care. *Online Journal of Issues in Nursing, 12.* Retrieved November 21, 2007, from http://nursingworld.org/ojin

Smeltzer, S. C., Bare, B. G., Hinkl, J. L., & Cheever, K. H. (2007). *Brunner & Suddarth's textbook of medical-surgical nursing* (11th ed.). Philadelphia: Lippincott Williams & Wilkins.

Sullivan, E. J., & Decker, P. J. (2005). *Effective leadership and management in nursing* (6th ed.). Upper Saddle River, NJ: Pearson Prentice Hall.

Wade, D. T., & Halligan, P. W. (2004). Do biomedical models of illness make for good healthcare systems [Electronic version]? *British Medical Journal, 329,* 1398–1401. Retrieved November 13, 2007, from http://www.bmj.com/cgi/content/full/329/7479/1398#BIBL

Wendt, A., Kenny, L., & Anderson, J. (2007). *National Council of State Boards of Nursing 2007 NCLEX-RN Detailed Test Plan.* Retrieved November 20, 2007, from https://www.ncsbn.org/2007_NCLEX_RN_Detailed_Test_Plan_Candidate.pdf

Clinical Judgment in Professional Nursing

Jill Rushing

LEARNING OBJECTIVES

After completing this chapter, the student should be able to:
1. Define critical thinking.
2. Describe important critical thinking skills.
3. Explore characteristics of critical thinking.
4. Describe the characteristics of a critical thinker.
5. Explain why critical thinking is important in nursing practice.
6. Explore the process involved in critical thinking.

Key Terms and Concepts

- Critical thinking
- Nursing process
- Mind mapping
- Journaling
- Group discussions
- Clinical judgment skills

The responsibilities of a professional registered nurse have increased significantly over the years. The impact of advanced technology, the increased acuity level and complexity of patients, combined with the accountability and responsibility nurses have in the delivery of safe and effective care, make it essential, more now than ever, for nurses to possess the ability to think critically. In nursing, critical thinking is the ability to think in a systematic and logical manner, solve problems, make decisions, and establish priorities

Critical thinking is the competent use of thinking skills and abilities to make sound clinical judgments and safe decision making.

in the clinical setting. Critical thinking is the competent use of thinking skills and abilities to make sound clinical judgments and safe decision making.

What Is Critical Thinking?

Although **critical thinking** is widely regarded as a component of clinical reasoning and decision making, it is difficult to define, and there is no single, simple definition that explains critical thinking. It is a complex and multifaceted process that includes logical, rhetorical, and humanistic skills that promote the ability to determine what one should believe and do. Critical thinking requires the nurse to actively process and evaluate information, to apply and validate existing knowledge, and to create new knowledge (Raingruber & Haffer, 2001). Critical thinking involves the ability to make your thinking more clear, precise, accurate, relevant, consistent, and fair. It is a disciplined, self-directed thinking that supports what we know and makes clear what we don't know (Wilkinson, 2007). Nurses should utilize critical thinking to determine which data are relevant and make inferences, solve problems, and make better decisions. Thus, critical thinking, problem solving, and decision making are processes that are interrelated, with creativity enhancing the result (Kozier, Erb, Berman, & Snyder, 2004). Other definitions of critical thinking are summarized in Box 9-1.

Nursing is not a superficial, meaningless activity. All acts in nursing are deeply significant and require the nurse's mind to be fully engaged (Heaslip, 2005).

Learning to be a nurse requires more than memorizing facts. It requires that you learn to think like a nurse, to think through and reason on a greater depth, and to draw a more sophisticated or deeper understanding of what you are doing in clinical practice so that you provide safe, effective patient care. Nursing is not a superficial, meaningless activity. All acts in nursing are deeply significant and require the nurse's mind to be fully engaged (Heaslip, 2005). The following illustration shows nursing is both thinking and doing: The physician has ordered an IV to be placed in a patient. How do you choose between a butterfly or an IV intracath? First, you have to consider why the line is being placed. You take into consideration whether it is a short-term, keep-open IV with limited medications; if so, then the butterfly IV is more comfortable and presents less of a threat of phlebitis. Doctors vary in their preferences as well, and this has to be considered. Also, the condition of the patient and his or her veins makes a great deal of difference. For example, with older patients special skill is required. The veins look as they are going to be easy to get because they look large, but they are very fragile. If you do not use a very slight tourniquet, the vein will pop open (Benner, 1984).

Characteristics of Critical Thinking

How do you know when critical thinking is taking place? Critical thinking has some of the following characteristics (Wilkinson, 2007):

BOX 9-1   DEFINITIONS OF CRITICAL THINKING

Critical thinking is:

"the art of thinking about your thinking while you're thinking so as to make your thinking more clear, precise, accurate, relevant, consistent, and fair" (Paul, 1988, pp. 2–3).

"the intellectually disciplined process of actively and skillfully conceptualizing, applying, analyzing, synthesizing, and/or evaluating information gathered from or generated by, observation, experience, reflection, reasoning, or communication, as a guide to belief and action" (Scriven & Paul, 2004).

"purposeful, informed, outcome focused thinking, that requires careful identification of specific problems and other physiological and psychological factors that affect the client's position on the health and wellness continuum" (Knapp, 2007).

"in nursing [it] is a logical, context-sensitive, reflective, reasoning process that guides the nurse in generating, implementing, and evaluating effective approaches to client care and professional concerns" (National League for Nursing, 2000).

"all or part of the process of questioning, analysis, synthesis, interpretation, inference, inductive and deductive reasoning, intuition, application, and creativity" (American Association of Colleges of Nursing [AACN], 1998, p.9).

"Critical thinking underlies independent and interdependent decision making" (AACN, 2008, p.36).

"taking in information, examine its important aspects by asking questions about it, and then put what you have learned to use through thinking processes such as problem solving, decision making, reasoning, opening your mind to new perspectives, and planning strategically" (Katz, Carter, Bishop, & Kravits, 2004).

- Critical thinking is rational and reasonable.
- Critical thinking involves conceptualization.
- Critical thinking requires reflection.
- Critical thinking involves cognitive (thinking) skills and attitudes (feelings).
- Critical thinking involves creative thinking.
- Critical thinking requires knowledge.

Critical thinking is rational and reasonable. Thinking is based on reasons rather than preferences, prejudice, or self-interest. It uses facts and observations to draw conclusions. For example, suppose during an election you decide to vote for the Democratic candidate because your family has always voted for Democrats. This decision is based on preference, prejudice, and, possibly, self-interest. By contrast, suppose you took time to reflect on what the candidate in the election said about the issues and based your choice on that. Even though you still might vote for the

CRITICAL THINKING QUESTION

You will be taking care of a patient in a nursing home for the first time. Your assignment will be caring for an older man who has heart disease. In addition, he has five other medical problems and takes 20 medications. While developing a plan of care for this patient, you can identify 8 to 10 nursing diagnoses. You have no previous experience with nursing homes, and most of what you have heard and read about them is negative. Will you find yourself dreading the clinical day and expecting a negative experience before you even begin?

Democrat, you would be thinking rationally, using facts and observations to draw your conclusions (Wilkinson, 2007).

Critical thinking involves conceptualization. Conceptual thinking is the ability to understand a situation by identifying patterns or connections, and focusing on key underlying issues and integrating them into a conceptual framework. It involves using professional training and experience, creativity, and inductive reasoning that lead to solutions or alternatives that may not be easily identified. Conceptual thinking involves a willingness to explore and having an openness to a new way of seeing things or "looking outside of the box." Consider, for example, a case in which a patient with heart failure is coughing up yellow sputum. If the nurse suspects that the patient is short of breath from infection, he or she will evaluate other indicators of infection. The nurse will check the patient for an elevated temperature and will assess the last white blood cell count in the patient's chart to see if it is elevated. The nurse will also consider factors that may place the patient at risk for infection, such as immobility, poor nutrition, or immune suppression (Craven & Hirnle, 2007).

Critical thinking uses reflection. Reflective thinking is deliberate thinking and careful consideration. It is the process of analyzing, making judgments, and drawing conclusions. Reflective thinking involves creating an understanding through one's experiences and knowledge and exploring potential alternatives—assessing what you know, what you need to know, and how to bridge that gap. Processes of reflective thinking involve the following:

- Determine what information is needed (what you need to know) for understanding the issue.
- Examine what you have already experienced about an issue.
- Gather the available information.
- Synthesize the information and opinions.
- Consider the synthesis from different perspectives and frames of reference.
- Create some meaning from the relevant information and opinions.

Reflective thinking is important during complex problem-solving situations because it provides an opportunity to step back and think about how to actually solve problems and how problem-solving strategies are used for achieving set goals.

Critical thinking involves cognitive (thinking) skills and attitudes (feelings). Critical thinking involves having thinking skills as well as the motivation to use them. It involves the willingness to utilize complex thought processes compared to easily understood ones. Critical thinkers do not oversimplify. Critical thinking is about being willing and able to think.

Critical thinking involves creative thinking. Creativity is the ability to produce something new through imaginative skill. Creativity is part of the thinking process. When you brainstorm potential problem solutions or possible decisions, you are using creativity. Creative and critical thinkers combine ideas and information in ways that form new solutions or innovative ideas (Katz, Carter, Bishop, & Kravits, 2004). A creative thinker is an open-minded thinker. Nurses may utilize creative thinking when encountering a patient situation in which traditional methods are not effective. For example, a pediatric nurse is caring for 9-year-old Pauline, who has ineffective respirations following abdominal surgery. The physician has ordered incentive spirometry breathing treatments, but Pauline is frightened by the equipment and she quickly tires during the treatments. The nurse offers Pauline a bottle of soap bubbles and a blowing wand. The nurse knows that the respiratory effort in blowing bubbles will promote alveolar expansion and suggests that Pauline blow bubbles between incentive spirometry treatments (Wilkinson, 2007).

Critical thinking requires knowledge. In most academic disciplines, the educational system uses an expert to deliver a body of knowledge to the unpracticed novice, who will later be expected to go out and apply the knowledge and rules learned in school to various work situations. In nursing, a specific educational knowledge base is required before applying that knowledge in patient care. It is important to know that the process is being applied correctly. In essence, to become a nurse you must learn the knowledge to think like a nurse. On the "flip side" of this, as the level of experience of the nurse increases, so will the scientific knowledge base that the nurse applies. For example, you are caring for a patient with heart failure. After obtaining the vital signs, what heart rate would prevent you from performing ambulation on this patient? If you did not have knowledge regarding heart failure or did not know that normal heart rate was 60–100 beats per minute, you could not make the good decision that ambulation should be postponed if the heart rate was above 100 beats per minute for this patient.

What Are the Characteristics of a Critical Thinker?

Nurses are required to think critically in all settings. Nurses' ability to think critically is one of their most important skills, and a commitment to think critically will benefit the nurse's ability to care for patients most effectively. A critical thinker has many characteristics, including the following:

- Critical thinkers are flexible—they can tolerate ambiguity and uncertainty.
- Critical thinkers base judgments on facts and reasoning, not personal feelings. They identify inherent biases and assumptions. Critical thinkers separate facts from opinions.
- Critical thinkers don't oversimplify.
- Critical thinkers examine available evidence before drawing conclusions.
- Critical thinkers think for themselves, and do not simply go along with the crowd.

- Critical thinkers remain open to the need for adjustment and adaptation throughout the inquiry stages.
- Critical thinkers accept change.
- Critical thinkers empathize; they appreciate and try to understand others' thoughts, feelings, and behaviors.
- Critical thinkers welcome different views and value examining issues from every angle.
- Critical thinkers know that it is important to explore and understand positions with which they disagree.
- Critical thinkers discover and apply meaning to what they see, hear, and read.

Approaches to Developing Critical Thinking Skills

As students develop within their nursing role, they learn and build critical thinking skills and apply them to real healthcare situations. Critical thinking requires conscious, deliberate effort (Craven & Hirnle, 2007). Critical thinking does not just come naturally, and people tend to believe what is easy to believe or what those around them believe (Wilkinson, 2007). With effort and practice, everyone can achieve some level of critical thinking to become an effective problem solver and decision maker (Kozier et al., 2004). Following are examples that can be used as approaches to developing critical thinking skills.

The Nursing Process

The nursing process is a systematic problem-solving approach toward giving nursing care that allows the nurse to be accountable by using critical thinking before taking actions.

The American Nurses Association (ANA) Standards have set forth the framework necessary for critical thinking in the application of the **nursing process**. The nursing process is the tool by which all nurses can become equally proficient at critical thinking. The nursing process contains the following criteria: (1) assessment, (2) diagnosis, (3) planning, (4) implementation, and (5) evaluation. It is in the application of each of these components that the nurse may become proficient at critical thinking. Nurses use critical thinking in each stage of the nursing process. This approach to critical thinking entails purposeful, informed, outcome-focused thinking, which requires identification of nursing and healthcare needs of clients (Knapp, 2007). The nursing process is a systematic problem-solving approach toward giving nursing care that allows the nurse to be accountable by using critical thinking before taking actions.

Assessment

The nursing assessment answers the questions: "What is happening?" or "What could happen?" It involves systematically collecting, organizing, and analyzing information about the client. Once data or information has been collected and it is determined that the data are accurate and complete, the nurse performs data analysis or data interpretation. What are the client's actual and/or potential problems? A problem list is then developed based on the data, and the nurse prioritizes the client's problems. The nurse performs an ongoing assessment throughout the implementation of the nursing process.

Diagnosis

The nurse analyzes and derives meaning from the assessment information and selects a diagnosis. Diagnosis is the identification of a problem. It is a statement that describes a specific response to an actual or potential health problem. The North American Nursing Diagnosis Association (NANDA) guides the classification of nursing diagnoses. A nursing diagnosis provides the foundation for selection of nursing interventions to achieve outcomes for which the nurse is responsible (NANDA, 2005). For example, a nursing diagnosis for a selected patient might be "decreased cardiac output related to inability of the heart to pump effectively, and occlusion and constriction of vessels impairing blood flow."

Planning

During planning, the nurse develops a plan to provide consistent, continuous care that will meet the client's unique needs. Planning includes developing expected outcomes and working with the client to identify goals and to determine appropriate nursing actions and interventions that will reduce the identified problem. The nurse uses critical thinking to develop goals and nursing interventions for problems that require an individualized approach. Nurses use judgment to determine which interventions have a probability of achieving desired outcomes (Wilkinson, 1996). To continue with the example from above, expected outcomes might include the following:

1. Patient will be free of chest pain during my shift.
2. Patient will maintain O_2 sat of 90% during my shift.
3. Vital signs will remain stable: $T < 99.0°F$, $HR > 60 < 110$ beats/min, $R > 12 < 24$ breaths/min, and $SBP > 90$ mm Hg while under my care.
4. Patient will have no further weight gain and have a decrease in edema during my shift.

Implementation

Implementation is carrying out the plan of care and depends upon the first three steps of the nursing process. These steps provide the basis for nursing actions performed during the implementation phase of the nursing process. The nurse carries out nursing interventions individualized to the patient, reassesses the client, and validates that the plan of care is accurate and successful. In this stage the nurse applies knowledge and principles from nursing and from related courses to each patient care situation. The ability to apply, not just memorize, principles is a component of critical thinking (Wilkinson, 2007). For the patient with decreased cardiac output the nurse could implement some of the following individualized interventions:

- Assess LOC—confusion, anxiety.
- Provide reassurance to the patient.
- Monitor vital signs every 4 hours.
- Assess heart rate and rhythm; monitor telemetry or ECG.
- Monitor for jugular vein distension.
- Monitor for chest pain.
- Monitor peripheral pulses; assess capillary refill.
- Auscultate lung sounds; monitor respiratory rate and rhythm; monitor oxygen saturation; assess for cough and sputum.
- Look at skin color and temperature.
- Monitor for fatigue and activity tolerance.
- Assess intake and output, daily weight, and edema in dependent areas.
- Assess abdomen for distension or bloating, ascites, and bowel function.
- Monitor lab and X-rays: CBC, PT/PTT, electrolytes, cardiac enzymes, arterial blood gases, and chest X-ray.
- Place patient with head of bed elevated while in bed to improve gas exchange.
- Administer oxygen as ordered to improve gas exchange.
- Administer morphine sulfate as prescribed to relieve chest pain, provide sedation and vasodilation, and monitor for respiratory depression and hypotension after administration.
- Administer diuretics as prescribed to reduce preload, enhance renal excretion of sodium and water, reduce circulating blood volume, and reduce pulmonary congestion; closely monitor potassium level, which may decrease as a result of diuretic therapy.
- Provide teaching: Identify precipitating risk factors of heart failure and prescribed medication regimen; notify physician if unable to take medications because of illness; avoid large amounts of caffeine; cardiac diet instruction; signs of exacerbation; monitor fluids; balance periods of activity and rest; avoid isometric activities that increase pressure in the heart.

Evaluation

During evaluation, the nurse compares the patient's current status to the patient goals. Were the goals achieved? The nurse analyzes outcomes to determine if the interventions worked, and if not, why? The information provided during evaluation may be used to begin another plan of care sufficient to meet patient needs. Continuing with the previous example, the evaluation might include:

- Patient denies chest pain on my shift. Patient rates pain "0" on pain scale.
- Patient's O_2 saturation dropped to 85% when oxygen at 3L nasal cannula was removed. With oxygen on, patient's O_2 saturation remained 92%.

- Vital signs were: T, 101.0°F; HR, 100–110 beats/min; R, 32 breaths/min and labored; BP, 90/50 mm Hg.
- Patient's weight was 241 lbs with 2+ edema in lower extremities.

Mind Maps

Mind mapping is the technique of arranging ideas and their interconnections visually and is a popular brainstorming technique. It is used to generate, visualize, structure, and classify ideas and is used as an aid in organization, problem solving, and decision making. A mind map is a visual learning tool that can help identify key elements in a situation and that can help you to understand their relationship with one another. A mind map is a visual record of your thoughts. They graphically depict associated thoughts and ideas, they help discover what might not have been clear previously, and they help generate solutions to problems (Rainburger & Haffer, 2001).

To begin a mind map, start in the center of the page with the main idea or central theme, and work outward in all directions, producing a growing organized structure composed of key words or pictures. Place words or pictures around the main idea to illustrate how they relate to each other and the central theme. Pictures, words, or a combination of both can be used to create a mind map. Key features of mind mapping include organization, key words, association, clustering, visual memory (print key words, use color, symbols, icons, arrows, pictures, or illustrations), outstandingness (every mind map needs a central theme), and conscious involvement (Russell, n.d.).

Mind maps are useful for summarizing information, consolidating information from different sources, thinking through complex problems, and presenting information in a format that shows an overall structure of your subject. Figure 9-1 illustrates mind mapping techniques used by students with a patient case.

Journaling

Keeping a journal of clinical experiences that were meaningful or troubling to you is a recommended way to help enhance and develop reasoning skills. Think about and record experiences that bother you, and consider what you could and would do differently in the future. This is a form of reflection and allows you to view your own thinking, reasoning, and actions. It helps create and clarify meaning and new understandings of a particular experience. When you encounter a similar situation, you should be able to recall what you did or would do differently as well as the reasoning behind your actions (Raingruber & Haffer, 2007). Some suggestions you should try to address when **journaling** your nursing experience include the following:

- What happened? What are the facts?
- What was my role in the event?
- What feelings and senses surrounded the event?
- What did I do?

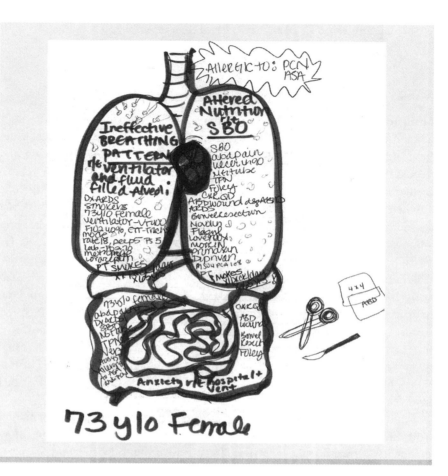

Figure 9–1
Student Example of Mind Mapping a Patient Case

- How and what did I feel about what I did? Why?
- What was the setting?
- What were the important elements of the event?
- What preceded the event, and what followed it?
- What should I be aware of if the event recurs?

It is important that you write in your journal as soon as possible after an event to capture the essence of what happened in the clinical experience. The following is an example of a journal excerpt that illustrates reflection upon events and the feelings elicited by those events over the course of many patient care encounters during the career of a nurse.

I have learned, not so easily, that my job is not just about saving a life, trying to keep people well, or helping them get well when they are ill, but importantly, it also entails providing that same dedicated care to them as they take their last breaths in life. It is my job, my duty, and I have learned, my privilege. As I care for a dying patient, listening to the rise and fall of methodical machines imitating life, I hope I never get calloused to the point that I say, "I do this every day. It is just another patient." I want to appreciate that every individual's life has been remarkable in some way— that they are remarkable in some way. I want to make my patient's journey through this last chapter in their life a little easier, provide comfort, recognize their fears, hold their hand, and always realize this is not another patient, but a person.

> **CRITICAL THINKING QUESTION**
>
> Think about a clinical experience that was troubling to you. Reflect on what bothered you about the experience. What could you have done differently? What were the reasons behind your actions? Try to create and clarify meaning or a new understanding of the particular situation.

Group Discussions

Another way to enhance critical thinking skills is by using **group discussions** to explore alternatives and arrive at conclusions. Group discussions between nursing students and teachers can take place in the classroom or following clinical experiences. During discussions, students are encouraged to formulate alternatives to clinical or ethical decisions. Teacher and learner group discussions over clinical and ethical scenarios should encourage questions, analysis, and reflection. Group discussions can assist nursing students in connecting clinical events or decisions with information obtained in the classroom. This form of cooperative learning occurs when groups work together to maximize their own and each other's learning. For example, following a clinical experience, students and teacher discuss a certain clinical experience that a student encountered. Together they discuss different scenarios of "What if?," "What else?," and "What then?" to encourage the formulation of alternatives or clinical decisions.

Why Is Critical Thinking Important in Nursing Practice?

Critical thinking is essential to providing safe, competent, and skillful nursing care. At times, the decisions that nurses must make about patient care forces them to think and act when there are not always clear answers or standard procedures. This turns decision making into a complex process. Nurses use critical thinking skills in the following various ways (Kozier et al., 2004):

- Nurses use knowledge from other subjects and fields. Nurses must draw meaningful information from other subject areas in order to make connections or understand the meaning of patient data and to plan effective nursing interventions. Nursing students take courses in biologic and social sciences such as physiology, chemistry, nutrition, and psychology to acquire a strong foundation on which to build nursing knowledge and skill.
- Nurses deal with change in stressful environments. Nurses work in rapidly changing environments where technology, medications, treatments, and a

patient's condition change constantly. Routine actions may not be adequate to deal with certain situations. For example, familiar routine medication administration does not help the nurse deal with a patient who may be frightened of injections or refuses a medication. During unexpected situations, critical thinking enables the nurse to respond quickly and adapt interventions to meet a patient's specific needs.

- Nurses must make important decisions. Nurses make vital decisions that often determine the well-being, and even survival, of patients. Nurses use critical thinking to collect and interpret information needed to make decisions. For example, the nurse must use good judgment to decide which observations need to be reported to the physician immediately.

New realities of health care require nurses to master complex information, to coordinate a variety of care experiences, to use advanced technology for healthcare delivery and evaluation of patient outcomes, as well as assist patients with managing and navigating an increasingly complex system of care. Some of the trends that have added to the complexities of the healthcare environment, and nursing specifically, include increases in longevity; markedly shortened hospital stays, which are moving patients out of the hospital "quicker and sicker"; scientific advances; major advances in technology; an increase in population; increased diversity in the US population; and an increased incidence of chronic diseases and infectious diseases (American Association of Colleges of Nursing, 1998).

To prepare nursing students for the multifaceted role of professional nurse, the learning process involves components that will provide a solid foundation for developing **clinical judgment skills**. One of these components or core competencies is critical thinking. Course work or clinical experience should provide the nursing student and graduate with knowledge and skills to do the following (American Association of Colleges of Nursing, 1998):

- Use appropriate nursing theories and models and appropriate ethical frameworks in practice.
- Use research-based knowledge from nursing and the sciences as the basis for practice.
- Use sound clinical judgment and decision-making skills.
- Engage in processes such as self-reflection and shared educational dialogue about professional practice.
- Evaluate nursing care outcomes through acquiring data and the questioning of inconsistencies, allowing for the revision of actions and goals.
- Engage in creative thinking and problem solving.

> ## CRITICAL THINKING QUESTIONS
>
> Beginning nursing students often tend to focus primarily on their routines, such as to get their list of tasks done, such as assessments, ordered treatments, daily care, and charting. What if an unexpected situation occurred during the day? Do you think you would be able to reason, plan, and take appropriate action—think critically? Look at the following situation (starting at the bottom of this page) and think about how you would react.

You are working in an acute care clinical situation. After receiving report, you have started your morning routines. Everything is going as planned, and you are about to start preparing your medications. The wife of one of your patients reports that the oxygen is burning his nose and wants you to get an oxygen humidifier. All of the sudden, the daughter of your other patient, Mr. Peary, rushes toward you and informs you that her father is spitting up blood. He looked fine when you observed him a few minutes ago. You walk rapidly toward the patient's room, thinking, "What am I going to do when I get there? I have to get the oxygen humidifier for room 202. His nose was burning, and his wife was waiting for me. What could be happening with Mr. Peary?"

You enter the room, and the first thing you think is: "He's lying flat," and you think to yourself, "I need to elevate his head. That is what I did on the respiratory unit where I recently worked." The daughter tells you that Mr. Peary coughed up some blood in the emesis basin. There is a small amount of bright red blood in it. You do not know what to do next. An RN stops by the room and tells you that the wife of the patient in room 202 is asking about the burning in her husband's nose again. Your mind doesn't seem to be able to think about anything. Do you feel scattered and things seem out of control at this point? Do you feel a little over-whelmed and can't think what to do next? The RN says she will take over with Mr. Peary while you follow up with the patient in room 202. Later, you recall the situation and can't believe you didn't think to take Mr. Peary's blood pressure, count respirations, ask about pain, or listen to his lungs or anything else. All you did was just raise his head. You wonder why you missed so many things (Raingruber & Haffer, 2001).

- What do you think was going on in the situation that influenced what was happening and caused you to lose your ability to think and plan what to do next?
- What would you do differently in this situation after having a chance to reflect on it? Prioritize the order in which you would have done things.
- If this had happened to you and no one helped you through it, what would you have done to mobilize yourself to think about what to do?

Conclusion

In nursing, critical thinking is the ability to think in a systematic and logical manner, solve problems, make decisions, and establish priorities in the clinical setting. Nurses need to develop critical thinking skills in order to make sound clinical judgments and to provide safe, competent patient care. Nursing requires constant decision making. What should I do first? What is the most important thing to do at this time? Prioritizing nursing actions involves recalling important nursing information as well as using complex problem-solving skills to make decisions in providing safe and effective patient care. As a nurse, you will constantly have to demonstrate good judgment in analyzing facts and situations and applying nursing knowledge.

CLASSROOM ACTIVITY 1

Critical thinking gives you the power to make sense of something by deliberately choosing how to respond to events that you encounter. You take in information, examine and ask questions about it, look at new perspectives, and identify a plan. You use problem-solving and decision-making strategies.

- Choose a decision that you need to make soon, and write it down.
- What goal or desired outcomes do you seek from this decision? Prioritize goals or desired outcomes, and write them down.
- Identify who and what will be affected by your decision, and indicate how your decision will affect them.
- Identify any available options you might have.
- Taking into account and evaluating your information, identify a plan or decide what you are going to do.
- After you have made your decision, evaluate the result.

CLASSROOM ACTIVITY 2

You are receiving morning reports on the following patients from the night-shift nurse. After receiving the following report, which patient would you choose to see first? As you make your decision, think about your thought processes and how you made your decision.

1. A woman who is scheduled to have a biopsy on a breast lump this morning, and who is scared and crying
2. An 85-year-old man who was admitted during the night because of increased confusion who remains disoriented this morning
3. A woman who had lung surgery the previous day, and who has two chest tubes in place with minimal drainage
4. A man who is scheduled to have a colon resection in two hours and is complaining of chills

Answer: You should have answered the client who is scheduled for surgery and is exhibiting symptoms of infection. This patient needs to be assessed immediately for infection, and the doctor notified. If an infection is present, the surgery needs to be postponed. The other patients are stable, and their needs do not have to be addressed immediately.

CASE STUDY   JIM FULLER

Jim Fuller is a 40-year-old male patient. He is currently in the recovery room following an inguinal hernia repair under general anesthesia. His vital signs are: T, 99.0°F; BP, 120/80 mm Hg; HR, 80 beats/min; R, 18 breaths per minute.

Two hours postoperative, Mr. Fuller begins to complain of abdominal pain. Vital signs at this time are: T, 99.5°F; BP, 90/60 mm Hg; HR, 122 beats/min; R, 24 breaths/min.

CASE STUDY QUESTIONS

- Are Mr. Fuller's vital signs within normal limits? List normal adult ranges.
- What factors might affect body temperature?
- List sites that a nurse might take a patient's pulse. What sites are most commonly used?
- What factors might influence respiratory rate?

CASE STUDY QUESTIONS

- What could Mr. Fuller's vital signs indicate?
- What nursing interventions are indicated? What should the nurse assess in Mr. Fuller at this time?
- What clinical signs associated with an elevated temperature might the nurse assess?
- If Mr. Fuller's fever persists and increases, what might the nurse suspect is happening, and what might be done?

References

American Association of Colleges of Nursing. (1998). *The essentials of baccalaureate education for professional nursing practice.* Washington, DC: Author.

American Association of Colleges of Nursing. (2008). *The essentials of baccalaureate education for professional nursing practice.* Washington, DC: Author.

Benner, P. (1984). *From novice to expert.* Menlo Park, CA: Addison-Wesley Publishing.

Craven, R. F., & Hirnle, C. J. (2007). *Fundamentals of nursing: Human health and function* (5th ed.). Philadelphia: Lippincott Williams & Wilkins.

Heaslip, P. (2005). *Critical thinking: To think like a nurse.* Retrieved July 21, 2005, from http://www.cariboo.bc.ca/nursing/faculty/heaslip/nrsct.htm

Katz, J., Carter, C., Bishop, J., & Kravits, S. L. (2004). *Keys to nursing success* (2nd ed.). Upper Saddle River, NJ: Pearson Education.

Knapp, R. (2007). *Nursing education—The importance of critical thinking.* Retrieved November 24, 2007, from http://www.articlecity.com/articles/education/article_1327.shtml

Kozier, B., Erb, G., Berman, A., & Snyder, S. (2004). *Fundamentals of nursing: Concepts, process, and practice* (7th ed.). Upper Saddle River, NJ: Pearson Education.

National League for Nursing. (2000). *Critical thinking in clinical nursing practice RN/ Examination.* Retrieved November 18, 2007, from http://www.nln.org/testproducts/pdf/ Ctinfobulletin.pdf

North American Nursing Diagnosis Association. (2005). *NANDA nursing diagnosis: Definitions and classification 2005–2006.* Philadelphia: Author.

Paul, R. W. (1988). *What then, is critical thinking?* Eighth Annual and Sixth International Conference on Critical Thinking and Educational Reform. Rohnert Park, CA: Center for Critical Thinking and Moral Critique, Sonoma State University.

Raingruber, B., & Haffer, A. (2001). *Using your head to land on your feet: A beginning nurse's guide to critical thinking.* Philadelphia: F. A. Davis

Russell, P. (n.d.) *How to mind map.* Retrieved November 27, 2007, from http://www.peterrussell.com/MindMaps/HowTo.php

Scriven, M., & Paul, R. (2004). *Defining critical thinking.* Retrieved November 13, 2007, from http://www.criticalthinking.org/page.cfm?PageID=410&CategoryID=51

Wilkinson, J. (2007). *Nursing process and critical thinking* (4th ed.). Upper Saddle River, NJ: Pearson Education.

Wilkinson, J. M. (1996). *Nursing process: A critical thinking approach* (2nd ed.). Menlo Park, CA: Addison-Wesley.

chapter 10

Evidence-Based Professional Nursing Practice

Kathleen Masters

LEARNING OBJECTIVES

After completing this chapter, the student should be able to:
1. Describe the importance of evidence-based nursing care.
2. Identify barriers to the implementation of evidence-based nursing practice.
3. Identify strategies for the implementation of evidence-based nursing practice.
4. Describe how and where to search for evidence.
5. Identify methods to evaluate the evidence.
6. Discuss approaches to integrating evidence into practice.
7. Identify models of evidence-based nursing practice.

Key Terms and Concepts

- Evidence-based practice
- Research utilization
- Quality improvement
- PICO
- Cochrane Library
- National Guideline Clearinghouse
- Clinical practice guideline
- AGREE instrument
- Academic Center for Evidence-Based Nursing (ACE) Star Model of Knowledge Transformation
- Iowa Model of Evidence-Based Practice

Evidence-Based Practice: What Is It?

Evidence-based practice—it is more than the most recent buzzword in nursing. **Evidence-based practice** allows nurses to provide high-quality patient care based upon research evidence and knowledge rather than tradition, myths, hunches, advice from peers, outdated textbooks, or even what the nurse learned in school 5, 10, or 15 years ago. Evidence-based practice provides a strategy to ensure that nursing care reflects the most up-to-date knowledge

Nursing practice that is based upon evidence is now the accepted standard for practice.

available. Nursing practice that is based upon evidence is now the accepted standard for practice.

Most nurses want to provide care based upon the most current knowledge for their patients, but for many nurses trying to integrate evidence-based practice into patient care in the clinical environment it raises many questions:

- What exactly is evidence-based practice, and how is it relevant to my practice?
- Is evidence-based practice different from research utilization?
- Is evidence-based practice different from quality improvement?

Although they may be widely used and related processes, evidence-based practice is not research utilization or quality improvement.

- **Research utilization** involves critical analysis and evaluation of research findings and then determining how these findings fit into clinical practice. In research utilization, the research findings are the only source of evidence. In evidence-based practice, research is only one of the sources of evidence (Levin, 2006a).
- **Quality improvement** focuses on systems, processes, satisfaction, and cost outcomes, usually within a specific organization. These projects may contribute to understanding best practices for the processes of care in which nurses are involved, but typically quality improvement efforts are not designed to develop nursing practice standards or nursing science.

Evidence-based practice assumes that evidence is used in the context of patient preferences, the clinical situation, and the expertise of the clinician.

Evidence-based practice is a framework for clinical practice that incorporates "the conscientious, explicit, and judicious use of the current best evidence in making decisions about the care of individual patients" (Beyea & Slattery, 2006). Put another way, evidence-based practice is "the integration of best research evidence with clinical expertise and patient values" (Sackett, Straus, Richardson, Rosenberg, & Haynes, 2000). In other words, evidence-based practice assumes that evidence is used in the context of patient preferences, the clinical situation, and the expertise of the clinician.

Evidence-based practice is relevant to nursing practice because it does the following:

- Helps resolve problems in the clinical setting
- Results in better patient outcomes
- Contributes to the science of nursing through the introduction of innovation to practice
- Keeps practice current and relevant by helping nurses deliver care based upon current best research
- Decreases variations in nursing care and increases confidence in decision making

- Supports JCAHO readiness as policies and procedures are current and include the latest research
- Essential for high-quality patient care and achievement of magnet status (Beyea & Slattery, 2006; Spector, 2007)

Barriers to Evidence-Based Practice

Because evidence-based practice is now the standard for professional nursing practice one would think that practice based upon evidence is commonplace. However, this is not the case. There are many barriers to evidence-based practice cited by practicing nurses. Common barriers to implementing evidence-based practice include:

- Lack of value for research in practice
- Difficulty in changing practice
- Lack of administrative support
- Lack of knowledgeable mentors
- Insufficient time
- Lack of education about the research process
- Lack of awareness about research or evidence-based practice
- Research reports and articles not readily available
- Difficulty accessing research reports and articles
- No time on the job to read research
- Complexity of research reports
- Lack of knowledge about evidence-based practice
- Lack of knowledge about the critique of articles
- Feeling overwhelmed by the process
- Lack of sense of control over practice
- Lack of confidence to implement change
- Lack of leadership, motivation, vision, strategy, or direction among managers (Beyea & Slattery, 2006; Spector, 2007)

Strategies to Promote Evidence-Based Practice

Despite barriers, nurses are making a difference in patient outcomes through the use of evidence-based practice. Strategies that can be useful in the promotion of evidence into practice generally fall into two categories: strategies for individual nurses and organizational strategies.

Strategies for individual nurses include the following:

- Educate yourself about evidence-based practice through avenues such as online sites, books, articles, and conferences.

- Conduct face-to-face or online journal clubs that can be used to educate yourself about critiquing articles, to share new research reports and guidelines with peers, and provide support to other nurses.
- Share your results through posters, newsletters, unit meetings, or a published article to support a culture of evidence-based nursing practice within the organization and the profession.
- Adopt a reflective and inquiring approach to practice by continuously asking yourself and others within your organization questions such as, "What is the evidence for this intervention?" or "How do my patients respond to this intervention?" (Beyea & Slattery, 2006)

Strategies for organizations include:

- Developing a center for evidence-based practice
- Administrative support for evidence-based practice by providing the time and the funds for necessary resources
- Access to electronic resources in the workplace
- Enhancement of job descriptions to include criteria related to evidence-based practice
- Offering incentives such as a paid registration to a conference for the best clinical question in a unit-wide or facility-wide contest
- Providing opportunities for nurses to collaborate with nurse researchers or faculty with nursing research expertise

CRITICAL THINKING QUESTION
How is new evidence disseminated to the bedside nurse in the organization in which you practice as a nursing student? How does the organization promote evidence-based practice? Do the nurses in the organization use current evidence in practice?

Whichever strategies are incorporated, it is important to note that passive dissemination of results within an organization is ineffective in changing practice. Multifaceted interventions are much more likely to be effective in facilitating evidence-based practice within an organization.

Searching for Evidence

Asking the Question

It is important that nurses learn to ask questions in a format that facilitates searching for evidence. It has been suggested that all nurses should learn how to use the **PICO** format to ask clinical questions. PICO is simply an acronym that assists in the formatting of clinical questions. Using this format helps the nurse to ask pertinent clinical questions, focus on asking the right questions, and choose relevant guidelines.

P = Patient, Population, or Problem
- How would I describe a group of patients similar to mine?
- What group do I want information on?

I = Intervention or Exposure or Topic of Interest
- Which main intervention am I considering?
- What event do I want to study the effect of?

C = Comparison or Alternate Intervention (if appropriate)
- What is the main alternative to compare with the intervention?
- Compared to what? Better or worse than no intervention at all, or than another intervention?

O = Outcome
- What can I hope to accomplish, measure, improve, or affect?
- What is the effect of the intervention? (Levin & Feldman, 2006)

After determining the patient, intervention, comparison, and outcome of interest, the nurse then combines these four elements into a single question in combinations such as the examples below:

- In (patient or population), what is the effect of (intervention or exposure) on (outcome) compared with (comparison)? (Levin, 2006b).
- For (patient or population), does the introduction of (intervention or exposure) reduce the risk of (outcome) compared with (comparison intervention)? (Levin, 2006b).

Resources to learn more about asking PICO questions are available at:

- www.urmc.rochester.edu/hslt/miner/resources/evidence_based/index.cfm
- ebling.library.wisc.edu/classes_tutorials/coursepages/pharm675/PICO.pdf
- www.studentbmj.com/back_issues/0902/education/313.html

Electronic Indexes

Electronic indexes provide options for narrowing or broadening a topic to identify relevant literature. Most electronic indexes provide citation information and will indicate if the selected articles are available locally in print form or if the items are available in an electronic format. Two of the most common electronic indexes used in health care are the Cumulative Index for Nursing and Allied Health (CINAHL), available at www.cinahl.com; Medline, available at www.nlm.hih.gov; or PubMed, a web-based format of Medline available at www.pubmed.gov.

Electronic Resources

There are many other helpful Internet resources available that will assist the nurse in uncovering the most current evidence for practice. Some of the most commonly used include:

- National Library of Medicine: www.nlm.nih.gov
- **Cochrane Library**: www.cochrane.org/reviews/clibintro.htm

- **National Guideline Clearinghouse**: www.ngc.gov
- Joanna Briggs Institute: www.joannabriggs.edu.au
- Netting the Evidence: www.shef.ac.uk/scharr/ir/netting
- Centre for Evidence-Based Medicine University Health Network: www.library.utoronto.ca/medicine/ebm
- Centre for Health Evidence: www.cche.net
- Registered Nurses Association of Ontario: www.rnao.org/bestpractices/about/bestPractice_overview.asp
- Other Web resources:
  - University of Minnesota: evidence.ahc.umn.edu/ebn.htm
  - Centre for Evidence-Based Nursing: www.york.ac.uk/healthsciences/centres/evidence/cebn.htm
  - McGill University Health Centre's Research and Clinical Resources for Evidence Based Nursing: www.muhc-ebn.mcgill.ca
  - University of North Carolina Health Science Library: www.hsl.unc.edu/Services/Tutorials/EBN/index.htm
  - Academic Center for Evidence-Based Nursing: www.acestar.uthscsa.edu

The **Cochrane Library** is a collection of databases that contain high-quality, independent evidence to inform healthcare decision making. Cochrane reviews represent the highest level of evidence on which to base clinical treatment decisions. In addition to the Cochrane systematic reviews, the Cochrane Library also offers other sources of information, including the Cochrane Database of Systematic Reviews, Database of Abstracts of Reviews of Effects, Cochrane Controlled Trials Register, Cochrane Methodology Register, NHS Economic Evaluation Database, Health Technology Assessment Database, and the Cochrane Database of Methodology Reviews (CDMR).

The **National Guideline Clearinghouse** includes structured summaries containing information about each guideline, including comparisons of guidelines covering similar topics that show areas of similarity and differences; full text or links to full text; ordering details for full guidelines; annotated bibliographies on guideline development, evaluation, implementation, and structure; weekly e-mail updates; and guideline archives.

Evaluating the Evidence

Regardless of the source, we always need to evaluate the evidence.

Regardless of the source, we always need to evaluate the evidence. Begin by asking such questions as:

- What is the source of the information?
- When was it developed?
- How was it developed?

- Does it fit the current clinical environment?
- Does it fit the current situation?

Best evidence for practice includes empirical evidence from randomized controlled trials; evidence from descriptive and qualitative research; as well as use of information from case reports, scientific principles, and expert opinion. When insufficient research is available, healthcare decision making is derived principally from nonresearch evidence sources such as expert opinion and scientific principles (Titler, 2008).

Several classification systems exist to evaluate the level or strength of the evidence. The Agency for Healthcare Research and Quality (AHRQ) serves as the recognized authority regarding the assessment of clinical research in the United States. The AHRQ levels of evidence include classifications 1–5 listed below (Melnyk & Fineout-Overholt, 2005). Other sources (Di Cesenso, Guyatt, & Ciliska, 2005) also include additional classifications or levels of evidence (6–7).

- 1A Meta-analysis or systematic reviews of multiple well-designed controlled studies
- 1 Well-designed randomized controlled trials
- 2 Well-designed nonrandomized controlled trials (quasi-experimental)
- 3 Observational studies with controls (retrospective, interrupted time, case-control, cohort studies with controls)
- 4 Observational studies without controls (cohort studies without controls and case series)
- 5 Systematic review of descriptive, qualitative, or physiologic studies
- 6 Single descriptive, qualitative, or physiologic study
- 7 Opinions of authorities, expert committees

Using this classification system, the strongest evidence comes from the first level, representing systematic reviews that integrate findings from multiple well-designed controlled studies. The weakest evidence is represented by the seventh level and is based upon opinion (Polit & Beck, 2008).

In addition, grading the strength of a body of evidence should incorporate three domains that include quality, quantity, and consistency. Quality has to do with the extent to which a study minimizes bias in the design, implementation, and analysis. Quantity refers to the number of studies that have evaluated the research question, as well as the sample size across the studies and the strength of the findings. The category of consistency refers to both the similarity and differences of study designs that investigate the same research question and report similar findings (Agency for Healthcare Research and Quality [AHRQ], 2002; LoBiondo-Wood, Haber, & Krainovich-Miller, 2006).

Using the Evidence

Clinical Practice Guidelines

Clinical practice guidelines are developed to guide clinical practice and represent an effort to put a large body of evidence into a manageable form. Clinical practice guidelines are usually based upon systematic reviews and give specific recommendations for clinicians. Guidelines usually attempt to address all the issues relevant to a clinical decision, including risks and benefits.

There is an ongoing collaboration that focuses on improving the quality and effectiveness of clinical practice guidelines. The group has established a framework for determining the quality of guidelines for diagnoses, health promotion, treatments, or clinical interventions. The instrument can be used with new, existing, or updated guidelines and is known as the **Appraisal of Guidelines for Research and Evaluation (AGREE) instrument**. The instrument is available at www.agreecollaboration.org. The AGREE instrument is composed of six categories comprising the 23 items listed below:

- Scope and purpose
  - Overall objectives of the guideline are specifically described.
  - Clinical questions covered by the guideline are specifically described.
  - Patients to whom the guideline is meant to apply are specifically described.
- Stakeholder involvement
  - Guideline development group includes individuals from all relevant professions.
  - Patient's views and preferences have been sought.
  - Target users of the guideline are clearly defined.
  - Guideline has been piloted among target users.
- Rigor of development
  - Systematic methods were used to search for evidence.
  - Criteria for selecting the evidence are clearly described.
  - Methods used for formulating the recommendations are clearly described.
  - Health benefits, side effects, and risks have been considered in formulating recommendations.
  - Explicit link exists between the recommendation and the supporting evidence.
  - Guideline has been externally reviewed by experts prior to publication.
  - Procedure for updating the guideline is provided.
- Clarity and presentation
  - Recommendations are specific and unambiguous.
  - Different options for management of the condition are clearly presented.

- Key recommendations are easily identifiable.
- Guideline is supported with tools for application.
- Application
  - Potential organizational barriers in applying the recommendations are discussed.
  - Possible cost implications of applying the recommendations have been considered.
  - Guideline presents key review criteria for monitoring or auditing purposes.
- Editorial independence
  - Guideline is editorially independent from the funding body.
  - Conflicts of interest of guideline development members have been recorded.

The usefulness of a guideline is dependent upon how meaningful and practical are the actual recommendations in the guideline. Recommendations should be practical in relation to implementation, be as unambiguous as possible, address frequency of screening and follow-up, and address clinically relevant actions. Other questions that the clinician must address in relation to guidelines must include such factors as the setting of care, the patient population, and the strength of the recommendations (Beyea & Slattery, 2006).

Models of Evidence-Based Nursing Practice

Differences exist between evidence-based practice models, but there are common elements between models that include selection of a practice topic, critique and synthesis of evidence, implementation, evaluation of the impact on patient care and provider performance, and consideration of the context in which the practice is implemented (Titler, 2008). No one model of evidence-based practice is a perfect fit for every organization. Some models focus upon the perspective of the individual clinician, or the researcher, while others focus on institutional efforts. Therefore, before embarking on this journey, several models should be reviewed and one selected or adapted that fits you or your organization.

ACE Star Model of Knowledge Transformation

The **Academic Center for Evidence-Based Nursing (ACE) Star Model of Knowledge Transformation**, developed by Dr. Kathleen Stevens, is available at www.acestar. uthscsa.edu/Learn_model.htm. The model involves five steps that include discovery, summary, translation, implementation, and evaluation. Discovery refers to the original research. During the second step the task is to synthesize all the related research into a meaningful whole. It is during this step that information is reduced to a manageable form. During the step of translation, the scientific evidence is considered in the context of clinical expertise and values. This results in clinical practice guidelines, best practices, protocols, standards, or clinical pathways. During the stage of implementation, changes take place in practice. During evaluation, the impact of the change is measured. Variables such as specific health outcomes, length of stay, or patient satisfaction are examples of possible outcomes that might be examined.

The Iowa Model of Evidence-Based Practice

The **Iowa Model of Evidence-Based Practice** resembles a decision-making tree that identifies either problem-focused or knowledge-focused triggers that initiate the process in the organization. Additional information and a diagram of the Iowa Model of Evidence-Based Practice are available at www.uihealthcare.com/depts/nursing/rqom/evidencebasedpractice/iowamodel.html.

Problem-focused triggers within an organization may include such things as risk management data, process improvement data, benchmarking data, financial data, or the identification of clinical problem. Knowledge-focused triggers within an organization may include such things as the publication of new research or literature, a change in organizational standards and guidelines, changes in philosophies of care within the profession or organization, or questions from an institutional standards committee.

Once there is either a problem-focused or knowledge-focused trigger within the organization, a team must first identify if the topic is a priority for the organization. If the topic is indeed a priority, evidence is examined, and the change in practice may be piloted. Depending upon the outcome, a change in practice may be instituted within the organization. This process is followed by monitoring and analysis of both the process and the outcome data and finally by dissemination of the results.

Agency for Healthcare Research and Quality Model

A model for maximizing and accelerating the transfer of research results from the Agency for Healthcare Research and Quality (AHRQ) patient safety research portfolio to healthcare delivery has recently been developed. There are three major stages of knowledge transfer in the AHRQ model that include: (1) knowledge creation and distillation, (2) diffusion and dissemination, and (3) organizational adoption and implementation. More specifically, knowledge creation and distillation refers to the conducting of research and then packaging relevant research findings into useable form such as practice recommendations. The diffusion and dissemination stage involves partnering with professional leaders, professional organizations, and healthcare organizations to disseminate knowledge to potential users such as nurses, physical therapists, or physicians. During the final stage of the process, the focus is upon organizational adoption and consistent implementation of evidence-based research findings and innovations in practice. In this model the stages of knowledge transfer are viewed from the perspective of the researcher or the creator of new knowledge and begin with decisions about what research findings ought to be disseminated (Titler, 2008).

Conclusion

Currently, the greatest challenge we face in fully implementing evidence-based practice in nursing as a profession is how to get the evidence to the practicing nurse. Nurses are very busy taking care of patients. From the perspective of the individual it can indeed be daunting; especially when many practicing nurses are not knowledgeable about evidence-based nursing practice. But daunting or not, the impetus for evidence-based practice will continue to grow. As healthcare costs continue to climb, the need for consistent, data-based answers to patient care problems will be an expectation. Patients will eventually demand evidence-based nursing care. Patients now have access to many computerized databases and reports, and they have the incentive and the time to read the reports. If patients are able to discern best practices, they will expect that nurses can as well (Simpson, 2004).

CLASSROOM ACTIVITY 1

Create clinical questions in PICO format for a patient in a case study provided by the instructor or a patient recently cared for in the clinical setting.

CLASSROOM ACTIVITY 2

Go to the computer lab and access evidence from resources such as CINAHL, the National Guideline Clearinghouse, or Cochrane Library in order to plan evidence-based care based upon the questions created in Classroom Activity 1.

References

Agency for Healthcare Research and Quality (AHRQ). (2002). *Systems to rate the strength of scientific evidence.* File inventory, Evidence Report/Technology Assessment No. 47, AHRQ Publication No. 02-E016. Rockville, MD: Author.

Beyea, S. C., & Slattery, M. J. (2006). *Evidence-based practice in nursing: A guide to successful implementation.* Marblehead, MA: The Healthcare Compliance Company.

Di Cesenso, A., Guyatt, G., & Ciliska, D. (2005). *Evidence-based nursing: A guide to clinical practice.* St. Louis, MO: Mosby.

Levin, R. F. (2006a). Evidence-based practice in nursing: What is it? In R. F. Levin & H. R. Feldman (Eds.), *Teaching evidence-based practice in nursing: A guide for academic and clinical settings.* New York: Springer.

Levin, R. F. (2006b). Teaching students to formulate clinical questions: Tell me your problems and then read my lips. In R. F. Levin & H. R. Feldman (Eds.), *Teaching evidence-based practice in nursing: A guide for academic and clinical settings.* New York: Springer.

In the previous 100 years great technological and medical advances have helped shape the world of bioethics, health care, and nursing practice. However, there has been a human price for the progress that has been made. New and intriguing moral dilemmas have surfaced related to professional healthcare practice, patient care, and the meaning of moral standing for individuals.

Relationships in Professional Practice

Although professional healthcare practices are made credible because of formal expert knowledge, relationships arising from natural human conditions, such as illness, are at the foundation of these practices.

Although professional healthcare practices are made credible because of formal expert knowledge, relationships arising from natural human conditions, such as illness, are at the foundation of these practices (Sokolowski, 1991). If nurses take seriously the guidance of the American Nurses Association's (ANA) 2001 *Code of Ethics for Nurses with Interpretive Statements,* patients are to be the central focus of nursing and nursing relationships. However, the quality of patient care that nurses render often depends on the existence of harmonious relationships between nurses and physicians, other nurses, and other healthcare workers. Nurses who are concerned about providing compassionate care to patients must be concerned about their relationships with colleagues as well as with their direct relationships with patients. If nurses view life as a network of interrelationships, all of a nurse's relationships can potentially affect patients' well-being. Therefore, these relationships have a moral nature.

Nurse–Physician Relationships

In 1967, Stein, a physician, wrote an article characterizing a type of relationship between physicians and nurses that he called "the doctor–nurse game" (Stein, Watts, & Howell, 1990). The game is based on a hierarchical relationship, with doctors being in the position of the superior. The hallmark of the game is that open disagreement between the disciplines is to be avoided. Avoidance of conflict is achieved when an experienced nurse, who is able to provide helpful suggestions to a doctor regarding patient care, cautiously offers the suggestions so that the physician does not directly perceive consultative advice as coming from a nurse. In the past, student nurses were educated about the rules of "the game" while attending nursing school. Over the years, other people have given credence to the historical accuracy of Stein's characterization of doctor–nurse relationships (Fry & Johnstone, 2002; Jameton, 1984; Kelly, 2000).

Stein, along with two other physicians, wrote an article revisiting the doctor–nurse game in 1990, 23 years after the phrase was first coined (Stein et al., 1990). They proposed that nurses unilaterally had decided to stop playing the game. Some of the reasons for this change and some of the ways the change was accomplished involved nurses' increased use of dialogue rather than gamesmanship, the profession's goal of equal partnership status with other healthcare professionals, the alignment of nurses with the civil rights and women's movements, the increased percentage of nurses who are receiving higher education, and the joint demonstration projects on collaboration between nurses and physicians. In conjunction with the dismantling of the doctor–nurse game, some nurses have taken an adversarial stance with physicians. These nurses believe that they need to continue fighting for freedom from physician domination in order to establish nursing as an autonomous profession.

However, rather than taking an adversarial stance that generates conflict, the nursing profession might be better served if nurses take a communitarian approach with physicians. It is within communities that morality in general and bioethics in particular receive their meaning (Engelhardt, 1996). A community works toward a common good and is held together by moral traditions. Nurses and physicians, as members of the healthcare community, must work together for the health and well-being of patients whether those patients are individuals, groups, or communities. When overt or covert battles are waged between nurses and physicians, moral problems arise, and patients may be the losers. Some ethicists have contended that the best approach for healing actually involves bringing patients into the community of healthcare providers (Hester, 2001). If nurses and physicians do not see themselves as members of a common community, the best interests of patients may not be served.

Nurse–Patient–Family Relationships

Unavoidable Trust

When patients enter the healthcare system, they are usually entering a foreign and forbidding environment (Chambliss, 1996; Zaner, 1991). Intimate conversations and activities, such as touching and probing, that normally do not occur between strangers, are commonplace between patients and healthcare professionals. Patients are frequently stripped of their clothes, subjected to sit alone in cold and barren rooms, and made to wait anxiously on frightening news regarding the continuation of their very being. When patients are in need of help from nurses, they frequently feel a sense of vulnerability and uncertainty. The tension that patients feel when accessing health care is heightened by the need for what Zaner (1991) called **unavoidable trust**. This concept represents Zaner's contention that patients, in most cases, have no option but to trust nurses and other healthcare professionals when the patient is at the point of needing care.

This unavoidable trust creates an asymmetrical, or uneven, power structure in nurse–patient and family relationships (Zaner, 1991). Professional nurses' responsiveness to this trust must include promising to be the most excellent nurses that they can be. According to Zaner, healthcare professionals must promise "not only to take care of, but to care for, the patient and family—to be candid, sensitive, attentive, and never to abandon them" (p. 54). It is paradoxical that trust is necessary before health

Nurses must never take for granted
the fragility of patients' trust.

care is rendered, but it only can be evaluated in terms of whether the trust was warranted after care is rendered. Nurses must never take for granted the fragility of patients' trust.

Boundaries

A discussion of professional boundaries is specifically covered in provision 2.4 of the *Code of Ethics for Nurses with Interpretive Statements* (ANA, 2001). In addition to the issues of trust discussed in the previous section, **boundaries** in nursing can be thought of in terms of appropriate professional behavior that serves to maintain trust between patients and nurses and to maintain nurses' good standing within their profession. Again, by keeping in mind that the primary concern of nurses' care is "preventing illness, alleviating suffering, and protecting, promoting, and restoring the health of patients," nurses can find guidance in maintaining professional boundaries (p. 11). The nature of nurses' work with both patients and colleagues has a very personal element but must not be confused with the common definition of friendship. Nurses are not discouraged from caring for patients, families, or colleagues. However, caring and jeopardizing professional boundaries are two distinct issues.

Concepts that underlie nurse–patient boundaries include power, choice, and trust (Maes, 2003). The asymmetry of power in favor of the nurse must prompt nurses to ask if they are inappropriately influencing the decisions of patients. Patients must be provided with complete information in order to make choices, and nurses must facilitate patients in receiving the information that they need. Patients trust nurses to have the knowledge and skill necessary to provide them with competent care; nurses must be faithful to that trust.

Potential violations of nurse–patient boundaries can involve gifts, intimacy, limits, neglect, abuse, and restraints (Maes, 2003). The gifts that patients give to nurses must be considered in terms of the implication of why the gift was given, its value, and whether the gift might provide therapeutic value for the patient but not influence the level of care provided by the nurse. Gifts generally lead to boundary violations and need to be discouraged most of the time. In addition to an obvious violation of intimacy through inappropriate sexual relationships, a violation of intimacy might occur if a nurse inappropriately shares information with other people in ways that violate patients' privacy. Nurses and patients must observe limits that prevent either person from becoming uncomfortable in their relationship. Nurses must take care to provide reasonable care to all patients according to appropriate ethical codes and state nurse practice acts so as not to be neglectful in the provision of nursing care, and they must do everything possible to prevent or intervene to stop patient abuse in whatever form it occurs. Finally, physically, chemically, and environmentally restraining patients can provide a major pitfall for nurses in terms of boundary violations. Nurses must know the policies of their employer as well as the standards set by accrediting agencies to safeguard patients.

Dignity

In the first provision of the *Code of Ethics for Nurses with Interpretive Statements*, the ANA (2001) included the standard that a nurse must have "respect for human dignity" (p. 7). However, Shotton and Seedhouse (1998) proposed that the term *dignity* has been used in vague ways. They characterized **dignity** as being related to persons being in a position to use their capabilities. In general terms, a person has dignity "if he or she is in a situation where his or her capabilities can be effectively applied" (p. 249). For example, nurses can enhance dignity when caring for elders by assessing their priorities and determining what the elder has been capable of in the past and what the person is capable of in the present.

A lack of or loss of capability is frequently an issue when caring for patients such as children, elders, and people who are physically and mentally disabled. Having absent or diminished capabilities is consistent with what MacIntyre (1999) was referring to in his discussion of human vulnerability. According to MacIntyre, people generally progress from a point of vulnerability in infancy to achieving varying levels of independent practical reasoning as they mature. However, all people, including nurses, would do well to realize that all persons have been or will be vulnerable at some point in their lives. Taking a "there but for the grace of God go I" stance may prompt nurses to develop what MacIntyre called the virtues of acknowledged dependence. These virtues include just generosity, *misericordia,* and truthfulness and are exercised in communities of giving and receiving. Just generosity is a form of giving generously without "keeping score" of who gives or receives the most; *misericordia* is a Latin word that signifies giving based on urgent need without prejudice; and truthfulness involves not withholding information from others that is needed for their own good. Nurses who cultivate these three virtues can move toward preserving patient dignity and toward the common good of the community.

Patient Advocacy

Nurses acting as patient advocates try to identify unmet patient needs and then follow up to address the needs appropriately (Jameton, 1984). **Advocacy**, as opposed to advice, involves the nurse's moving from the patient to the healthcare system rather than moving from the nurse's values to the patient. The concept of advocacy has been a part of the International Council of Nursing's (ICN) *Code of Ethics* and the ANA's code since the 1970s (Winslow, 1988). In the *Code of Ethics for Nurses with Interpretive Statements,* the ANA (2001) continues to support patient advocacy in elaborating on the "primacy of the patient's interest" (p. 9) and requiring nurses to work collaboratively with others to attain the goal of addressing the healthcare needs of patients and the public. Nurses are called on to ensure that all appropriate parties are involved in patient care decisions, that patients are provided with the

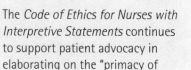

The *Code of Ethics for Nurses with Interpretive Statements* continues to support patient advocacy in elaborating on the "primacy of the patient's interest."

information needed to make informed decisions, and that collaboration is used to increase the accessibility and availability of health care to all patients who need it. The International Council of Nursing (2006), in the *Code of Ethics for Nurses*, affirms that the nurse must share "with society the responsibility for initiating and supporting action to meet the health and social needs of the public, in particular those of vulnerable populations" (p. 2).

Nurse–Nurse Relationships

As in the case of nurse–physician relationships, nurse–nurse relationships can be thought of as relationships within a community. Nurses in a nursing community might be what Engelhardt (1996) called moral friends. According to Wildes (2000), moral friends exist together within communities and use similar moral language. They "share a moral narrative and commitments [and] common understandings of the foundations of morality, moral reason, and justification" (p. 137). Communities are strongest when moral friends share "common moral traditions, practices, and [a] vision of the good life" (p. 137). In putting patients first in nurses' priorities, nurses in a community work together for a common good, using professional traditions to guide the communal narrative of nursing.

Unfortunately, nurses often treat other nurses in hurtful ways through what some people have called lateral or horizontal violence (Kelly, 2000; McKenna, Smith, Poole, & Coverdale, 2003). Lateral or horizontal violence involves interpersonal conflict, harassment, intimidation, harsh criticism, sabotage, and abuse among nurses. Some people believe that this oppression among nurses occurs because nurses feel oppressed by other dominant groups such as physicians or institutional administrators. Kelly (2000) reported that some nurses have characterized the violence perpetrated against nurses who excel and succeed as the "tall poppy syndrome." Nurses who succeed are ostracized, thereby creating a culture among nurses that discourages success.

Lateral violence in nursing is very counterproductive for the profession. A more productive path for nurses might be to cultivate the virtue of sympathetic joy. Sympathetic joy refers to experiencing happiness in regard to the good things experienced by others. The nursing community does not benefit from lateral violence, but nurses who cultivate the virtue of sympathetic joy can strengthen the sense of community among nurses. Nurses must support other nurses' success rather than treating colleagues as "tall poppies" that must be cut down.

However, there are occasions when unpleasant action must be taken in regard to nursing colleagues. In addition to advocating directly for patients' unmet needs, nurses are advocates when they take appropriate action to protect patients from the unethical, incompetent, or impaired practice of other nurses (ANA, 2001). When nurses are aware of these situations, they must deal compassionately with the offending coworkers while ensuring that patients receive safe, quality care. Concerns must be expressed to the offending nurse when personal safety or patient safety is not jeopardized in doing so and appropriate guidance must be obtained from supervisory personnel and institutional policies. Although action must be taken to safeguard patients' care, the manner in which a nurse handles situations involving unethical, incompetent, or impaired colleagues must not be a matter of gossip, condescension, or unproductive derogatory talk.

Moral Rights and Autonomy

In a society that is perfectly just, moral rights and legal rights would overlap; however, the two types of rights are not the same in our society (Brannigan & Boss, 2001). A **moral right** can be defined as "the right to perform certain activities (a) because they conform to the accepted standards or ideas of a community (or of a law, or of God, or of conscience), or (b) because they will not harm, coerce, restrain, or infringe on the interests of others, or (c) because there are good rational arguments in support of the value of such activities" (Angeles, 1992, p. 264).

Generally, moral rights are separated into welfare rights and liberty rights (Brannigan & Boss, 2001). Welfare rights allow persons to pursue their legitimate interests or those personal interests that do not interfere with the interests of other persons' that are similar and equal to one's own. "Welfare (positive) rights entail the right to receive basic goods such as education, medical care, and police protection, as well as a duty on the part of others such as the government to provide these social goods" (p. 33).

As opposed to welfare rights, liberty (negative) rights involve the right to noninterference from any person or governmental entity when pursuing one's legitimate interests (Brannigan & Boss, 2001). "Liberty or negative rights include autonomy, privacy, freedom of speech, and freedom from harassment, confinement, unwanted medical treatment, or participation in experiments without our informed consent" (p. 33). Although the World Health Organization has proposed that every person has a fundamental right to health without prejudice, in the United States, liberty rights are emphasized over welfare rights, except in cases of elders and the poor.

Informed Consent

Considerations of informed consent fall within the overview of respect for autonomy, or self-direction (Beauchamp & Childress, 2001; Veatch, 2003). Although nurses often facilitate informed consent and have a role in terms of patient advocacy, the actual responsibility for ensuring informed consent historically has belonged to the physician. However, with the increased numbers of advanced practice nurses and the increased complexity of nurses' roles, informed consent has become more of a direct ethical issue for nurses. A liberally applied concept of **informed consent** includes the rule that "meaningful information must be disclosed even if the clinician does not believe that it [the information] will be beneficial" (Veatch, 2003, p. 75). This definition is in contrast to the rule applied under the Hippocratic Oath that allowed for healthcare professionals to withhold information if they believed that it would harm or upset a patient.

It must be noted that a patient's signature on a consent form proves neither that a patient read the form nor that the patient understands what is written on it (Veatch, 2003). It would be impossible to inform each patient of everything about a procedure. In an attempt to deal with this reality, two standards are often applied. The first is the reasonable person standard that states the healthcare professional will disclose information that a reasonable person would want to know. The second is the subjective standard that states that disclosure must be based on the subjective interests of a particular patient rather than a hypothetical reasonable person. The ideal standard, therefore, adjusts what a reasonable person would want to know with what the healthcare professional knows that a particular patient is or might be interested in knowing.

Patient Self-Determination Act

The **Patient Self-Determination Act** of 1990, enacted in 1991, was designed to facilitate the knowledge and use of advance directives (Guido, 2001). Under the act, healthcare providers must ask patients if they have advance directives and must provide patients with advance directives information according to patients' wishes. This act provides nurses with a good opportunity to take an active role in facilitating the moral rights of patients in regard to end-of-life decisions. In addition to responding to the direct questions that patients ask about advance directives and end-of-life options, nurses would do well to "listen" for the subtle cues that patients give that signal their anxieties and uncertainty about end-of-life care. It would be a practice of compassion for nurses to listen deeply to patients and to actively try to alleviate patients' suffering and fears in regard to end-of-life decision making.

Advance Directives

An **advance directive** is "a written expression of a person's wishes about medical care, especially care during a terminal or critical illness" (Veatch, 2003, p. 119). Said another way, individuals lose control over their lives when they lose their decision-making capacity, and advance directives become instructions about health care for the future (Devettere, 2000). Advance directives may be self-written instructions or may be prepared by someone else as instructed by the patient.

There are three types of advance directives: living will, medical care directive, and durable power of attorney (Devettere, 2000). A **living will** is a formal legal document that provides written directions concerning medical care that is to be provided in specific circumstances (Beauchamp & Childress, 2001; Devettere, 2000). The living will gained recognition in the 1960s, but the Karen Ann Quinlan case in the 1970s brought public attention to the living will and subsequently prompted legalization of the document (Devettere, 2000). Although at the time, they were a good beginning, today living wills are inadequate. Living wills often consist of vague language, only instructions for unwanted treatments, and a lack of legal penalties for people who choose to ignore to follow the living wills. Also, living wills may be legally questionable in regard to their authenticity.

A **medical directive** is not a formal legal document but provides specific written instructions concerning the type of care and treatments that individuals want to receive if they become incapacitated (Devettere, 2000). One advantage to medical directives is that physicians can use them as a guide to know what the incapacitated patient wants in terms of specific healthcare treatments. Some attorneys believe that medical directives are only a minimal improvement over living wills. Their rationale is that they think that medical directives are only an elaborate informed consent. Also, other weaknesses of medical directives are that people cannot possibly anticipate every medical problem that may occur in their future, and people change over time and may change in regard to their future wishes. A **durable power of attorney**, the legal document with the most strength, is a written directive in which a designated person is allowed to make either general or healthcare decisions for a patient (Devettere, 2000).

Families and healthcare professionals may experience fear about making the wrong decisions regarding a patient who is incapacitated (Beauchamp & Childress, 2001). Advance directives may help to reduce emotional stress but at the same time may produce ethical dilemmas.

Social Justice

Definition and Theories of Social Justice

A Sicilian priest first used the term *social justice* in 1840, and then in 1848, the term was more popularized by Antonio Rosmini-Serbati (Novak, 2000). Since then, **social justice** has been defined as (Center for Economic & Social Justice, n.d.):

> A virtue that guides us in creating those organized human interactions we call institutions. In turn, social institutions, when justly organized, provide us with access to what is good for the person, both individually and in our associations with others. Social justice also imposes on each of us a personal responsibility to work with others to design and continually perfect our institutions as tools for personal and social development. (p. 2)

A large portion of the use of the term has been related more to competing powers of social systems and regulative principles on an impersonal basis, such as "high unemployment," "inequality of incomes," "lack of a living wage," and "social injustice" (Novak, 2000, p. 1). The term also has been related to the question of what makes the common good for everyone (Brannigan & Boss, 2001). People who take a communitarian approach will put common goods of the community over individual freedoms.

In his social contract book, *A Theory of Justice,* John Rawls (1971) viewed fairness and equality under a "veil of ignorance." This concept means that if people had a veil to shield their own or others' economic, social, and class standing, each person would be more likely to make justice-based decisions from a position that is free from all biases and would view the distribution of resources in impartial ways. Under the veil, people would view social conditions neutrally because they would not know what their own position might be at the time the veil is lifted. This "not knowing" or ignorance of persons about their own position means that they cannot gain any type of advantage for themselves by their choices. Based on this "ignorance" principle, Rawls stated that this view is just (cited in Brannigan & Boss, 2001). Rawls (1971) advocated two principles of equality and justice: everyone should be given equal liberty no matter what adversities exist for people, and differences should be recognized among people by making sure that the least advantaged people are given their desert for improvements.

Nozick (1974, cited in Brannigan & Boss, 2001) presented the idea of an entitlement system in his book, *Anarchy, State, and Utopia,* meaning that if individuals could pay for insurance, only then are they entitled to health care. Nozick emphasized that in order for a system to be just and fair, it must reward people who contribute to the system (Brannigan & Boss, 2001). Then later, Daniels explored Rawls's concept of justice further by basing his book, *Just Health Care* (1985; cited in Brannigan & Boss, 2001), on the liberty principle, as he espoused that every person should have equal opportunity. Daniels emphasized equal health care and reasonable access to healthcare services and recommended national healthcare reform.

Allocation and Rationing of Healthcare Resources

The cost of health care is spiraling out of control worldwide, and therefore, healthcare resources and deciding how to allocate them remain at the forefront of peoples' concerns. The unfortunate and troublesome experiences with healthcare reimbursements are played out through narratives on the front page of almost every newspaper. A central question that healthcare professionals, economists, and politicians have asked themselves for years is what makes up a just and equitable healthcare system? The question continues to be unanswered.

The health care of people in the United States is not the best in the world, yet in 2005, United States healthcare expenditures were $2 trillion (Kaiser Family Foundation, 2007). The federal government's second major goal in *Healthy People 2010* is to eliminate health disparities, yet the disparities continue to occur without much, if any, improvement in the health of people in the United States (U.S. Department of Health & Human Services, 2000). It is believed that inequalities in health care exist because of complex differences in socioeconomic status, racial and ethnic backgrounds, education levels, and healthcare access. These differences underlie many of the health disparities in the United States. As a result, health-promoting behaviors are not as likely to be practiced.

As healthcare costs increase, resources become more limited for people. Distributive justice has become a critical issue in the healthcare system. Guidelines in how scarce resources are distributed must be clearly delineated. Some guiding questions that members of society need to explore in terms of distributive justice include the following:

- Does every person have a right to health care?
- Is health care a right or a privilege that must be earned?
- How should resources be distributed so that everyone receives a fair and equitable share for health care?
- Should healthcare rationing ever be considered as an option in the face of scarce healthcare resources? If so, how?

There may never be clear and concise answers to these complex questions. Brannigan and Boss (2001) outlined criteria that could be used when rationing is considered. The criteria include standards of distribution by market or according to people who could afford to pay, social worth, medical needs, age, a first-come, first-served basis, and randomization. From the 1990s to the present, systems of managed care have been operating in the United States as one strategy to improve the use of services based on needs and to maximize health and well-being while reducing overall healthcare costs to individuals (Sugarman, 2000). However, the public has responded very poorly to managed care. Some people have labeled managed care as an ethical disaster. Before such complaints are made, however, healthcare professionals and nurses need to address the sources of the problems.

Sugarman (2000) discussed the enormous travesty that occurred with the Medicaid and Medicare systems from 1965 to 1990. Big money was made available by the United States federal government based on the autonomous practice of physicians— meaning that physicians could redirect large amounts of money from taxpayers to the care of sick people via Medicaid and Medicare. Sugarman termed this period as "the good old days," when physicians were not required to justify or show evidence for their medical care for sick people. Since 1990, however, times have changed, and criticism is plentiful. Sugarman contended that no matter what healthcare system is in place, physicians and the public would be critical. Engelhardt (1996), a bioethicist, stated this about the current healthcare system:

> Concepts of adequate care are not discoverable outside of particular views of the good life and of proper medical practice. In nations encompassing diverse moral communities, an understanding of what one will mean by an adequate level or a decent minimum of health care will need to be fashioned, if it can indeed be agreed to, through open discussion and by fair negotiation. (p. 400)

Promoting open dialogue for expressing moral views in the community and in institutions, negotiating policy change for better allocation and an improved healthcare system, and maintaining a firm commitment for better patient health outcomes are just a few ways that nurses can assist with supporting good health for the common good of the community.

CRITICAL THINKING QUESTION

Think about the questions posed above in relation to the distribution of scarce healthcare resources under a "veil of ignorance," and then think about the same questions considering your own circumstances. Do you come up with the same answers to the questions?

Ethics and Organ Transplantation

A dramatic social allocation issue that involves scarce resources is organ transplantation. In the United States, patients may "opt in" by signing a donor card as potential donors of one or more organs in the event of their death (Perrin & McGhee, 2001). If patients choose not to sign donor cards, they are free from any obligation to donate organs. There are three ethical issues that are involved with organ transplantation: the moral acceptability of transplanting an organ from one person to another, procurement, and allocation of the organs (Veatch, 2003).

For the first ethical issue, Veatch (2003) posed this question: "Is performing transplants 'playing God'?" (p. 136). This phrase has become quite common in the last couple of decades with transplants, genetics, and human reproduction technologies being so popular. Many people view transplantations as unacceptable based on religious or cultural beliefs, or just basic beliefs, such as the association that the human heart has with romance and as the "seat of the soul" (Veatch, 2003, p. 137).

The second ethical issue is procurement of organs. In some countries other than the United States, organs can be routinely salvaged without the consent of the patient or anyone in the family with the basic belief that organs, once the person is dead, become the property of the state or country (Veatch, 2003). In the United States, it is believed that donation and informed consent are based on the rights and autonomy of each person.

The third ethical issue is organ allocation, which is one of the most debated issues in health care today because of the scarcity of donor organs. There is a national waiting list established by the United Network for Organ Sharing (UNOS) Committee (U.S. Department of Health & Human Services, 2003). At least 98,151 people in the United States are awaiting organs for transplant (Organ Procurement and Transplantation Network, 2007). Because of the demand for organs and the prospect of money that can be made, the organ black market is thriving. The U.S. organ donor system is organized so that allocation decisions are coordinated by UNOS, and the system is designed to be driven by the principle of justice. UNOS or the organ transplant team should never deny organs based on perceived social worth; rather, allocation of resources should be distributed fairly and equally based on need.

There are five major focus areas of health disparities that are known to affect racial and ethnic groups in all ages: cardiovascular disease, diabetes, HIV infections and AIDS, cancer screening and disease management, and immunizations (U.S. Department of Health & Human Services, 2000). People who suffer the most from health disparities between populations often have diseases that eventually result in a need for organ transplants. For instance, a health conditions report from the Office of Minority Health (2007) revealed in 2004 that high blood pressure occurs 1.5 times more in African Americans than in non-Hispanic whites and in 2002, African-American men were 2.1 times as likely to start treatment for end-stage renal disease related to diabetes, compared to non-Hispanic white men. One primary role for nurses is to assist with attempting to eliminate health disparities. Education programs with substantive content that target particular populations provide a beginning role for nurses, who function on a broad community level.

Other roles for nurses include encouraging patients and families to express their feelings and attitudes about donations and transplantations, especially in regard to ethical issues involving death and dying; supporting, listening, and maintaining confidentiality with patients and families; assisting in monitoring patients for organ needs; continually being aware of inequalities and injustices in the health-care system, which may affect the care of patients; and assisting in the care of surgical organ transplant and donation patients and their families.

Death and End-of-Life Care

Defining Death

The last words of the great composer Frédéric Chopin were, "The earth is suffocating. . . . Swear to make them cut me open, so that I won't be buried alive" (Death: The Last Taboo, 2003). In the 1700s and 1800s, especially in Europe, there was widespread fear of premature burial or being buried alive because of the inadequate methods for detecting when a person was dead and because of actual accounts of people being buried alive (Bondeson, 2001). In those days, when a body was exhumed, claw marks sometimes were found on the inside of coffin lids (Mappes & DeGrazia, 2001). Because of the widespread fear, a variety of special safety coffins were invented with detailed devices to help the dead, once they were buried, to communicate with others above the ground (Death: The Last Taboo, 2003). The devices included such things as a rope extending to the surface of the ground with a bell on the other end, a speaking tube to the outer coffin, a shovel, and food and water. In addition to a new law that prevented premature burial, funeral home attendants even went to the extent to have their employees monitor dead bodies for any signs of life during the "wait" time.

For several centuries, when a person became unconscious, physicians or other people would palpate for a pulse, listen for breath sounds with their ears, look for condensation on an object when it was held close to the body's nose, and check for fixed and dilated pupils (Mappes & DeGrazia, 2001). In 1819, fear was reduced when the stethoscope was invented because physicians could listen with greater certainty for a heartbeat through a magnified listening device on the chest of the body. In 1903, Willem Einthoven, a Dutch physician, discovered the existence of the electrical properties of the heart with his invention of the electrocardiograph, which provided sensitive information about whether the electrical activity of the heart was functioning. The artificial respirator of the 1950s brought about more uncertainty of death as physicians kept patients alive in the absence of a natural heartbeat (Death: The Last Taboo, 2003). By the 1960s, when transplants were being performed, it was becoming apparent that a diagnosis of death would not depend necessarily on the absence of a heartbeat. Rather, the definition of death would need to include brain death criteria in the future.

The first attempt to redefine death was made in the United States by the Harvard Medical School ad hoc committee in 1968. The definition was based on the committee members' attempt to identify reliable clinical criteria for respirator-dependent patients who had no brain function (Youngner & Arnold, 2001). Then, in 1981, the President's Commission members sanctioned a definition of death, which included brain death, and recommended its adoption by all states (Mappes & DeGrazia, 2001). The 1981 definition led to the Uniform Determination of Death Act (UDDA), in which death is defined as:

> An individual who has sustained either (1) irreversible cessation of circulatory and respiratory functions or (2) irreversible cessation of all functions of the entire brain, including the brain stem, is dead. A determination of death must be made in accordance with accepted medical standards. (President's Commission, 1981; cited in Mappes & DeGrazia, 2001, p. 318)

Since this definition was adopted, criteria for brain death have been integrated in almost every state but have been continually debated. A provocative thought that Veatch (2003) has contributed to the debate on the definition of death concerns the loss of full moral standing of human beings. This statement triggers the question as to when humans should be treated as full members of the human community. Although almost every person has reconciled the thought that some persons have full moral standing and others do not, there is continued controversy about when full moral standing ceases to exist and what characteristics qualify the cessation of full moral standing.

Losing full moral standing is equivalent to ceasing to exist. Presently, various groups have proposed and debated the following four conceptions of death since the enactment of the UDDA in 1981 (Munson, 2004, pp. 692, 693):

- Traditional—A person is dead when he is no longer breathing and his heart is not beating (cardiopulmonary).
- Whole-brain—Death is regarded as the irreversible cessation of all brain functions . . . no electrical activity in the brain, and even the brain stem is not functioning (brain death).
- Higher brain—Death is considered to involve the permanent loss of consciousness. Someone in an irreversible coma would be considered dead, even though the brain stem continued to regulate breathing and heartbeat (persistent vegetative state).
- Personhood—Death occurs when an individual ceases to be a person. This may mean loss of features that are essential to personal identity or for being a person.

With whole-brain death, a patient physically may survive for an indeterminate period of time with a mechanical ventilator. With higher brain death, a patient lives in a persistent vegetative state indefinitely but without the need for mechanical ventilation. It is because of these situations that the question exists regarding when a person should be treated as one who has full moral standing within the human community. Society, physicians, and nurses have had difficulty in defining *death* by the UDDA definition, which includes the traditional and the whole-brain concepts. However, the greatest difficulty has been when they have tried to incorporate the concepts of higher brain death and personhood death (Munson, 2004). No definite criteria for either of these concepts—higher brain or personhood—have been established for defining death. The debate continues, and questions continue about when life begins, when life ends, and what it is that ceases to exist when someone is dead (Benjamin, 2003; Veatch, 2003).

Euthanasia

Most people do not want prolonged agony and suffering before their death and would like to keep their emotional, financial, and social burdens to a minimum and their dignity intact. However, dying the "good death" is not always possible (Munson, 2004). Euthanasia, meaning "good death" in Greek, has come to mean "easy death" and has developed a

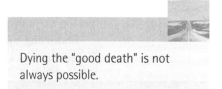

Dying the "good death" is not always possible.

strong appeal in recent years. A patient may ponder options of euthanasia if suffering and pain become too much for the person to bear. There are two major types of euthanasia: active and passive. **Active euthanasia** occurs when a person takes an action to end a life (including one's own life). Active euthanasia may include a lethal dose of medication, such as in physician-assisted suicide. **Passive euthanasia** means that a person allows another person to die by not acting to stop death or prolong life. An example of this type of euthanasia may include withholding treatment that is necessary to prevent death at a point in time.

Euthanasia also is recognized by the categories of voluntary and nonvoluntary (Brannigan & Boss, 2001). **Voluntary euthanasia** occurs when persons with a sound mind authorize another person to take their life or to assist them in achieving death. Also, this type may include the taking of one's own life. **Nonvoluntary** euthanasia occurs when persons are not able to express their decision about death. A blending of these types of euthanasias may occur, such as voluntary active, nonvoluntary active, voluntary passive, and nonvoluntary passive.

A vigorous debate in the United States continues about whether there is a real moral difference between active euthanasia, such as the intentional taking of someone's life, and passive euthanasia, such as withholding or withdrawing life-sustaining treatments (Brannigan & Boss, 2001; Jonsen, Veatch, & Walters, 1998). The action versus omission distinction many times causes nurses and physicians to ponder this troublesome question: "Is there a moral difference between actively killing and letting die?"

professionals make certain that the patient's decision is noncoercive and autonomous and that the decision has been made based on the patient's mentally competent decision-making capacity (Mappes & DeGrazia, 2001). Although nurses and other healthcare professionals may have the assurance of the patient's autonomous and competent decision making, sometimes the patient's decision is difficult to accept. Refusal of medical treatments may occur at any time in life, whether at the end of life or not, such as times when patients may refuse treatment based on religious or cultural beliefs.

Deciding for Others

When patients are no longer able to make competent decisions, families may experience problems in trying to determine a progressive right course of action. The ideal situation is for patients to be autonomous decision makers, but when autonomy is no longer possible, decision making falls to a surrogate (Beauchamp & Childress, 2001). The surrogate, or proxy, is either chosen by the patient, is court appointed, or has other authority to make decisions.

There are three types of surrogate decision makers (Beauchamp & Childress, 2001; Veatch, 2003). The **standard of substituted judgment** is used to guide medical decisions that involve formerly competent patients who no longer have any decision-making capacity. This standard is based on the assumption that incompetent patients have the exact rights as competent patients to make judgments about their health care (Buchanan & Brock, 1990). Surrogates make medical treatment decisions based on how the surrogates believe that the patients would have decided were the patients still competent and able to express their wishes. In making decisions, the surrogates use their understanding of the patients' previous overt or implied expressions of their beliefs and values (Veatch, 2003). Before losing competency, the patient could have either explicitly informed the proxy of treatment wishes by oral or written instruction or implicitly made clear treatment wishes through informal conversations with the proxy.

Decisions based on the **pure autonomy standard** are made on behalf of an incompetent person and are based on decisions that the formerly competent person made. This type of decision also is called the *principle of autonomy extended* meaning that a person's autonomy continues to be honored even when the person cannot exercise autonomy through normal channels.

The **best interest standard** is based on the goal of the surrogate's doing what is best for the patient or what is in the best interest of the patient (Veatch, 2003). This standard is applied when the patient who the proxy represents has never been competent, such as a child.

Withholding and Withdrawing Treatment

People in society and healthcare professionals have accepted and ethically justified withholding and withdrawing treatments that have been deemed as futile or extraordinary. When a treatment has no physiologic benefit for a terminally ill person, the treatment is considered to be **futile care** (Beauchamp & Childress, 2001). Medical treatments may include cardiopulmonary resuscitation, medications, mechanical ventilation, artificial feeding and fluids, hemodialysis, chemotherapy, and other life-sustaining technologies. Futility issues need to be discussed among nurses, physicians, family members, and patients when possible. A court-appointed or family surrogate decision maker may be the spokesperson for the patient. Nurses need to ensure that a decision-making process between the healthcare team and the decision makers for the patient takes place so that everyone has a chance to express feelings and concerns (Ladd, Pasquerella, & Smith, 2002).

There are three legal cases that generated landmark decisions about withholding and withdrawing treatments. In 1975, Karen Ann Quinlan's case established the right to discontinue mechanical ventilation (Jonsen et al., 1998; *In re Quinlan,* New Jersey). In 1990, the U.S. Supreme Court established through Nancy Cruzan's case three conditions: the patient has a right to refuse medical treatment; artificial feeding constitutes medical treatment; and if the patient is mentally incompetent, then each state has to document clear and convincing evidence that the patient's desires were for discontinuance of medical treatment (Jonsen et al.; *In re Cruzan,* Missouri).

The third case is a more recent one. It is the case of Terri Schiavo, a young woman in a persistent vegetative state, who died on March 31, 2005. There were a total of 21 legal suits, but the last few cases involved Terri's husband Michael's request to have her feeding tube discontinued, which also would end her artificial nutrition and hydration. Terri's parents fought this request. According to Florida law, Michael Schiavo as a spouse and guardian had a legal right to serve as a surrogate decision maker for Terri Schiavo. In conjunction with this legal standard, substituted judgment was used as the appropriate ethical standard. Because Terri Schiavo had no written advance directive, her surrogate was charged with making an unbiased substituted judgment about her care. The judgment should be based on an understanding of what she would decide for herself and *not* the values of the surrogate. Michael Schiavo and other people testified that Terri had stated that she did not want to live in a condition in which she would be a burden to anyone else. This evidence served as the basis for many of the court's denials of the Schindlers' requests to continue Terri's artificial nutrition and hydration.

In the *Code of Ethics for Nurses with Interpretive Statements,* Provision 1.3, the ANA (2001) has taken the position that nurses ethically support the provision of compassionate and dignified end-of-life care as long as nurses do not have the sole intention of ending a person's life. A special statement concerning the Terri Schiavo case was released to the press by the ANA on March 23, 2005, that upheld the decision for the right of a patient or surrogate to choose forgoing artificial nutrition and hydration. No matter what the outcome of difficult end-of-life decisions, family members and patients need to feel a sense of confidence that nurses will maintain moral sensitivity and good judgment.

Terminal Sedation

Legally permissible yet ethically controversial, **terminal sedation** (TS) seems to be moving toward a social and an ethical acceptance (Quill, 2001). TS is defined by Quill as follows:

> When a suffering patient is sedated to unconsciousness, usually through the ongoing administration of barbiturates or benzodiazepines. The patient then dies of dehydration, starvation, or some other intervening complication, as all other life-sustaining interventions are withheld. (p. 181)

When the word *terminal* is used, there is an understanding among the health-care team members and family that the outcome, and possibly a desired outcome, is death (Sugarman, 2000). TS has been used in situations when patients need pain relief that requires being sedated to the point of unconsciousness. The ANA (2001) did not address TS directly in the *Code of Ethics for Nurses with Interpretive Statements* but did state that nurses are to give compassionate care at the end of life. There is an emphasis in the code that nurses are not to have the sole intent of ending a person's life.

Physician-Assisted Suicide

Moral outrage toward social acceptance regarding **physician-assisted suicide** has occurred in society. Physician-assisted suicide is defined as the "the act of providing a lethal dose of medication for the patient to self-administer" (Sugarman, 2000, p. 213). Oregon is the only state in the United States that currently allows physician-assisted suicide. The legal basis in Oregon is the Death with Dignity Act, which was passed in 1994. With certain restrictions, patients who are near death may obtain prescriptions to end their lives in a dignified way.

Although the ANA (2001), in the *Code of Ethics for Nurses with Interpretive Statements,* plainly stated that nurses are not to act with the sole intent of ending a person's life, the Oregon Nurses Association issued special guidelines for nurses that relate to the Death with Dignity Act (Ladd et al., 2002). The guidelines include maintaining support, comfort, and confidentiality; discussing end-of-life options with the patient and family; and being present for the patient's self-administration of medications and during the death. Nurses may not administer the medications themselves; breach confidentiality; subject others to any type of judgmental comments or statements about the patient; or refuse care to the patient.

End-of-Life Decisions and Moral Conflicts

Nurses first must sort out their own feelings about the various types of euthanasia before appropriate guidance and direction can be offered to patients and families. In one Japanese study of 160 nurses, Konishi, Davis, and Toshiaki (2002) studied withdrawal of artificial food and fluid from terminally ill patients. The majority of the nurses supported this act only under two conditions: if the patient requested the withdrawal of artificial food and fluids, and if the act relieved the patient's suffering. Nurses agreed that comfort for the patient was a great concern. One nurse in the study stated this: "[Artificial food and fluid] AFF only prolongs the patient's suffering. When withdrawn, the patient showed peace on the face. I have seen such patients so many times" (Konishi et al., 2002). In the same study, another nurse who was experiencing moral conflict with the decision to withdraw the artificial food and fluid stated this: "Withdrawal is killing and cruel. I feel guilty" (Konishi et al.).

Other end-of-life issues may generate moral conflicts, as well. Georges and Grypdonck (2002) conducted a literature review on the topic of ethical issues in terms of how nurses perceive their care to dying patients. They outlined some of the moral dilemmas that are particularly related to nurses and end-of-life care. Some of the moral problems of nurses found in the literature were:

- Communicating truthfully with patients about death because they were fearful of destroying all hope among the patient and family
- Managing pain symptoms because of fear of hastening death
- Feeling forced to collaborate with other health team members about medical treatments that in nurses' opinions are futile or too burdensome
- Feeling insecure and not adequately informed about reasons for treatment
- Trying to maintain their own moral integrity throughout relationships with patients, families, and coworkers because of feeling that they are forced to betray their own moral values

Although the conscientious nurse has an obligation to provide compassionate and palliative care, the nurse also has a right to withdraw from treating and caring for a patient as long as another nurse has assumed care for the dying patient. When care is such that the nurse perceives it as violating personal morality and values, the professional nurse must seek alternative approaches to achieve patients' goals.

Conclusion

Nurses' involvement with bioethical issues becomes more complicated as time passes. Nurses must learn to cultivate good professional relationships while also ensuring that the stresses of their job do not distract them from delivering direct or indirect patient care that is ethical and patient centered. Practicing nursing ethically cannot be based merely on intuitive functioning. To be advocates for patients during difficult and sensitive times, nurses must understand key ethical concepts and seek active involvement in being valuable members of healthcare teams.

CASE STUDY   END-OF-LIFE CARE

Gertrude, an 85-year-old woman, was diagnosed with end-stage renal disease, long-standing adult-onset diabetes, and aortic stenosis. Her renal disease now has led to a terminal condition. Still conscious, she told her youngest daughter that she wanted no life-sustaining measures done. On the next day, she lost consciousness. Then, her other two daughters arrived at the hospital from out of town. The three daughters argued about the treatment for their mother; the youngest wanted to honor the wishes of her mother and the other two wanted full medical treatment to be initiated. The physician and nurse discussed the treatment options and the futility issue with the family. To avoid further disagreement, the youngest daughter decided to go along with the decision of the other two sisters.

CASE STUDY QUESTIONS

1. Explain the reason that the physician and nurse discussed futile treatment with the daughters.
2. Do you believe that the mother had a right to choose her course of treatment? Explain.
3. Discuss the end-of-life options that the daughters could have chosen for their mother's care had they chosen the "no treatment" option.
4. Discuss the different types of surrogate decision making. Was there a surrogate decision maker in this family? Explain.
5. What specific nursing support and care could you offer to this family and patient?

References

American Nurses Association. (2001). *Code of ethics for nurses with interpretive statements.* Washington, DC: Author.

Angeles, P. A. (1992). *The HarperCollins dictionary of philosophy* (2nd ed.). New York: HarperCollins Publishers.

Beauchamp, T. L., & Childress, J. F. (2001). *Principles of biomedical ethics* (5th ed.). New York: Oxford University Press.

Benjamin, M. (2003). Pragmatism and the determination of death. In G. McGee (Ed.), *Pragmatic bioethics* (2nd ed.). London: Bradford Book-MIT Press.

Bondeson, J. (2001). *Buried alive: The terrifying history of our most primal fear.* New York: W. W. Norton & Company.

Brannigan, M. C., & Boss, J. A. (2001). *Healthcare ethics in a diverse society.* Mountain View, CA: Mayfield.

Buchanan, A. E., & Brock, D. W. (1990). *Deciding for others: The ethics of surrogate decision making.* New York: Cambridge University Press.

Center for Economic Justice and Social Justice. (n.d.). *Defining economic justice and social justice.* Washington, DC: Author. Retrieved December 6, 2003, from http://cesj.org/thirdway/economicjustice-defined.htm

Centers for Disease Control and Prevention. (2007). *Suicide: Facts at a glance.* Retrieved December 29, 2007, from http://www.cdc.gov/ncipc/dvp/suicide/SuicideDataSheet.pdf

Daniels, N. (1985). *Just health care.* Cambridge, England: Cambridge University Press.

Death: The last taboo. (2003). *What is death?* Australian Museum. Retrieved December 5, 2003, from http://www.deathonline.net/what_is

Devettere, R. J. (2000). *Practical decision making in health care ethics: Cases and concepts* (2nd ed.). Washington, DC: Georgetown University Press.

Engelhardt, H. T. (1996). *Rights to health care, social justice, and fairness in health care allocations: Frustrations in the face of finitude: The foundations of bioethics* (2nd ed.). New York: Oxford University Press.

Finnerty, J. L. (1987). Ethics in rational suicide. *Critical Care Nursing Quarterly, 10*(2), 86–90.

Fry, S., & Johnstone, M. J. (2002). *Ethics in nursing practice: A guide to ethical decision making* (2nd ed.). Oxford, UK: Blackwell Science.

Georges, J. J., & Grypdonck. M. (2002). Moral problems experienced by nurses when caring for terminally ill people: A literature review. *Nursing Ethics, 9*(2), 155–178.

Guido, G. W. (2001). *Legal and ethical issues in nursing* (3rd ed.). Upper Saddle River, NJ: Prentice-Hall.

Hester, D. M. (2001). *Community as healing: Pragmatist ethics in medical encounters.* Lanham, MD: Rowman & Littlefield Publishers.

International Council of Nurses. (2006). *The International Council of Nurses code of ethics for nurses.* Geneva: Author.

Jameton, A. (1984). *Nursing practice: The ethical issues.* Englewood Cliffs, NJ: Prentice-Hall.

Jonsen, A. R., Siegler, M., & Winslade, W. J. (2002). *Clinical ethics* (5th ed.). New York: McGraw-Hill.

Jonsen, A. R., Veatch, R. M., & Walters, L. (1998). *Source book in bioethics.* Washington, DC: Georgetown University Press.

Kaiser Family Foundation. (2007). *U.S. health care costs.* Retrieved December 28, 2007, from http://www.kaiseredu.org/topics_im.asp?imID=1&parentID=61&id=358

Kelly, C. (2000). *Nurses' moral practice: Investing and discounting self.* Indianapolis, IN: Sigma Theta Tau International Center Nursing Press.

Konishi, E., Davis, A. J., & Toshiaki, A. (2002). The ethics of withdrawing artificial food and fluid from terminally ill patients: An end-of-life dilemma for Japanese nurses and families. *Nursing Ethics, 9*(1), 7–19.

Ladd, R. E., Pasquerella, L., & Smith, S. (2002). *Ethical issues in home health care.* Springfield, IL: Charles C. Thomas.

MacIntyre, A. (1999). *Dependent rational animals.* Chicago: Open Court Publishing.

Maes, S. (2003). How do you know when professional boundaries have been crossed? *Oncology Nursing Society News, 18*(8), 3–5.

Mappes, T. A., & DeGrazia, D. (2001). *Biomedical ethics* (5th ed.). Boston: McGraw-Hill.

McKenna, B. G., Smith, N. A., Poole, S. J., & Coverdale, J. H. (2003). Horizontal violence: Experiences of registered nurses in their first year of practice. *Journal of Advanced Nursing, 42*(1), 90–96.

Munson, R. (2004). *Intervention & reflection: Basic issues in medical ethics* (7th ed.). Victoria, Australia: Wadsworth-Thomson.

Novak, M. (2000). Defining social justice. *First Things First, 108,* 11–13. Retrieved December 6, 2003, from http://www.freerepublic.com/forum/a3a42c6be4e23.htm

Nozick, R. (1974). *Anarchy, state and utopia.* New York: Basic Books.

Office of Minority Health. (2007). *Data statistics African American profiles: Health conditions.* Retrieved December 28, 2007, from http://www.omhrc.gov/templates/browse.aspx?lvl=2&lvlID=51

Organ Procurement and Transplantation Network. (2007). *Waiting list candidates.* Retrieved December 28, 2007, from http://www.optn.org

Perrin, K. O., & McGhee, J. (2001). *Ethics and conflict.* Thorofare, NJ: Slack.

President's Commission for the Study of Ethical Problems in Medicine and Biomedical and Behavioral Research. (1981). *Defining death, 73*. Washington, DC: Government Printing Office.

Quill, T. E. (2001). *Caring for patients at the end of life: Facing an uncertain future together.* New York: Oxford University Press.

Rawls, J. (1971). *A theory of justice.* Cambridge, MA: Harvard University Press.

Shotton, L., & Seedhouse, D. (1998). Practical dignity in caring. *Nursing Ethics, 5*(3), 246–255.

Siegel, K. (1986). Psychosocial aspects of rational suicide. *American Journal of Psychotherapy, 40*(3), 405–418.

Sokolowski, R. (1991). The fiduciary relationship and the nature of professions. In E. D. Pellegrino, R. M. Veatch, & J. P. Langan (Eds.), *Ethics, trust, and the professions: Philosophical and cultural aspects* (pp. 23–43). Washington, DC: Georgetown University Press.

Stein, L. I., Watts, D. T., & Howell, T. (1990). The doctor–nurse game revisited. *Nursing Outlook, 38*(6), 264–268.

Sugarman, J. (2000). *20 Common problems: Ethics in primary care.* New York: McGraw-Hill.

U.S. Department of Health & Human Services. (2000, November). *Healthy people 2010: Understanding & improving health* (2nd ed.). Washington, DC: U.S. Government Printing Office.

U.S. Department of Health & Human Services. (2003). *Organ donation and transplantation.* Retrieved December 6, 2003, from http://www.4woman.gov/faq/organ_donation.htm

Veatch, R. M. (2003). *The basics of bioethics* (2nd ed.). Upper Saddle River, NJ: Prentice Hall.

Wildes, K. W. (2000). *Moral acquaintances: Methodology in bioethics.* Notre Dame, IN: University of Notre Dame Press.

Winslow, G. R. (1988). *Ethical issues in professional life.* New York: Oxford University Press.

World Health Organization. (2003). *WHO definition of palliative care.* Retrieved December 10, 2003, from http://www.who.int/cancer/palliative/definition/en/print.html

World Health Organization. (2007). *Mental health: The bare facts.* Retrieved December 29, 2007, from http://www.who.int/mental_health/en

Youngner, S. J., & Arnold, R. M. (2001). Philosophical debates about the definition of death: Who cares? *Journal of Medicine & Philosophy, 26*(5), 527–537.

Zaner, R. M. (1991). The phenomenon of trust and the patient-physician relationship. In E. D. Pellegrino, R. M. Veatch, & J. P. Langan (Eds.), *Ethics, Trust, and the professions: Philosophical and cultural aspects* (pp. 45–67). Washington, DC: Georgetown University Press.

Law and the Professional Nurse

Kathleen Driscoll and Evadna Lyons

LEARNING OBJECTIVES

After completing this chapter, the student should be able to:

1. Discuss why an understanding of the legal profession is necessary for the nurse.
2. Discuss the functions and sources of law as they relate to health care and professional nursing practice.
3. Discuss what the term *standard of care* means for the nurse.
4. Discuss the elements of malpractice and negligence and how they relate to nursing practice.
5. Describe the trial process in regard to civil procedures including the nurse's role as an expert witness.
6. Examine the functions of the state boards of nursing in relationship to education, practice, and discipline.
7. Discuss the importance of the Nurse Practice Act in regard to safe and effective nursing practice.
8. Apply the concept of professional accountability to professional and legal standards in relationship to informed consent, confidentiality, and privacy.
9. Critique the legal aspects of delegation.
10. Examine strategies for avoiding legal problems.

Key Terms and Concepts

- Statutory law
- Lobbyist
- Administrative or regulatory law
- Case law
- Civil law
- Tort
- Expert witness
- Negligence
- Malpractice
- *Respondeat superior*
- Licensure
- Alternative program
- Informed consent
- Privacy
- Confidentiality
- Delegation

The professions of law and nursing are both devoted to helping patients, clients, and society. A harmonious interaction between the areas of law and nursing is necessary for achieving effective outcomes for both the nurse and the patient. Nurses must understand how the legal system works in order to be safe and effective practitioners. The advanced state of medical technology creates new legal, ethical, moral, and financial problems for the consumer and the healthcare practitioner. Patients are more aware of their legal rights; hence, nurses must make a concerted effort to practice by the legal and professional standards set forth by federal and state entities.

Law serves as a guiding force for relationships between persons, persons and groups, and groups and other groups. Note the words *guiding* and *force*. For guidance to occur, law must be developed. For implementation to occur, the law must be enforced.

Law evolves by accommodating to changes in society while adhering to the basic principles set forth in a nation's guiding document, which in the United States is the Constitution. Principles set forth in the Constitution include freedom of religion and assembly, freedom from undue interference by government, and the right to trial by jury in criminal cases. Three sources of law are built on the fundamental law of the federal Constitution. They are statutory law, administrative law or regulatory law, and case law. It is important to note that federal law is administered the same in all states. However, each state may vary on how it interprets and implements laws. Hence, interpretation of legal issues for nurses varies from state to state.

Nursing and healthcare law set forth nursing and health policy goals. A nurse practice act has the goal of protecting the safety of the public who receive nursing care. Each state has statutes that govern the practice of nursing, while some differences exist from state to state, in general the nurse practice acts define who must be licensed, requirements for licensure, duties of the licensed nurse, and grounds on which the license may be revoked or taken away. This chapter discusses the three sources of law, nurse practice acts, delegation standards of care, civil procedures, and professional and legal accountability in nursing practice.

The Sources of Law

Statutory Law

In a democratic society such as the United States, the people elect representatives to governing bodies that consider proposed legislation. Each state and the federal government have a legislative body that is composed of two houses. The federal government has the House of Representatives and the Senate. Most state legislatures have similar names for their legislative bodies. Together the federal legislative body is termed Congress. Most state legislatures also have inclusive names for their legislative bodies; for example, the combination of two state bodies may carry a designation such as General Assembly.

Statutory law consists of ever-changing rules and regulations created by the US Congress, state legislators, local governments, and constitutional law. The statutes are the rights, privileges, or immunities secured and protected for each citizen by the U.S. Constitution (Fremgen, 2002).

The process of creating legislation is complex. The process may begin with a legislator responding to the interests of a group of persons. A legislator may also initiate action on a problem by convening a group of interested persons or other legislators to consider legislative options for resolving the problem. Interested persons or groups may represent specific concerns. Since the turn of the 21st century, nursing organizations such as the American Nurses Association (ANA) and the American Association of Colleges of Nursing (AACN) have focused on legislation addressing patient safety, such as specific staffing levels and controlling mandatory overtime. Such organized groups often hire lobbyists rather than relying on group members to promote their interests to legislators.

Lobbyists develop expertise on proposed legislation and learn to present that information to legislators clearly and concisely. Conscientious legislators and their staffs listen to both sides before voting on an issue. On a very important issue, however, organizations will also encourage their members to write letters supporting the organization's position or to make an appointment to speak with the legislator or talk with the legislator's staff.

Generally, no action will be taken on bills introduced to legislative bodies unless there is a confluence of problems, solutions, and political circumstances that create a climate for passing legislation (Longest, 2002). Many more bills are introduced into Congress and the state legislatures than are passed. Legislative action alone is insufficient for a bill to become law. Congressional bills require the president's signature, and state bills require the signature of the state's governor in order to be enacted into law. The president and state governors may also choose to veto legislation. This check on legislative power by the executive branch of government is part of the system of balances among the branches of government ensured by the nation's founders.

Administrative Law (Regulations)

Once a bill becomes law, that law is subject to further refinement by federal or state agencies, which are part of the executive branch of government. Enacted statutory law states what Congress or a state legislature wants to accomplish and what activities should occur in order to accomplish the legislative goal. Federal or state agencies carry out that activity by developing regulations that further define the law and establish the procedures for administering the law. For example, a state nurse practice act may provide that advanced practice nurses develop a formulary of medications they may prescribe. The process for developing the formulary will be done through the rule-making or regulatory process.

The regulatory process is itself governed by statutory law called administrative procedure acts at both federal and state levels. These acts provide that before regulations can be adopted a published notice of the proposed rules and where they are available must occur. The published notice and availability of the proposed rules provide concerned persons with the opportunity to comment on and suggest changes to the rules before final adoption. When rules are adopted they become administrative law within a set period of time. Thus, the process has three steps: (1) proposal of regulations, (2) consideration of proposed regulations, and (3) adoption of regulations with or without changes.

Staffs of executive branch agencies develop proposed regulations. In the case of federal regulations, notice of the proposed regulations is provided through a publication called the *Federal Register.* An example is Medicare regulations that describe conditions for healthcare facilities to receive reimbursement. This is a serious concern for hospitals because a high percentage of hospital revenue comes from Medicare reimbursement. Information on federal statutory and **administrative law** is available at http://thomas.loc.gov. Information on state law can be found at state Web sites. These can be accessed by entering terms such as *State of Ohio* or *State of California* in a search.

Case Law

Case law is established from court decisions, which may explain or interpret the other sources of law. For example, a court case may explain what the constitution, a statute, or a regulation means. Case law or common law also defines legal rights and obligations. For example, a nurse's obligation to practice as a reasonably prudent nurse is a legal obligation stemming from actual court decisions. Case law is based on precedent, meaning a ruling in one case that is then subsequently applied to later similar cases. When case law is applied, it must be reviewed by the court to determine if it is still relevant; hence, many case laws are changed and updated over the years. The prevailing ruler over case law is ultimately the state supreme court for state laws and the US Supreme Court for federal statutes. When the judicial branch of government becomes involved, it creates case law. The judicial branch of government is the third component of the balance of power in government at both federal and state levels.

Classification and Enforcement of the Law

When people choose not to follow the law, courts have the obligation to enforce the law. Enforcers of the law also include police and prosecutors. The justice department at the federal level and the attorney general's offices at the state level represent federal and state government interests. Judges are also enforcers of the law. In jury trials, they instruct jurors to apply the facts of a case to the law; in cases in which there is no jury, trial judges both examine the facts and apply the law.

Case law is both civil and criminal. Civil law involves relationships between individuals or between individuals and the government. Civil laws are divided into six categories: tort, contract, property, inheritance, family, and corporate law. Criminal law protects the public from the harmful acts of others.

Civil Law

Civil laws that commonly affect nurses include tort and contract laws. **Tort** law refers to acts that result in harm to another. Contract law includes enforceable agreements between two or more persons. A tort is a wrongful act that is committed against another person or property that results in harm.

To sue for a tort, a patient must have suffered a mental or physical injury that was caused by the nurse. Torts may be intentional or accidental and the patient may recover monetary damages. According to Fremgen (2002), intentional torts may include assault, battery, false imprisonment, defamation, fraud, and invasion of privacy:

- Assault—The threat of bodily harm to another. There does not have to be actual touching (battery) for an assault to take place. For example, threatening to harm a patient or to perform a procedure without the informed consent (permission) of the patient.
- Battery—Actual bodily harm to another person without permission. This is also referred to as unlawful touching or touching without consent. For example, performing surgery or a procedure without the informed consent (permission) of the patient.
- False imprisonment—A violation of the personal liberty of another person through unlawful restraint. For example, refusing to allow a patient to leave an office, hospital, or medical facility when they request to leave.
- Defamation of character—Damage caused to a person's reputation through spoken or written word. For example, making a negative statement about another nurse's ability.
- Fraud—Deceitful practice, such as promising a miracle cure.
- Invasion of privacy—The unauthorized publicity of information about a patient. For example, allowing personal information, such as test results for HIV, to become public without the patient's permission.

An **unintentional tort** usually occurs when the nurse does not act within the reasonable standards of nursing care. A "reasonable standard of care" means that the nurse must implement the type of care that a "reasonably prudent nurse would use in a similar circumstance." Oftentimes unintentional torts result from negligence. Negligence is the failure to perform professional duties to an accepted standard of care. Nurses should focus on preventing negligence rather than trying to defend it during a civil case.

The Trial Process for Civil Procedures

Nurses are most often involved in civil cases related to malpractice or negligence. The patient brings the case against the healthcare facility or nurse who becomes the defendant. If the defendant loses, the plaintiff receives monetary damages as compensation for the injury. For a civil case to be won, the judge or jury must find a preponderance of evidence for the winning side.

Nurses should have a basic understanding of the proceedings involved in a civil trial since this is the type of trial that involves the nursing profession. In a civil case, if the judge or jury finds in favor of the plaintiff, the defendant will be ordered to pay the plaintiff a monetary award. A plaintiff or defendant may appeal the decision to a higher court (Havinghurst, 1998). See Figure 12-1 for an illustration of a civil trial procedure.

Nurses as Expert Witnesses

Nurses with advanced degrees and clinical knowledge are often called as **expert witnesses** during civil trials. An expert witness has complex knowledge beyond the general knowledge of most people in the court or on the jury. Most nurses who testify as experts are called to testify as to what the "standard of care" for a patient is in a similar circumstance. Expert witnesses generally do not testify about the exact facts of the case, rather clarifying points of knowledge using charts, models, and diagrams.

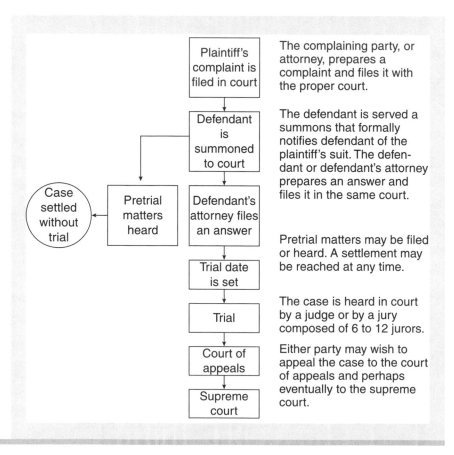

Figure 12-1

Procedure for a Civil Trial

Source: Adapted from *A Citizen's Guide to Washington Courts.* State Office of Administrator for the Courts, 1997.

Criminal Law

Criminal laws protect society from the harmful acts of others. Criminal acts are classified as felonies or misdemeanors. A felony carries a punishment of death or imprisonment in a state or federal facility. Felonies often involve murder, rape, robbery, or practicing without a license. Misdemeanors are less serious and may include theft, traffic violations, and disturbing the peace. A nurse's license may be revoked by the state board if he or she is convicted of a crime.

A nurse selling or stealing drugs results in a criminal case. In a criminal case, society is the plaintiff, and the nurse becomes the defendant. If the nurse defendant loses, the nurse will have restrictions placed on his or her liberty. Restrictions can include a prison term, probation, or treatment in lieu of conviction. In the last situation, the restriction is compliance with a drug treatment program that includes random drug testing. Failure to comply with the treatment program may result in a criminal punishment such as probation or even incarceration. Criminal cases have a higher standard of evidence. Juries must find the defendant guilty beyond a reasonable doubt. The US justice system is based on the premise that people are innocent until proven guilty. Because the plaintiff is claiming that the nurse violated the law, the burden of proof is placed upon the plaintiff to prove that the defendant is liable.

Boards of nursing also act as enforcers of the law when they discipline a nurse for violation of a provision of the law or rules of the state's nurse practice act. Boards use the preponderance-of-evidence standard.

> **CRITICAL THINKING QUESTION**
>
> What measures are taken when a nurse is summoned to court for a legal action? Is a nurse more responsible than a doctor in that situation if both were involved with the patient's care?

Malpractice and Negligence

The public generally has a very positive view of nurses. Nurses are expected to be of good moral and ethical character as the public has a great deal of trust for nurses. Furthermore, the privilege of obtaining a nursing license is often overlooked as an opportunity, and the right to practice nursing is frequently perceived as an "incidental entitlement" after completing a nursing education (Clevette, Erbin-Rosenmann, & Kelly, 2007). The nurturing aspect of nursing supports a "good will" profile with little, if any, intention of wrongdoing. However, when nurses fail to follow the standards of practice this may result in claims of malpractice or negligence.

What are standards? The ANA defines standards as "authoritative statements by which the nursing profession describes the responsibilities for which its practitioners are accountable" (American Nurses Association [ANA], 2004, p. 1). ANA standards of practice are broad and are formatted according to the steps of the nursing process, which is the critical thinking tool of nursing. The steps include assessment, diagnosis, outcomes identification, planning, implementation, and evaluation. The ANA elected to incorporate measurement criteria for each step of the process, thus making the measurement criteria part of the standard. The consistent themes of the measurement criteria permit determining whether the standards are met. They include culturally and ethnically sensitive care, maintaining a safe environment, education of patients, continuity of care, coordination of care, management of information, effective communication, and using technology. Carry out the steps of the nursing process, incorporating the application of the measurement criteria, and the standard of care will be met.

A legal nurse consultant or nurse expert scrutinizing a healthcare record at issue in a lawsuit can use these standards to determine whether there is reason to go forward with a malpractice suit. The nurse will also apply the more specialized and specific standards developed by specialty groups in nursing. For example, the Neonatal Nursing Association, the American Association of Women's Health and Obstetrical and Neonatal Nursing, and the American Association of Critical Care Nurses have their own standards. Standards come from other sources as well. A good example is the Blood-Borne Pathogen Standard promulgated by the Occupational Safety and Health Administration. This standard is an example of a standard for all healthcare providers, not just nurses. Standards evolve over time as practice incorporates research findings into practice.

Standards of practice are critical, but there are also standards that are expectations of a professional. Recognizing these expectations, the ANA elected to add professional performance standards to its 1991 standards document. These standards address quality of practice, education, professional practice evaluation, collegiality, collaboration, ethics, research, resource use, and leadership. Because standards of care evolve, one of the ANA's professional performance standards speaks directly to the nurse attaining knowledge and competency that reflects current nursing practice (ANA, 2004). Practice and professional standards may also appear in state practice acts and rules. The legal nurse consultant will expect that the nurses documenting in the medical record demonstrate current knowledge and competency based on general and specialized standards in their area of practice.

Most nurses are very familiar with the terms *negligence* and *malpractice*. What is the difference between malpractice and negligence?

Negligence is defined as the failure to act as a reasonably prudent person would have acted in a specific situation.

- **Negligence** is defined as the failure to act as a reasonably prudent person would have acted in a specific situation (Finkelman, 2006). For example, an elderly obese patient needs assistance ambulating to the bathroom. The patient tells the nurse that she feels "weak and dizzy." The nurse assists the patient to the bathroom without additional assistance. The patient falls and fractures her femur. The nurse may be liable for this injury because he or she failed to ambulate the client with the proper assistance.

■ **Malpractice** is the failure of a professional to use such care as a reasonably prudent member of the profession would use under similar circumstances, which leads to harm. For example, a nurse administers an intravenous dose of 0.5 mg Lanoxin. The patient informs the nurse that she is nauseated, weak, and has blurred vision. The nurse failed to check the patient's Lanoxin level prior to administering the daily dose. The patient's pulse drops to 20 beats per minute followed by a full cardiac arrest. Upon inspection of the patient's daily lab work for the digoxin level, the nurse discovers that the client had digitalis toxicity. The client expired the following day.

> Malpractice is the failure of a professional to use such care as a reasonably prudent member of the profession would use under similar circumstances, which leads to harm.

Nurses can be both negligent and guilty of malpractice. According to Finkelman (2006), in order to prove negligence or malpractice the following four elements must be met:

■ There was a duty owed to the patient.
■ There was a breach of duty or standard by the healthcare professional.
■ There was harm caused by the breach of duty or standard.
■ The person (plaintiff) experienced damages or injuries.

Some examples of potential risks for nurses are failure to adequately assess, monitor, and communicate; failure to act as a patient's advocate (for example, not providing proper education for a client with congestive heart failure); or failure to protect the patient when suicidal or at risk for falls. All nurses need to consider these risks when caring for patients.

A question that often comes up with nurses is who is ultimately responsible for the malpractice or negligence: the nurse or the employing institution? *Respondeat superior* is the doctrine that indicates the employer may also be responsible if the nurse was functioning in the employee role at the time of the incident (Grossman, 2005). This implies that both the healthcare organization and the nurse can be sued.

The US Department of Health and Human Services (2003) conducted a study to determine the types of malpractice acts commonly reported to the National Practitioners Data Bank. The results of the study indicated about 1 out of 50 malpractice reports are made for nurses. The report is publicly available at www.npdbhipdb.com. The nursing specializations included in this study were RNs, nurse anesthetist, nurse midwife, nurse practitioner, advanced practice nurse, and LVN/LPN (Bolin, 2005). The types of malpractice codes reported are listed in Table 12-1.

Can a nurse be brought to court for negligence? Yes. A finding of negligence occurs when the nurse owes a duty to a patient and breaches an ordinary standard of care known by laypersons, and the patient is harmed. An example would be the nurse leaving the side rail down on the bed of a 2-month-old infant. An ordinary person

---

TABLE 12-1   MALPRACTICE ACT OR OMISSION CODES

Diagnosis: Failure, wrong, improper performance, unnecessary, delay, lack of informed consent

Anesthesia: Failure to properly assess, monitor, test, and use equipment, improper choice, intubation, positioning, and failure to obtain informed consent

Surgery: Failure to perform, improper positioning, foreign body, wrong body part, improper performance, unnecessary surgery, delay, improper management, and lack of informed consent

Medication: Wrong med, dosage, improper administration, improper technique, and lack of informed consent

IV and Blood: Failure to monitor, wrong solution, wrong type, improper administration and management

Obstetrics: Improper delivery, delay in delivery, failure to properly manage, delay, abandonment

Treatment: Wrong treatment, improper instruction, improper performance, failure to supervise, failure to refer or seek consult

Monitoring: Failure to monitor, failure to respond and report

Equipment/Product: Improper maintenance, improper use, failure to instruct patient, malfunction or failure

Miscellaneous: Breach of confidentiality, injury to third parties, improper behavior, breach of institutional policies

Source: US Department of Health and Human Services, 2003.

---

would know that leaving the side rail down was unsafe. Findings of either malpractice or negligence result in the nurse being liable to compensate the harmed person. A malpractice lawsuit requires an expert witness, and a negligence lawsuit does not.

Nurses are rarely individually sued. Malpractice insurance of the facility for which the nurse works will most often cover damages. Nurses, however, can and should purchase malpractice insurance to avoid the risk of losing their personal assets. The nurse might be in a situation in which he or she is viewed as practicing as a nurse and harm occurs. An example might be poor advice given to a friend in failing to recommend further assessment by a healthcare provider when a child is injured in a fall.

Malpractice and negligence are not intentional actions or inactions. They are careless actions or inactions that are more likely to occur in stressful circumstances or because the nurse has not maintained knowledge and competency in an area of practice. Montgomery (2007) examined basic principles of human error and sleep physiology and evaluated the evidence for potential effects of fatigued healthcare workers and workload on medical errors. The researchers conducted the study in a pediatric intensive care unit, which is a highly complex environment in which fatigue and excessive workload may allow errors to occur. The results indicated that nursing fatigue and workload have documented effects on increasing intensive care unit error, infections, and cost. Specific environmental factors such as distractions and communication barriers were also associated with greater error. The researchers concluded that fatigue, excessive workload, and the pediatric intensive care environment could adversely affect the performance of physicians and nurses working in this type of setting. Castledine (2006) reviewed a nursing negligence case in which a registered nurse with 6 months experience performed a bladder irrigation using a can of cola. The patient suffered major distress and the nurse was reported to the board of nursing for breach of the code of professional conduct and negligence. The nurse claimed that she thought the cola would break down the "debris" in the bladder. Obviously, this nurse did not follow professional standards of practice relating to bladder irrigation. Due to her inexperience and lack of knowledge the nurse was only required to receive additional education and support. Nurses must be accountable for their actions while providing patient care. The nurse has a duty to practice competently and possess knowledge, skills, and abilities required for lawful, safe, and effective practice.

Murphy (2004) examined a case (*Logsdon v. Miller*) in which the plaintiff developed reflex sympathetic dystrophy in her left arm and hand after a 7-hour reconstructive jaw surgery in 1999. The circulating nurse positioned, supported, and padded the plaintiff. Postoperatively, the plaintiff woke with numbness and pain in her left arm. The plaintiff suffered permanent nerve damage and sued the physician and the nurse's employer hospital alleging negligence for failure to properly position the patient. The court ruled that the nurse was not liable because she had followed the appropriate standard of care in positioning the patient. These cases indicate that all nurses need to comply with the guidelines and standards of nursing practice.

> **CRITICAL THINKING QUESTION**
>
> What does "reasonable and prudent" mean as it relates to standards of care?

Prevention requires learning how to manage stress and adhering to current standards of care. Nurses should learn to leave their personal life stresses at the door of their workplace. They should resist the temptation to self-medicate their stresses with alcohol or other drugs. When they find themselves doing so, they should seek help before their professional practice is affected.

Nurses should also seek to practice in work environments that encourage examination of incidents that may have caused or do cause harm to patients. Often, systems in which the nurse works can be changed to make the environment safer for nurses and patients. Changing systems to lower the risk of malpractice has been recommended in several reports from the Institute of Medicine (IOM). These include *To Err Is Human: Building a Safer Health System, Crossing the Quality Chasm: A New Health System for the 21st Century,* and *Keeping Patients Safe: Transforming the Work Environment of Nurses* (Institute of Medicine, 2000, 2001, 2004).

CRITICAL THINKING QUESTION

You have been asked by a charge nurse on a medical surgical unit to discuss the importance of the legal system for nurses. What are the important aspects regarding law and nursing that you will include in your presentation?

In addition the IOM has released a report entitled *Informing the Future: Critical Issues in Health* that addresses quality of patient care in the United States (Institute of Medicine, 2007). Changing systems is not the sole solution. Patterns of substandard practice still require the facility to either help the nurse improve practice or make a complaint to the state board of nursing so that disciplinary action can remove the nurse from being in a position to harm patients either through revocation, suspension, or a monitored practice improvement program.

Nursing Licensure

History of Licensure

Nursing has evolved on a track parallel with other healthcare providers. The education of nurses particularly parallels that of medicine. Both disciplines first experienced apprenticeship education followed by gradual evolution to education within educational institutions. Even today, a critical piece of this education remains the opportunity for clinical practice in healthcare facilities. Increasingly, however, understanding of human physiology has been refined to examination at the cellular and molecular levels. Advances in diagnostic and treatment technology have also occurred. These changes have bred the need for an increasing knowledge base at both the foundational and specialization levels of education in both medicine and nursing (Kalisch & Kalisch, 1995).

Licensure was not always a requirement for nursing practice. In fact, the acknowledged founder of modern nursing, Florence Nightingale, did not believe nurses should have recognition by a government body (Kalisch & Kalisch, 1995). Both medicine and nursing eventually thought otherwise. An increasing knowledge base led to increasing risk for patients. Evidence of a basic education with recognized components led to nurses first being registered and later being licensed. The term *registered nurse* is of historical vintage. The use of the term reflects the period of permissive licensure for nurses. Permissive licensure meant anyone could practice nursing, but only a person with a recognized foundation of nursing education could use the title "registered nurse." During this time, which in some states spanned the 60 years from the first to the sixth decade of the 1900s, the education of nurses primarily took place within hospital schools of nursing. Because hospitals were not recognized as institutions of higher learning, state licensure boards set the standards for nursing education. This involvement for boards of nursing remains true today despite the advent of accreditation bodies for nursing education. One reason for continued involvement is a lack of accreditation for practical nursing programs or simply practical nursing programs' reluctance to seek accreditation, often because of lack of funds.

The advent of practical nursing education (known as vocational nursing in some states) was also the reason for the change from permissive to mandatory licensure. Permissive licensure provides for title recognition. Mandatory licensure provides for a scope of practice. Two levels of nursing practice necessitated defining a scope of practice. Today there are also advanced practice nurses who have specified scopes of practice under the titles of nurse practitioner, nurse midwife, nurse anesthetist, and clinical specialist.

Nursing licensure boards contrast with medical boards in licensing or certifying at multiple levels rather than a single basic level. In medicine, board certification is obtained by passing a professional examination that then allows a physician to practice in a specialty area. There is only one level of licensure. Nurse licensure boards require passing a certification exam generated by a recognized nursing professional organization prior to nurses with master's degrees in that area being recognized as advanced practice nurses.

Nurses initially licensed in one state can acquire licensure in another state through a process called endorsement. Endorsement requires verification that the nurse's license has not been disciplined in another state. Previous discipline may or may not preclude licensure by endorsement depending on the circumstances of the discipline. The nurse seeking endorsement will also have to meet licensure requirements in the endorsing state. Criminal background checks and continuing education requirements are two examples of requirements.

In the late 1990s, the National Council of State Boards of Nursing developed the Nurse Licensure Compact. The compact is a statutory agreement between and among states to permit nurses who are residents of one state to have the privilege of practice in another state without acquiring a license in the second state. The nurse does become subject to the provisions of the law and rules of the second state. In this respect, compact state nurses enjoy the same privileges provided by a state driver's license. Drivers in one state can travel through others subject to the vehicular laws of other states. If, however, the driver becomes a resident of another state, the driver must obtain a license in that state. In the case of the compact, until all states adopt the compact, the nurse will have to determine whether the state in which he or she seeks to practice requires licensure by endorsement or is a member of the compact along with the nurse's current state of licensure. A major advantage of the compact is the facilitation of practice in border areas of states.

The National Council of State Boards of Nursing (2007) generates the initial licensure exam for both the licensed practical nurse and registered nurse. Initial licensure measures competence at a minimal level to ensure safe practice. Clearly, the changing nature of practice demands acquisition of knowledge consistent with continuing competence. The content of the NCLEX-RN test plan is organized into four major client needs categories: safe and effective care environment, health promotion and maintenance, psychosocial integrity, and physiological integrity.

The category that relates to legal aspects of nursing is found primarily under the category of safe and effective care. The related content includes:

- Advance directive
- Advocacy
- Client rights
- Collaboration with interdisciplinary team
- Confidentiality and information security
- Delegation
- Ethical practice
- Informed consent
- Legal rights and responsibilities

Although continuing education has never been clearly demonstrated to be evidence of continuing competence in nursing, many states require continuing education for licensure renewal. It is argued that conscientious nurses would undertake continuing education voluntarily, and mandatory continuing education adds only reluctant nurses to program attendance with perhaps little impact on the reluctant nurses' competence (Hall, 1996). Current competence is also of concern for nurses reentering practice. Mandatory refresher courses seem desirable but have the drawback of high cost for persons who may be reentering practice for economic reasons. Ideally, the burden of maintaining competence rests with the nurse and the nurse's workplace. The workplace should provide and support opportunities for gaining new knowledge and determine its application in practice.

The state boards of nursing possess all the information related to the nurses licensed within their state through the nursing application process, thus providing a convenient database of information that could be studied. The general areas identified in the nursing licensure discipline literature were age, education, gender, nursing experience, and areas of practice concern. Overall, an experienced middle-aged registered staff nurse with an associate's degree who has recently changed jobs is profiled as the practicing nurse who will commit an error that will likely result in nursing board discipline (Green, Fitzpatrick, & Waddil, 1994). The nurses' lack of knowledge regarding the nursing role, including the components of ethics and theory, could be a result of their minimal level of educational preparation and also potentially explain the increased frequency of associate-degree nurses receiving discipline (Delgado, 2002). Registered nurses with an associate's degree constitute a large proportion of employed registered nurses. Preliminary findings in the 2004 National Sample of Registered Nurses revealed 42.2% of employed registered nurses had associate's degrees (US DHHS Health Resources and Services Administration, 2004). Data reviewed from available profiles in Arizona, Colorado, Louisiana, New York, Ohio, Tennessee, and Texas revealed that males are disciplined more than females. Additionally, several general areas of nursing practice concern were acknowledged, with chemical dependency, substance abuse, and records management most prevalent.

The Function of Boards of Nursing

Composition and Role of Boards

The statutory law governing nursing practice in all states and territories of the United States is known as the Nurse Practice Act. Boards of nursing are the state or territorial agencies that administer the law. Members of boards of nursing represent various types of nursing expertise and various geographic areas within the state or territory. A recent trend has been for boards to include consumer members to represent the public. Board members are generally appointed by the governor of the state or territory.

The overriding obligation of all board members is to protect the safety of the public by initially and continuously licensing only competent nurses. Board members direct the activities of the agency through providing direction to the executive director of the board, who in turn directs the activities of board staff. Board staffs may be as small as 2 or as many as 50 or more, depending on the number of licensees in the state or territory. Boards set standards of practice and delegation and often standards for nursing education through the rule-making process. Other board rules govern the disciplinary process and programs such as alternative programs for drug and alcohol abuse and practice intervention improvement.

Boards meet at regularly scheduled intervals during the year to act on disciplinary matters, approve nursing education programs, and review and update the nurse practice act and regulations governing practice as nursing practice evolves. A trend among nursing boards has been to assume the legal oversight of other types of healthcare providers as well. These include nursing assistants, dialysis technicians, community health workers, and medication technicians.

Discipline of Nurses

In legal terms, licensure is a privilege not a right. Not surprisingly, a privilege can be withdrawn or withheld from a person if the behavior of the person does not merit the privilege. Thus, a board of nursing holds legal authority to discipline a nurse who holds a license or to act to withhold licensure from a person seeking initial licensure within a state or territory.

In recent years, boards of nursing have moved to bar from initial licensure persons who have been convicted of, who have plead guilty to, or who had a judicial finding of guilt for felonies involving potential or actual physical harm to persons. Examples of such felonies include murder, robbery, kidnapping, rape, sexual battery, or sexual imposition. Because a large proportion of board disciplinary actions is related to alcohol and substance abuse, boards are concerned about previous histories of drug abuse and drug treatment. Uncontrolled psychiatric illness is also often associated with incompetent practice and substance abuse. Persons seeking initial licensure in a state with a history of drug-related and psychiatric health problems may be allowed to practice but are required to enter into an agreement to be monitored for a period of time under a set of prescribed conditions to ensure that they are safe practitioners. The monitoring would not constitute a disciplinary action. However, if monitoring conditions are violated or the person's practice is unsafe, the board may consider the full range of disciplinary actions. According to Clevette, Erbin-Rosenmann, and Kelly (2007), common disciplinary categories reviewed by boards of nursing include:

- Substandard nursing practice not involving medications including verbal abuse, using force to administer medications, or failing to respond to changes in patient condition
- Destruction or alteration of patient records including fraudulent charting and/or signatures and/or replacement of records with intent to mislead or deceive
- Physical patient abuse, such as when a nurse hits, strikes, or performs similar physical acts of aggression involving physical contact
- Failure to follow policy such as violation of an employer's policy statements
- Medication "errors," including inaccurate documentation, discarding meds and charting them as given, wrong dosages, wrong route, wrong time, and/or incorrect medication technique
- Controlled substance violations or chemical dependency including diversion of drugs from facility or patient for self-use or sale, prescription fraud, doctor-shopping to obtain prescriptions, or practicing under the influence
- Impaired mental or physical competency. For example, practice is negatively impacted by mental or physical incapacity
- Inappropriate management decision such as when a supervisor or manager makes a decision contrary to acceptable nursing standards such as permitting practice without a license
- Practice beyond the authorized scope such as administering medications without a physician's order
- Sexual misconduct including nurse and client communication or contact of a sexual nature or convictions related to sexual misconduct not with clients but related to the practice of nursing
- Patient or employer abandonment such as leaving or not arriving for a patient care assignment
- Unethical actions with a rational relationship to nursing practice, including actions not directly related to nursing care such as falsification of licensure or employment applications, diversion of third-party payments, embezzlement, or distribution of a controlled substance
- Actions demonstrating poor judgment, including irrational behavior not described under the other categories

Boards of nursing have a number of disciplinary choices: denying a license, imposing a fine, issuing a reprimand, placing restrictions on a license, and suspending or revoking a license. Boards must follow a designated process before taking action against a license. First, the board must receive a complaint. Complaints are investigated by board staff. If board staff concludes that the evidence merits action against the nurse's license, a consent agreement may be offered. This procedure is a disciplinary action that bypasses the hearing process, and the nurse agrees to conditions placed on her license. An example would be a period of suspension with random drug testing and treatment for drug abuse. Compliance with the agreement would lead to returning to practice with a person in the workplace assigned to report on the nurse's practice at regular intervals. The nurse might also be expected to provide evidence of attendance at a support group for persons with addictions. Consent agreements must be approved by the state's board of nursing before being implemented.

In the absence of a consent agreement, the nurse receives a notice of opportunity for a hearing. When a timely response requesting a hearing is not received, the board members decide the disciplinary action at a subsequent board meeting. Hearings may be conducted by a board or a hearing examiner. In both instances, board members must make the final decision with respect to action against a nursing license.

Reasons for disciplinary action are described in the nurse practice act. Some common examples include conviction of a misdemeanor in the course of practice, conviction of any felony, self-administering a prescription medication without a prescription, impairment of ability to practice safely because of habitual or excessive use of drugs or alcohol, and assaulting or causing harm to a patient. Nurses working in long-term care and home health are at risk for violations of the practice act such as theft and crossing professional boundaries, often resulting in sexual offenses (Driscoll, 2004).

Alternative Programs for Nurses

In many states, an **alternative program** for persons with drug and alcohol addictions exists. Nurses must qualify for the program. A criterion is likely to be that the nurse turns herself in to the board because the nurse recognizes the addiction and no person or facility has made a complaint to the board. These programs grew as addiction became viewed as a disease resulting in calls for state boards and nurse employers to provide support for the addicted nurse (Caroselli-Karinja & Zboray, 1986; Daniel, 1984). Successful completion of a monitoring program results in no disciplinary action by a board. The nurse's license remains unscathed. Data from these programs are emerging. Haack and Yocom (2002) found similar rates of relapse in a 6-month period after admission to both alternative and disciplinary programs, although disciplinary action was more likely with criminal convictions, and those persons were less likely to be employed or hold an active license. Although not generalizeable, the study does provide support for the rehabilitative approach provided by the alternative program.

Other data come from Trinkoff and Storr (1998), who addressed substance use among nurses and found choice of substance varied by specialty in the population they studied. Emergency nurses were more likely to choose marijuana and cocaine. Oncology nurses and nurses in administrative positions were more likely to binge drink. Psychiatric nurses were more likely to smoke. Another study found that among nurses their greatest dependence was on tobacco and caffeine. The same study reported a greater percentage of never-married nurses used marijuana and cocaine (Collins, Gollnisch, & Morshemier, 1999). Storr, Trinkoff, and Anthony (1999) found that high-strain jobs were more likely to result in nonmedical drug use. Using legal drugs inappropriately and using illegal drugs set the stage for violations of the practice act. With substance use remaining the leading cause of disciplinary action for boards of nursing, prevention appears the key to reduction. Following public health principles of education as an early intervention is most likely a major key to providing a safe environment for patients.

> **CRITICAL THINKING QUESTION**
>
> What are the differences between nursing disciplinary action by a board of nursing and legal ramifications set forth by state and federal laws?

Intervention programs as an alternative to discipline are not limited to substance abuse. Practice intervention improvement programs are also emerging as an alternative to discipline.

Professional Accountability: Informed Consent, Privacy and Confidentiality, and Delegation

Informed Consent

Informed consent "mandates to the physician or independent healthcare practitioner the separate legal duty to disclose needed material facts in terms that patients can reasonably understand so that they can make an informed choice" (Guido, 2001, p. 129). The practitioner is required to inform the patient who will perform the procedure or treatment, discuss available alternatives to the recommended treatment, and identify possible complications of the procedure in terms that the patient can understand.

Informed consent is more than simply getting a patient to sign a written consent form.

The AMA (2007) states that informed consent is more than simply getting a patient to sign a written consent form. It is a process of communication between a patient and physician that results in the patient's authorization or agreement to undergo a specific medical intervention.

In the communications process, the physician providing or performing the treatment and/or procedure (not a delegated representative), should disclose and discuss with the patient:

- The patient's diagnosis, if known
- The nature and purpose of a proposed treatment or procedure

- The risks and benefits of a proposed treatment or procedure
- Alternatives (regardless of their cost or the extent to which the treatment options are covered by health insurance)
- The risks and benefits of the alternative treatment or procedure
- The risks and benefits of not receiving or undergoing a treatment or procedure

This communication process is both an ethical obligation and a legal requirement spelled out in statutes and case law in all 50 states.

Informed consent cases are a type of malpractice suit. An informed consent case can be brought by a patient when a risk of a procedure occurs that should have been divulged but was not or alternatives to the procedure were not provided that the patient would have chosen had he or she known the particular risk. Informed consent cases arise with invasive procedures and complicated treatment regimens such as those for cancer. Central to informed consent is ensuring that the patient is capable of comprehending the information; otherwise, the consent is invalid.

Information components of informed consent include explanation by the physician of the nature of the procedure, its risks, its benefits, and alternatives to the procedure, including the risks and benefits of the alternatives. The information to be provided is generally described as what is material to the patient's decision to go forward with the procedure, decline the procedure, or select an alternative to the proposed procedure. Material risks are expected serious risks such as death, hemorrhage, infection, or any other risk that would seriously compromise the functioning of a person, such as a stroke or paralysis. Failure to meet these standards of disclosure puts the physician at risk for a malpractice suit resulting from failure to provide informed consent if the undisclosed risk occurs and the patient is harmed (*Nickell v. Gonzalez*, 1985). In a leading case that helped establish this type of malpractice suit, the physician did not inform the patient of the risk of paralysis with back surgery (*Canterbury v. Spence*, 1972). In an Ohio case, a patient's incapability to express himself because of temporary aphasia led to the signing of a consent form for a procedure that in his individual case put him at high risk for a stroke, and a stroke occurred (*Greynolds v. Kurman*, 1993). In a California case (*Truman v. Thomas*, 1980), a physician was sued for failing to warn the patient of the risks of not consenting to a diagnostic test.

The standards used for determining whether consent information is sufficient vary from state to state. The first is the medical standard—what are regarded as material risks in the medical community. The second is what a reasonable patient would need to know. The third is what a particular patient needs to know. The first errs in favor of the medical community. The second is considered objective because it provides a standard favoring the patient community. The third is clearly subjective and essentially leaves physicians in the dark as to what information to give patients.

Is there a role for nurses when informed consent is required? There is an advocacy role. When a nurse obtains a signature on a hospital or ambulatory facility consent form, that interaction provides an opportunity to ascertain whether the patient has questions about a procedure. When a conversation reveals that the patient has misconceptions about the procedure or its risks and benefits, the nurse should contact the physician so that additional communication regarding the procedure can occur. The advocacy role of the nurse in this situation is not a legally defined role. It falls in the realm of professional performance standards and a code of ethics responsibility to collaborate with other healthcare providers and the patient to ensure appropriate care. The legal role of the nurse in this situation is acting as a witness to the patient's signature.

> **CRITICAL THINKING QUESTION**
>
> Are there differences in the responsibility related to informed consent for the nurse and physician. If so, what are the differences?

Privacy and Confidentiality

Privacy is the right of a person to be free from unwanted intrusion into the person's personal affairs. To receive appropriate health care, however, a person often must disclose very personal information. Sexual activity and acknowledgment of alcohol or drug abuse are examples of such personal information. Because of the stigma attached to mental illness, patients may also be reluctant to disclose a family or personal history of mental illness. To fulfill their social contract to provide nursing care, nurses must often gather such sensitive information from patients. Thus, the nurse, along with other caregivers, has the obligation to keep healthcare information confidential. Privacy is the right of the patient. **Confidentiality** is the obligation of all healthcare providers.

The *Code of Ethics for Nurses* addresses privacy and confidentiality under provision 3, "The nurse promotes, advocates for, and strives to protect the health, safety, and rights of the patient" (ANA, 2001). Rules of boards of nursing may also spell out the nurse's duty of confidentiality.

In 2000, final federal rules protecting patient privacy were issued. The rules affect health plans, healthcare clearinghouses, and healthcare providers who engage in electronic transactions. The rules were a response to concerns that patient privacy would be compromised without legal standards for the scope of information that could be shared. The rules required all of these groups (called entities) to be in compliance with the rules by April 14, 2003, with the exception of small health plans. The small health plan compliance date was April 14, 2004. The rules were promulgated by the Department of Health and Human Services under provisions of the Health Insurance Portability and Accountability Act (HIPAA) of 1996.

The rules assure patients that only necessary information will be shared with groups such as insurers and third-party intermediaries who administer insurance plans by engaging in functions such as claims processing and membership tracking. The rules also ensure access to patient records by patients themselves, although a reasonable period of time may be needed to copy those records, and the patient may be charged for the cost of copying and sending records. The rules prohibit patient information from being shared for marketing purposes without the patient's consent. The rules require employee training on the provisions of the rules for employees of all healthcare employers.

HIPAA protection of patient privacy highlights the traditional value placed on patient privacy by the healthcare professions. Nurses should remember that conversations in healthcare facilities about patients should occur only among healthcare providers. Elevators and cafeterias are not appropriate sites for such discussions. Pictures of patients and specific healthcare information should be shared with family members only with the express permission of the patient. Generally, medical records cannot be sent to anyone without written consent except when the record is subpoenaed.

Each nurse needs to be aware of and follow the policies and procedures related to oral, written, or electronic patient-identifiable data set up by the healthcare organization regarding issues where the nurse practices; however, there are some key areas that are affected by these new privacy regulations:

- Patients must be informed of their privacy rights.
- Patients must be informed as to who will see their records and for what purpose.
- Patients have the right to inspect and obtain a copy of their medical records. (There are some exceptions to this that each organization should make clear to staff.)
- Valid authorization to release health information must contain certain information, such as a copy of the signed authorization given to the patient, in understandable language, and how the patient may revoke authorization.
- Although information may be used for research purposes to assess outbreak of a disease, all individual identifiable data must be removed.
- Personal data may not be used for marketing (for example, pharmacies may not share this information with others for this purpose) (Finkelman, 2006).

Delegation

Today, nurses face many work-related issues, such as the nursing shortage, the increasing need for services, and constant changes within the environment and government. "In an effort to reduce labor costs by decreasing registered nurse positions, hospitals have increasingly turned to a new kind of healthcare worker, unlicensed assistive personnel (UAP)" (Kleinman & Saccomano, 2006, p. 164). The use of UAPs helps fill the chasm caused by the nursing shortage and helps decrease the cost of patient care. However, in the past, "nurses were educated in practice settings where the model of care was primary nursing or a similar model in which the registered nurses were responsible for most of the direct care needs of the patients" (Kleinman & Saccomano, 2006, p. 166). Therefore, many nurses are not familiar with how to delegate tasks to UAPs because they were not taught these skills. Thus, legal **delegation** has become an increasing challenge for registered nurses (RNs).

As licensed professionals, RNs are responsible to the community for providing safe, competent, and effective care for patients in a variety of healthcare settings. In each setting, RNs work beside other licensed professionals and assign and delegate tasks to these other licensed professionals in order to give efficient care to patients. Additionally, RNs remain accountable or answerable for patient outcomes and are responsible for supervising delegated tasks. The American Nurses Association (ANA) and the National Council of State Boards of Nursing (NCSBN) define delegation as "the process for a nurse to direct another person to perform nursing tasks and activities" (National Council of State Boards of Nursing, 2006, p. 1). Delegation may be direct (i.e., verbal instructions) or indirect (i.e., tasks verified by hospital policy) in the healthcare setting (Trappen, Weiss, & Whitehead, 2004). The RN or nurse manager judges which staff member is competent to perform an assigned duty; however, permitted tasks may depend upon the organization or institution.

RNs remain accountable or answerable for patient outcomes and are responsible for supervising delegated tasks.

In terms of accountability, nurses must take responsibility for their actions and the actions of others involved in the delegation process. When allegations of unethical, illegal, and inappropriate conduct occur, nurses "must answer to patients, nursing employers, the board of nursing, and the civil and criminal court system when the quality of patient care provided is compromised" (American Nurses Association (ANA), 2005, p. 4). Therefore, it is important for RNs and nurse managers to be knowledgeable of the delegation guidelines within each state's nurse practice act, job descriptions, and the scope of practice of all personnel.

Delegation is part of the language of management. Work may be within the job description of a healthcare worker, but this does not automatically make delegation of a particular task appropriate. The nurse making an assignment is acting as a manager of care. The nurse must carefully select the person to whom a task is assigned because ultimately the nurse as manager is accountable for whether the task is accomplished and whether the desired outcome is achieved. Complete independence in caring for a complex critical care patient would not be an appropriate assignment for a newly licensed registered nurse. Licensed practical nurses cannot shoulder complete responsibility for acting on assessment of a newly admitted patient. Unlicensed assistive personnel may take blood pressures, but they should do so with clear parameters established for communicating deviance from those parameters.

Certain activities cannot be delegated. An advanced practice nurse may delegate the drawing of blood to a nursing assistant but cannot delegate the decision for the types of lab tests to be performed (ANA, 2004). Only the advanced practice nurse can make the judgment as to what tests are necessary. Furthermore, the advanced practice nurse could not delegate the blood draw to a nursing assistant if the nursing assistant had not learned the proper technique for drawing blood and had not received sufficient supervision in carrying out the procedure to determine the nursing assistant's competence.

Unlicensed assistive personnel cannot delegate a task delegated to them by a nurse because that would be engaging in the practice of nursing without a license. Similarly, a nurse cannot delegate a task if the nurse does not know how to do the task. That would be delegating beyond the nurse's scope of practice.

The nurse delegating any task must provide supervision to the unlicensed person. This means determining the competence of the person to carry out the task properly. If the unlicensed person does not properly carry out the task, the unlicensed person should not again be delegated the task until further education ensures that the person has reached a level of competence. Demonstrated competence does not eliminate the supervisory role.

The five rights of delegation as outlined by the National Council of State Boards of Nursing in 2006 are as follows:

- The right task—One that is delegable for a specific patient
- The right circumstances—An appropriate patient setting, available resources, and consideration of other relevant factors
- The right person—The right person is delegating the right task to the right person to be performed on the right person
- The right direction and communication—A clear, concise description of the task, including objectives, limits, and expectations
- The right supervision and evaluation—Appropriate monitoring, intervention, and as needed, feedback

Keeping this rights mantra in mind will help the nurse to delegate care according to the legal standard of acting as a reasonable prudent nurse would do in similar circumstances. However, authority to delegate varies, so licensed nurses must check the jurisdiction's statutes and regulations. RNs may need to delegate to the LPN the authority to delegate to the UAP.

Barriers to Delegation

Nurses face many challenges when trying to delegate to others. Contributing factors leading to delegation barriers "range from not having had educational opportunities to learn how to work with others effectively to not knowing the skill level and abilities of nursing assistive personnel to simplify the work pace and turnover of patients" (National Council of State Boards of Nursing (NCSBN), 2006, p. 4). Also, the scope of the nursing practice is changing and the tasks performed by UAPs are increasing in complexity. This may make many nurses apprehensive in delegating tasks because of a fear of endangering their own licensure. Plus, due to the nursing shortage, many inexperienced nurses are being placed at the helm. Thus, many nurses are not knowledgeable of how to communicate effectively and how to use the institution's resources efficiently. Ultimately, barriers that lead to ineffective delegation place a strain on the quality of patient care.

In 2005, Kalisch conducted a qualitative study to examine the care missed on medical-surgical units. By interviewing 107 RNs, 15 LPNs, and 51 nursing assistants (NAs) from two hospitals in the United States, Kalisch (2006) found that the following activities were frequently missed: "ambulation, turning, feedings, patient teaching, discharge planning, emotional support, hygiene, intake and out-put documentation, and surveillance" (p. 307). There were several contributing factors as to why hospital employees missed these important measures; however, ineffective delegation was cited as one of the major factors. Kalisch (2006) discovered that many NAs were not present during routine nursing reports, and neither did the nurses report to the NAs. "Even when NAs received report, there was a lack of collaborative planning for patient care" (Kalisch, 2006, p. 310). Therefore, lack of communication may have been a problem.

Also, many nurses had difficulty retaining accountability. "Many nurses considered the work delegated to NAs as no longer the RN's responsibility" (Kalisch, 2006, p. 310). This is a major misconception, because the nurse remains accountable for the care given to the patient. Another problem was that many staff members did not feel that it was their job to perform a particular task. "Nurses stated that certain tasks such as vital signs were the NA's responsibility, and if the NA did not complete these tasks, it was the 'fault' of the NA, not the RN" (Kalisch, 2006, p. 310). State nurse practice acts define the scope of practice and what nurses can delegate. Also, hospitals and institutions have policies and procedure that help define which tasks can be delegated.

Kalisch (2006) also cited that many nurses had difficulty with conflict management. "Many nurses reported limited authority and influence over the NAs and expressed reluctance to confront NAs who did not 'do their job' (Kalisch, 2006, p. 310). In several cases, staff members tried to avoid confrontation and had difficulty engaging in conflict management to strive for a solution. "If delegates are resistant, the delegator may simply choose to do the task him or herself to avoid confrontations; instead, the situation should be reevaluated from the UAP's point of view" (Quallich, 2005, p. 122). In some cases, a UAP may lack the confidence or knowledge to perform a task; however, if a UAP refuses to perform a task due to defying authority, guidelines for delegation should be clearly reinstituted. Also, if a nurse lacks confidence and does not trust the abilities of other staff members, delegation is unlikely to occur. "Similarly, delegation will be unsuccessful if the only tasks that are delegated are those that are time-consuming or unpleasant; this approach risks exhausting staff that are otherwise capable" (Quallich, 2005, p. 122).

Regardless of the institution, delegation has a strict chain of command among employees. Nurses sometimes may experience feelings of guilt among those that they delegate tasks to. The RN also may worry about being labeled as lazy when delegating a task to other employees. "But working in an organizational hierarchy should not result in the delegator taking on disproportionate amounts of responsibility in order to respect the feelings of other delegatees" (Quallich, 2005, p. 122).

Some nurses may also feel that they should show loyalty to other nurses and should only delegate to student and graduate nurses. However, this loyalty or discrimination is not cost-efficient and only acts as another delegation barrier. Plus, if a nurse refuses to delegate a task as instructed by the employer, the nurse may face disciplinary actions by the employer (Hauslaer & Jones, 2003). If a nurse has concerns regarding the implementation of a task or activity, it is important to document concerns for patient safety and to inform the employer. After the staff becomes comfortable with their skill at delegation, the next challenge is making sure they have the skills necessary to assess the competence of their UAP for individual tasks.

Delegation Decision-Making Tree

In 1997, the National Council of State Boards of Nursing (NCSBN) developed a delegation decision-making tree, which identifies several steps nurses can take to help them make delegation decisions. In 2006, the American Nurses Association (ANA) and the NCSBN published a joint paper on the topic of delegation that includes the ANA principles of delegation and the NCSBN decision-making tree. The delegation decision-making tree assists nurses with the delegation decision-making process. The decision-making tree is a useful tool or "grid that may be used by staff education specialists to provide orientation and education to staff nurses and UAP" (Kleinman & Saccomano, 2006, p. 168). The decision-making tree is available online at www.ncsbn.org/Joint_statement.pdf.

Preventing Legal Problems

Preventing legal problems intentionally runs as a theme through this chapter. In summary, prevention requires consistently following the nursing process—the decision-making process of nursing in all nursing care situations. Because nurses act as managers of care, following management principles will also reduce the risk of legal problems. This is especially true with delegation of care, an activity that predictably will increase as care systems adjust to the nursing shortage.

Communication with patients, families, nursing staff, and other healthcare providers also reduces the risk of legal problems. A once-a-year commitment to reviewing the state nurse practice act and rules as well as professional standards of care and code of ethics will enhance the nurse's appreciation of legal accountability in care. Beyond these general activities the nurse should tailor her risk prevention to being aware of the law and rules that affect the nurse's particular practice situation. Hospital and long-term care settings will be affected by different law and rules. Nurses holding administrative positions should know the law and rules affecting their area of practice. In turn, they should educate nursing staff in their responsibilities to carry out the law in their practice setting.

The practice of nursing is never static. Practice is a continuous quest involving adaptation to the current healthcare environment with a commitment to making that environment as safe as possible for the patients for whom the nurse cares.

Conclusion

Nurses are generally law-abiding citizens who have a positive relationship and respect for their profession. However, nurses must develop a clear understanding of the legal system, sources of law, nurse practice acts, delegation, standards of care, and strategies for avoiding legal problems. Every effort should be made by nurses to provide high-quality care for patients that will not only help them recover their health, but will also avoid lawsuits. Nurses have a legal and ethical duty to be knowledgeable about their scope of practice and legal issues.

CLASSROOM ACTIVITY

A mock trial is a fun way to explore some of the concepts in this chapter. Assign roles to students and use a graduation gown for the judge to increase the realism. Make up your own case or use one already prepared such as the excellent mock trial presented in *Nurse Educator* by Haidinyak (2006).

References

American Medical Association. (2007). *Informed consent.* Chicago: Author.

American Nurses Association. (2001). *Code of ethics for nurses with interpretive statements.* Washington, DC: Author.

American Nurses Association. (2004). *Nursing: Scope and standards of practice.* Washington, DC: Author.

American Nurses Association. (2005). *Principles for delegation* [Brochure]. Retrieved June 28, 2007, from http://www.healthsystem.virginia.edu/internet/e-learning/principlesde legation.pdf

Bolin, J. N. (2005). When nurses are reported to the national practitioner's data bank. *Journal of Nursing Law, 10*(3), 141–148.

Canterbury v. Spence, 464 F. 2d 772 (D.C. Cir 1972).

Caroselli-Karinja, M. F., & Zboray, S. D. (1986). The impaired nurse. *Journal of Psychosocial Nursing and Mental Health Services, 24*(6), 14–19.

Castledine, G. (2006). Nurse whose inexperience and negligence in bladder washout put her patient at risk. *British Journal of Nursing, 15*(3), 141–143.

Clevette, A., Erbin-Rosenmann, M., & Kelly, C. (2007). Nursing licensure: An examination of the relationship between criminal convictions and disciplinary actions. *Journal of Nursing Law, 11*(1), 5–8.

Collins, R. L., Gollnisch, G., & Morshemier, E. T. (1999). Substance use among a regional sample of female nurses. *Drug and Alcohol Dependence, 55,* 145–155.

Daniel, I. Q. (1984). Impaired professionals: Responsibilities and roles. *Nursing Economics, 2,* 190–193.

Delgado, C. (2002). Competent and safe practice: A profile of disciplined registered nurses. *Nurse Educator, 27*(4), 159–161.

Driscoll, K. (2004). Current issues: Crossing professional boundaries: Ethical, legal, and case perspectives. *Rehabilitation Nursing, 29*(3), 78–79.

Finkelman, A. W. (2006). *Leadership and management in nursing.* Upper Saddle River, NJ: Pearson Prentice Hall.

Fremgen, B. F. (2002). *Medical law and ethics.* University of Notre Dame. Upper Saddle River, NJ: Prentice Hall.

Green, A., Fitzpatrick, O., Crismon, C., & Waddil, L. (1994). *Disciplined professional nurses in the state of Texas: A profile and comparison to the nondisciplined RN.* Austin, TX: Texas State Board of Nurse Examiners.

Greynolds v. Kurman, 91 Ohio App.3d 389 (1993).

Grossman, S. C. (2005). *The new leadership challenge.* Philadelphia: F. A. Davis.

Guido, G. (2001). *Legal and ethical issues in nursing* (3rd ed.). Upper Saddle River, NJ: Prentice Hall.

Haack, M. R., & Yocom, C. J. (2002). State policies and nurses with substance abuse disorders. *Journal of Nursing Scholarship, 34,* 89–94.

Haidinyak, G. (2006). Try a mock trial. *Nurse Educator, 31*(3), 119–123.

Hall, J. K. (1996). *Nursing ethics and law.* Philadelphia: W. B. Saunders.

Haslauer, S., & Jones, D. (2003). Delegation: Concept, art, skill, process. *Arkansas State Board of Nursing Update,* Winter, 22–24.

Havinghurst, C. (1998). *Health care law and policy: Readings, notes and questions.* Westbury, NY: Foundation Press.

Institute of Medicine. (2000). *To err is human: Building a safer health system.* Washington, DC: National Academy Press.

Institute of Medicine. (2001). *Crossing the quality chasm: A new health system for the 21st century.* Washington, DC: National Academy Press.

Institute of Medicine. (2004). *Keeping patients safe: Transforming the work environment of nurses.* Washington, DC: National Academy Press.

Institute of Medicine. (2007). *Informing the future: Critical issues in health.* Washington, DC: The National Academies Press.

Kalisch, B. J. (2006). Missed nursing care: A qualitative study. *Journal of Nursing Care Quality, 21*(4), 306–313.

Kalisch, P. A., & Kalisch, B. J. (1995). *The advance of American nursing* (3rd ed.). Philadelphia: J. B. Lippincott.

Kleinman, C. S., & Saccomano, S. J. (2006). Registered nurses and unlicensed assistive personnel: An uneasy alliance. *Journal of Continuing Education in Nursing, 37*(4), 162–170.

Longest, B. B. (2002). *Health policymaking in the United States* (3rd ed.). Chicago: Health Administration Press.

Montgomery, V. L. (2007). Effect of fatigue, workload, and environment on patient safety in the pediatric intensive care unit. *Pediatric Critical Care Medicine, 8*(Suppl. 2), S11–6.

Murphy, E. K. (2004). Implications for perioperative nurses. *American Operating Room Nurse, 80*(2), 314–317.

National Council of State Boards of Nursing. (2006). *Joint statement on delegation.* American Nurses Association (ANA) and the National Council of State Boards of Nursing (NCSBN). Retrieved June 28, 2007, from http://www.ncsbn.org/Joint_statement.pdf

National Council of State Boards of Nursing. (2007). *NCLEX-RN test plan.* Chicago: Author.

Nickell v. Gonzalez, 17 Ohio St.3d 136, 477 N.E.2d 1145 (1985).

Quallich, S. A. (2005). A bond of trust: Delegation. *Urologic Nursing, 25*(2), 120–123.

State Office of Administration for the Courts. (1997). *A citizen's guide to Washington courts. The procedure for a civil trial.* Washington, DC: Author.

Storr, C. L., Trinkoff, A. M., & Anthony, J. C. (1999). Job strain and non-medical drug use. *Drug and Alcohol Dependence, 55,* 45–51.

Trappen, R. M., Weiss, S. A., & Whitehead, D. K. (2004). *Essentials of nursing leadership and management* (3rd ed., pp. 91–103). Philadelphia: F. A. Davis.

Trinkoff, A. M., & Storr, C. L. (1998). Substance use among nurses: Differences and specialties. *American Journal of Public Health, 88,* 581–585.

Truman v. Thomas, 27 Cal 3d 285, 611. P2d (1980).

US Department of Health and Human Services. (2003). *Survey of the national practitioner's data bank.* Washington, DC: Author.

US Department of Health and Human Services Health Resources and Services Administration. (2004). *Preliminary findings: 2004 National Sample Survey of Registered Nurses.* Retrieved April 28, 2006, from http://bhpr.hrsa.gov/health-workforce/reports/mpopulation/preliminaryfindings.htm

chapter 13

The Role of the Professional Nurse in Patient Education

Kathleen Masters

LEARNING OBJECTIVES

After completing this chapter, the student should be able to:

1. Differentiate between patient education and patient teaching.
2. Discuss the purposes of patient education.
3. Describe the process of patient education.
4. Identify three domains of learning.
5. Discuss two theoretical frameworks related to the learning process.
6. Demonstrate use of a readability formula to assess reading grade level.
7. Discuss strategies to accommodate for age-related barriers to learning in older adults.
8. Discuss the development of culturally appropriate patient education.

Key Terms and Concepts

- Patient education
- Patient teaching
- Learning domains
- Andragogy
- Health Belief Model
- Social learning theory
- Self-efficacy
- Readiness to learn
- Health literacy
- Age-related changes

Patient education has formally been a part of nursing care since the time of Florence Nightingale (1860/1969). During the 1900s, patient education increasingly became identified as a role of the professional nurse; however, it was not until 1973 that the American Nurses Association (ANA, 1973) defined patient education as a component of the practice of the registered nurse. Beginning in 1976, the Joint Commission on Accreditation of Healthcare Organizations (JCAHO, 1995) included patient and family education as a function critical to patient care. The American Association of Colleges of Nursing (1998) also recognized that the implementation of the professional nursing role requires that nurses are prepared to effectively teach patients.

Today, patient education is both an expectation and legal obligation of the professional nurse.

Patient Education: What Is It?

"**Patient education** is any set of planned, educational activities designed to improve patients' health behaviors, health status, or both" (Lorig, 2001, p. xiii). There is nothing in this definition about improving knowledge, although a change in knowledge may be necessary to reach the goal of changing health status or health behaviors. In contrast, activities aimed at improving knowledge are known as **patient teaching** (Lorig, 2001, p. xiv). The point is that the purpose of patient education involves more than a change in knowledge.

The purposes of patient education are to maintain health, to improve health, or to slow deterioration of health. These purposes are met through changes in health-related behaviors and attitudes (Lorig, 2001). These changes are not easily achieved. Effective patient education requires the nurse to have the ability to communicate effectively with patients in order to assess the individual needs, attitudes, and preferences of the patient that may affect health behaviors before any changes can be expected (Falvo, 2004).

> The purposes of patient education are to maintain health, to improve health, or to slow deterioration of health. These purposes are met through changes in health-related behaviors and attitudes.

In addition to communication and assessment skills, if the nurse is to be effective as a patient educator, the nurse must also have sufficient knowledge of the information that needs to be taught. If the knowledge base of the nurse is insufficient, the nurse risks providing inadequate or inaccurate information to the patient (Falvo, 2004).

Finally, to be an effective patient educator, it is important that the nurse have an understanding of how to conduct patient education. The remainder of this chapter provides a foundation for the conduct of patient education.

Theories and Principles of Learning

There are many educational theories and principles that can be used to guide the patient education process. Some of those that are most commonly used in the health-care setting are presented here.

Domains of Learning

First, we should examine the nature of learning in relationship to **learning domains**. Identification of the learning domain reflects the type of learning desired as a result of the patient education process. Learning occurs in three domains: the cognitive, the psychomotor, and the affective (Bloom, 1956). Each domain has levels, and each level builds on the previous one in a hierarchical fashion. In the cognitive and psychomotor domains, levels are arranged in the order of increasing complexity. In the affective domain, levels are organized according to the degree of internalization of a value or attitude.

Cognitive learning encompasses the intellectual skills of remembering, understanding, applying, analyzing, evaluating, and creating. Psychomotor learning refers to learning of motor skills and performance of behaviors or skills that require coordination. Affective learning requires a change in feelings, attitudes, or beliefs (Anderson & Krothwohi, 2001).

Understanding which domain is the target of learning will help guide the planning, implementation, and evaluation of learning. For example, if based on assessment you know that a patient is knowledgeable about insulin administration and is committed to administering the injection but has not yet been able to manipulate correctly the syringe to administer the injection, then you know that your target domain for learning is the psychomotor domain, and the focus of your objectives, planning, learning activities, and evaluation will be on the performance of the identified behaviors.

Andragogy

Andragogy, initially defined as "the art and science of helping adults learn" (Knowles, 1970), has taken on a broader meaning over the past 35 years and is currently used to refer to learner-focused education for people of all ages (Conner, 2004). The andragogic model asserts that four issues be considered and addressed in learning. These include (Knowles, Swanson, & Holton, 1998):

- Letting learners know why something is important to learn
- Showing learners how to direct themselves through information
- Relating the topic to the learners' experiences
- Realizing that people will not learn until they are ready and motivated

Adults learn best when there is immediate opportunity for application. Adults in particular are motivated to learn when they recognize a gap between what they know and what they want to know or what they need to know (Knowles, 1970). Therefore, the adult learner is rarely interested in learning detailed anatomy and physiology related to their chronic disease, but they are motivated to learn how to care for themselves after discharge from the hospital. Effective patient education will be based on principles that capitalize on these characteristics of the adult learner.

Health Belief Model

The **Health Belief Model** (HBM) is one of the most widely used frameworks in research and programs related to health promotion and patient education. This model was originally developed to predict the likelihood of a person following a recommended action and to understand the person's motivation and decision making regarding seeking health services (Hochbaum, 1958). According to the HBM, the likelihood of a person acting in response to a health threat is dependent on six factors:

- The person's perception of the severity of the illness
- The person's perception of susceptibility to illness and its consequences
- The value of the treatment benefits (i.e., do the cost and side effect of treatment outweigh the consequences of the disease?)
- Barriers to treatment (i.e., expense, complexity of treatment)
- Costs of treatment in physical and emotional terms
- Cues that stimulate taking action toward treatment of illness (i.e., mass media campaigns, pamphlets, advice from family or friends, and postcard reminders from healthcare providers)

The HBM can provide a framework for assessing areas where patients have gaps in knowledge, such as severity of illness or susceptibility to illness, and then address those areas to increase the potential for compliance with the treatment regimen. Through use of the HBM, you can easily categorize and cover the essential components of your educational message, thus providing the patient with a basic understanding of the severity of the illness, the risk and consequences of the illness, the value of treatment, the barriers to treatment, and the costs of treatment.

> **CRITICAL THINKING QUESTION**
>
> Think about your own life. Do you act to prevent a disease or accident when you perceive that you are not susceptible to the disease or at risk for the accident?

Social Learning Theory

According to Bandura's **social learning theory**, if a person believes that he or she is capable of performing a behavior (**self-efficacy**) and also believes that the behavior will lead to a desirable outcome, the person will be more likely to perform the behavior (Bandura, 1997). In contrast, if a person does not believe that he or she is capable of performing a behavior, he or she will have no incentive to do so, even if the person is actually capable. Perceptions of self-efficacy are particularly important in relationship to a patient's learning complex activities or long-term changes in behavior (Prohaska & Lorig, 2001, p. 33).

There are four methods for developing or enhancing efficacy expectations if assessment reveals a need for such enhancement. These methods include:

- Performance accomplishments
- Vicarious experience or modeling
- Verbal persuasion
- Interpretation of physiological state

Performance accomplishment is the most direct and influential way to enhance self-efficacy. In this method, the patient first performs tasks that he or she can easily perform. By succeeding with these first tasks, the patient develops a sense of competence and enhancement of self-efficacy before proceeding to more difficult tasks. Along these same lines, it is also important to set short-term goals that are measurable so that patients can see their success and the impact of the change in their behavior. A patient who can see the benefits of a behavior change within a reasonable time is more likely to continue practicing the behavior.

The second method for enhancing self-efficacy is through modeling where the patients observe others who appear to be similar and who are successfully performing behaviors. Modeling can also be achieved through the use of illustrations in pamphlets or in programming materials by using illustrations and models that are of various cultures, body shapes, and ages (Prohaska & Lorig, 2001).

Verbal persuasion can also be an effective method of enhancing self-efficacy expectations. The content of the message needs to include basic factual information that emphasizes the importance of performing the behavior. It is usually better to ask for incremental changes or ask the patient to do just slightly more than they are currently doing (Prohaska & Lorig, 2001). Encouragement and support not only from the nurse but also from family and friends will help the patient to be successful.

Most illnesses present with symptoms, and most new behaviors will cause some physiologic changes. Addressing the meaning of symptoms and physiologic states can influence self-efficacy. For example, a patient who is trying to quit smoking may expect withdrawal symptoms. If the patient understands the reasons for the symptoms and the limitation in the duration of the symptoms, the patient may decide that he or she has the ability to make the change. Without that knowledge, the patient may give up because he or she experiences physiologic changes that are not understood.

The Patient Education Process

According to Redman (2001), the process of patient education may be viewed as parallel to the nursing process. Each of these processes begins with assessment, negotiation of goals and objectives, planning, intervention, and finally evaluation (Rankin & Stallings, 2001; Rankin, 2005).

The process of patient education may be viewed as parallel to the nursing process.

Assessment

The goal of the nurse in the process of patient education is to assist the patient in obtaining the knowledge, skills, or attitude that will help them develop behaviors to meet their needs and maximize their potential for positive health outcomes (Falvo, 2004). Because no patient or situation is exactly the same, an assessment is required.

There are many guides available that are helpful in assessing the learning needs of patients (Redman, 2003). Some nurses construct their own assessment tools to meet specific needs. Observation, interviews, open-ended questions, focus groups, and the patient's medical record are additional ways to gather information for the assessment of learning needs.

to use is the SMOG formula, which predicts the reading grade level of materials within 1.5 grades 68% of the time (McLaughlin, 1969). The procedure for using the SMOG readability formula is outlined in Box 13-1, and an example of the use of the formula is provided in Box 13-2.

Low health literacy can be a barrier to effective patient education, but the patient with low health literacy skills is capable of learning if the nurse is willing to invest

---

BOX 13-1 SMOG READABILITY FORMULA

1. Choose 10 consecutive sentences near the beginning, 10 consecutive sentences from the middle, and 10 consecutive sentences from the end of the material.
2. In these 30 sentences, count the number of words containing three or more syllables, including repetitions. Consider hyphenated words as one word. Proper nouns are also counted. Numerals and abbreviations should be counted as they would if the words were written out. When a colon divides words, each portion of the sentence is considered a separate sentence.
3. Estimate the square root of the number of polysyllabic words counted.
4. Add three to the square root. This gives the SMOG grading, which is the reading grade level that a person must have achieved to fully understand the material.
5. The quickest way to assess reading grade level is to use the SMOG conversion table. Simply compare the total number of words containing three or more syllables in the 30 sentences with the SMOG Conversion Table.

SMOG Conversion Table

Word Count	Grade Level	Word Count	Grade Level
0–2	4	73–90	12
3–6	5	91–110	13
7–12	6	111–132	14
13–20	7	133–156	15
21–30	8	157–182	16
31–42	9	183–210	17
43–56	10	211–240	18
57–72	11		

However, not all written patient education materials contain 30 sentences. To assess materials with fewer than 30 sentences:
1. Count all of the polysyllabic words.
2. Count the number of sentences.
3. Find the average number of polysyllabic words per sentence.
4. Multiply that average by the number of sentences short of 30.
5. Add that figure to the total number of polysyllabic words.
6. Find the square root of the number you obtained in Step 5 and add the constant of three. This procedure also gives you the SMOG grading.

Source: Data are from Office of Cancer Communications, National Cancer Institute, 1989.

BOX 13-2   USING THE SMOG READABILITY FORMULA (FOR MATERIALS WITH FEWER THAN 30 SENTENCES)

Check Your Weight and Heart Disease IQ

The following statements are either true or false. The statements test your knowledge of overweight and heart disease. The correct answers can be found on the back of this sheet.

1. Being *overweight* puts you at risk for heart disease. 2. If you are *overweight*, losing weight helps lower your high blood *cholesterol* and high blood pressure. 3. Quitting smoking is healthy, but it *commonly* leads to *excessive* weight gain, which *increases* your risk for heart disease. 4. An *overweight* person with high blood pressure should pay more *attention* to a *low-sodium* diet than to weight *reduction*. 5. A reduced intake of *sodium* or salt does not always lower high blood pressure to normal. 6. The best way to lose weight is to eat fewer *calories* and to *exercise*. 7. Skipping meals is a good way to cut down on *calories*. 8. Foods that are high in complex *carbohydrates* (starch and fiber) are good choices when you are trying to lose weight. 9. The single most *important* change most people can make to lose weight is to avoid sugar. 10. *Polyunsaturated* fat has the same number of *calories* as *saturated* fat. 11. *Overweight* children are very likely to become *overweight* adults.

$$\frac{\text{Total number of polysyllabic words}}{\text{Total number of sentences}} = \frac{21}{11} = 1.91 - (30 - 11) = 36.3$$

36 + polysyllabic words (21) = 57

Nearest square root of 57 = 8

8 + constant 3 = 11th-grade level

Source: US DHHS, 1993.

---

the extra time that is required. It is important for the nurse to take extra care to present information in terms that the patient is familiar with rather than using medical jargon, to use alternate formats such as pictographs when possible, to restate information using simple words, and to verify the patient's understanding by having him or her convey the information in his or her own words. The dividends for the extra effort include the patient who is able to manage his or her own illness, make informed health decisions, and make health-related behavior changes as a result of a patient education process that has accommodated for their weaknesses.

Planning

The patient and the nurse share the planning process for patient education, but it is the responsibility of the nurse to guide the process. The nurse guides the process through the use of goals and objectives. Learning goals are derived from the learning assessment, and nursing diagnosis and objectives are developed based on goals in collaboration with the patient. The use of goals and objectives helps the nurse to focus on what is important for the patient to learn and keep patient education focused on outcomes (Rankin & Stallings, 2001).

Patient education is directed toward behavioral change. Therefore, the objectives for patient education are stated as behavioral objectives. There are three components of behavioral objectives that include performance, conditions, and criteria (Mager, 1997). Performance refers to the activity that the patient will engage in and answers this question: "What can the learner do?" The condition refers to special circumstances of the patient's performance and answers this question: "Under what conditions will the learner perform the behavior?" The criteria or evaluation component refers to how long or how well the behavior must be performed to be acceptable and answers this question: "What is the performance standard?" (Rankin & Stallings, 2001).

The learning objectives should be specific, measurable, and attainable (Rankin & Stallings, 2001; Rankin, 2005). Learning objectives are also written in a manner that is learning domain specific. Recognizing the targeted domain of learning as cognitive, psychomotor, or affective will help guide the process of writing behavioral learning objectives and thus guide the selection of learning activities.

Implementation

The next stage of the process involves the actual intervention. Whether the teaching will occur in a group or with an individual patient, learning activities need to be consistent with learning objectives.

Using various learning activities can make learning more fun and more effective. Some common learning activities include lectures, demonstrations, practice, games, simulations, role playing, discussions, and self-directed learning through computer-assisted instruction or self-directed workbooks.

Patient education materials are frequently used in the implementation stage of the patient education process. Patient education materials may be designed to be used alone or to supplement other types of patient education activities but should be previewed before use and only used if consistent with learning objectives. There are many types of patient education materials currently on the market, or you may opt to produce your own materials.

Patient education materials generally include audiovisual materials, computer programs, Internet resources, posters, flip charts, charts, graphs, cartoons, slides, overhead transparencies, photographs, drawings, patient education newsletters, or written patient materials such as handouts, brochures, or pamphlets. These materials, even if designed to be used alone, should not be used without some verbal instruction as to why the patient is being instructed to view the videotape or read the brochure (Falvo, 2004). Additionally, the nurse should keep the door of communication open by inviting questions that the patient might have as a result of exposure to the teaching materials.

A variety of factors will need to be examined as you look at the appropriateness of patient education materials. Three important criteria for judging patient education materials include the following (Doak, Doak, Gordon, & Lorig, 2001, p. 184):

- The material contains the information that the patient wants.
- The material contains the information that the patient needs.
- The patient understands and uses the material as presented.

It is an expectation of JCAHO that the right educational materials are used in patient and family education and that the materials are accurate, age specific, easily accessible, and appropriate to patient needs (JCAHO, 1999, 2003). To address all of these criteria, the nurse needs to conduct a needs assessment before preparing or choosing patient education materials.

Considerations: Patient Education with Older Adults

When caring for older adults, one of the primary considerations related to the patient education process is accommodation for age-related barriers to learning. The age-related barriers particularly important in the patient education process include age-related changes in cognition, vision, and hearing. Research has demonstrated that teaching is not as effective if it does not accommodate for age-related cognitive and sensory changes (Donlon, 1993; Masters, 2001; Weinrich, Weinrich, Boyd, Atwood, & Cervenka, 1994).

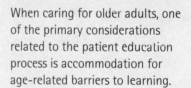

When caring for older adults, one of the primary considerations related to the patient education process is accommodation for age-related barriers to learning.

Age-related changes in cognitive function occur slowly and are thought to begin at approximately 60 years of age in healthy adults (Miller, 2004). Age-related visual changes are the most prevalent physical impairments affecting older adults. Hearing impairment ranks as one of the four most prevalent chronic conditions affecting the older population, occurring in 30–35% of the US population between the ages of 65 and 75 years and in 40% of the population over the age of 75 years (National Institute on Deafness and Other Communication Disorders, 1997). Each of these age-related changes can have a profound effect on the teaching and learning process. Specific age-related changes in cognition, vision, and hearing are listed in Box 13-3.

Specific strategies can be used during the patient education process to help overcome the age-related learning barriers in cognition, vision, and hearing. Some of these strategies are included in Box 13-4.

Cultural Considerations

Developing an educational program that is culturally appropriate is not much different from creating any other patient education program. You begin with a needs assessment; then you write objectives and design the program. The difference is that you must be culturally sensitive and incorporate cultural information that you

BOX 13-3   AGE-RELATED BARRIERS TO LEARNING

Category of Age-Related Change	Cognitive and Sensory Changes
Cognitive	• Changes in encoding and storage of information • Changes in the retrieval of information • Decreases in the speed of processing information*
Visual	• Smaller amount of light reaches the retina • Reduced ability to focus on close objects • Scattering of light resulting in glare • Changes in color perception results in difficulty distinguishing colors such as dark green, blue, and violet • Decrease in depth perception and peripheral vision[†]
Hearing	• Reduced ability to hear sounds as loudly • Decrease in hearing acuity • Decrease in ability to hear high-pitched sounds • Decrease in the ability to filter background noise[†]

Sources: *Merriam & Caffarella, 1999; [†]Miller, 2004.

have learned about the target group into the patient education process (Gonzalez & Lorig, 2001; Bastable, 2006; Lengetti, Ordelt, & Pyle, 2007).

How important is it that you incorporate cultural information in the patient education process? Cultural awareness and sensitivity of nurses can influence the ability of patients to receive and apply information regarding their health care (Campinha-Bacole, Yahle, & Langenkamp, 1996). The way that information is communicated can influence a patient's perception of the healthcare system and affect their adherence to prescribed treatments. In a recent study, patients who received care from nurses with cultural sensitivity training not only showed improvement in use of social resources but also improvement in overall functional capacity (Majumdar, Browne, Roberts, & Carpio, 2004).

In addition to the difference that it can make in relationship to patient outcomes, JCAHO standards require not only that the patient's learning needs, abilities, and readiness to learn are assessed but also that the patient's preferences are assessed. This assessment must consider cultural and religious practices, as well as emotional and language barriers (JCAHO, 1999, 2003).

How do you incorporate cultural information into the patient education process? Gonzalez and Lorig (2001, p. 172) suggest the following:

- Change the information into more specific or more relevant terminology.
- Create descriptions or explanations that fit with different people's understanding of key concepts.

BOX 13-4   STRATEGIES TO ACCOMMODATE FOR AGE-RELATED BARRIERS TO LEARNING

Category of Age-Related Change	Strategies to Accommodate for Cognitive and Sensory Changes
Cognitive	• Slow the pace of the presentation. • Give smaller amounts of information at a time. • Repeat information frequently. • Reinforce verbal teaching with audiovisuals, written materials, and practice. • Reduce distractions. • Allow more time for self-expression of learner. • Use analogies and examples from everyday experience to illustrate abstract information. • Increase the meaningfulness of content to the learner. • Teach mnemonic devices and imaging techniques. • Use printed materials and visual aids that are age specific*
Visual	• Make sure patient's glasses are clean and in place. • Use printed materials with 14- to 16-point font and serif letters. • Use bold type on printed materials, and do not mix fonts. • Avoid the use of dark colors with dark backgrounds for teaching materials, but instead use large, distinct configurations with high contrast to help with discrimination. • Avoid blue, green, and violet to differentiate type, illustrations, or graphics. • Use line drawings with high contrast. • Use soft white light to decrease glare. • Light should shine from behind the learner. • Use color and touch to help differentiate depth. • Position materials directly in front of the learner.[†]
Hearing	• Speak distinctly. • Do not shout. • Speak in a normal voice, or speak in a lower pitch. • Decrease extraneous noise. • Face the person directly while speaking at a distance of 3 to 6 feet. • Reinforce verbal teaching with visual aids or easy to read materials.[†]

Sources: *Weinrich, Boyd, & Nussbaum, 1989; [†]Oldaker, 1992; Weinrich, Boyd, & Nussbaum, 1989.

■ Incorporate a group's cultural beliefs and practices into the program content and process.

In addition, any visual aids that are used should reflect the target group or population. The use of culturally relevant analogies can also help people to understand complex, abstract, or foreign concepts (Gonzalez & Lorig, 2001).

Evaluation

Evaluation determines worth by judging something against a standard. The standard used in the patient education process is the learning objective. Thus, the term *evaluation* as used here implies measuring the outcomes resulting from systematically planned activities implemented as a part of a patient education program or patient education process against the learning objectives.

Initiation of the patient education evaluation process is the responsibility of the nurse, and according to Rankin and Stallings (2001, p. 326), the evaluation process should include the following:

- Measuring the extent to which the patient has met the learning objectives
- Identifying when there is a need to clarify, correct, or review information
- Noting learning objectives that are unclear
- Pointing out shortcomings in patient teaching interventions
- Identifying barriers that prevented learning

Nurses commonly use several methods to evaluate patient learning. These methods include direct observation, records of health-related behaviors that the patients documented, interviews, questionnaires, and critical incidents (such as readmission, emergency room visits, and mortality).

Documentation of Patient Education

It is essential that the process of patient education be documented. Documentation functions to promote communication among members of the healthcare team, to provide a legal record, to support quality assurance efforts, to promote continuity of care, to promote reimbursement, and to meet JCAHO standards.

Documentation of patient education should be concise, organized, and focused on patient outcomes. Documentation systems will vary by setting, but the following elements of the patient education process should be included in documentation (Rankin & Stallings, 2001, p. 336):

- Initial assessments and reassessments
- Nursing diagnoses, patient needs, and priorities
- Interventions planned and interventions provided
- Patient's response and outcomes of care
- Patient and family ability to manage needs after discharge

Conclusion

This chapter has provided an introduction to some of the major concepts related to the process of patient education. There is no recipe for patient education that will fit everyone, but if you mix the basic principles discussed in this chapter with some practice, you will be on your way to providing your patients with effective education.

CLASSROOM ACTIVITY 1

Provide students with a copy of printed patient education materials. These can be obtained from a local healthcare organization or from online sources such as the American Heart Association. Ask students to evaluate the materials for readability using the SMOG formula in Box 13-1. Next ask students to evaluate the materials for use with older adults using the information presented in Box 13-3 and Box 13-4. Finally, have students evaluate the materials for use with a population of a different culture. Ask students to share findings during informal presentations to classmates.

CLASSROOM ACTIVITY 2

In small groups ask students to create a patient education brochure that conforms to recommended reading levels, considers age-related learning barriers, and accommodates cultural differences. The group may choose a fictitious case scenario or an actual scenario from a recent clinical experience.

For this activity several students will either need to bring laptops to class or the class will need to have access to a computer lab or the students will need colored pencils and paper. Alternately, this activity could be assigned to students to complete outside of class to be shared with the class or submitted for a grade.

References

American Association of Colleges of Nursing. (1998). *The essentials of baccalaureate education for professional nursing practice.* Washington, DC: Author.

American Nurses Association. (1973). *Standards of nursing practice.* Kansas City, MO: Author.

Anderson, L. W., & Krothwohl, D. R. (2001). *A taxonomy for learning, teaching and assessing: A revision of Bloom's taxonomy of educational objectives.* New York: Addison Wesley.

Baker, D. W., Parker, R. M., Williams, M. V., & Clark, W. S. (1998). Health literacy and the risk of hospital admission. *Journal of General Internal Medicine, 13,* 791–798.

Baker, D. W., Parker, R. M., Williams, M. V., Pitkin, K., Parikh, N. S., Coates, W., & Imara, M. (1996). The health care experience of patients with low literacy. *Archives of Family Medicine, 5,* 329–334.

Bandura, A. (1997). *Self-efficacy: The exercise of control.* New York: W. H. Freeman.

Bastable, S. B. (2006). *Essentials of patient education.* Sudbury, MA: Jones and Bartlett Publishers.

Bloom, B. (1956). *Taxonomy of educational objectives.* New York: Addison Wesley.

Campinha-Bacole, J., Yahle, T., & Langenkamp, M. (1996). The challenge of cultural diversity for nurse educators. *Journal of Continuing Education in Nursing, 27*(2), 59–64.

Conner, M. (2004). Andragogy and pedagogy. *Ageless Learner.* Retrieved June 18, 2004, from http://www.agelesslearner.com/intros/andragogy.html

Davis, T. C., Long, S. W., Jackson, R. H., Mayeaux, E. J., George, R. B., & Murphy, P. W. (1993). Rapid estimate of adult literacy in medicine: A shortened screening instrument. *Family Medicine, 25,* 391.

Doak, C., Doak, L., Gordon, L., & Lorig, K. (2001). Selecting, preparing, and using materials. In K. Lorig (Ed.), *Patient education: A practical approach* (3rd ed., pp. 183–197). Thousand Oaks, CA: Sage.

Doak, C. C., Doak, L. G., & Root, J. H. (1996). *Teaching patients with low literacy skills.* Philadelphia: J. B. Lippincott.

Doak, L. G., & Doak, C. C. (Eds.). (2002). *Pfizer health literacy principles.* Retrieved September 12, 2002, from http://www.pfizerhealthliteracy.com

Donlon, B. C. (1993). The effect of practical education programming for the elderly (PEPE) on the rehospitalization rate of older congestive heart failure patients: A quasi-experimental study. Unpublished doctoral dissertation. University of Southern Mississippi.

Falvo, D. (2004). *Effective patient education: A guide to increased compliance* (3rd ed.). Sudbury, MA: Jones and Bartlett Publishers.

Flesch, R. (1948). A new readability yardstick. *Journal of Applied Psychology, 32*(3), 221–233.

Fry, E. (1968). A readability formula that saves time. *Journal of Reading, 11,* 513–577.

Gonzalez, V. M., & Lorig, K. (2001). Working cross-culturally. In K. Lorig (Ed.), *Patient education: A practical approach* (3rd ed., pp. 163–182). Thousand Oaks, CA: Sage.

Hochbaum, G. M. (1958). *Public participation in medical screening programs: A socio-psychological study.* Public Health Service Publication No. 572. Washington, DC: US Government Printing Office.

Jastak, S., & Wilkinson, G. S. (1993). *Wide-range achievement test: Review 3.* Wilmington, DE: Jastak Associates.

Joint Commission on Accreditation of Healthcare Organizations. (1995). *Comprehensive accreditation manual for hospitals,* Vols. 1 and 2. Oakbrook Terrace, IL: Author.

Joint Commission on Accreditation of Healthcare Organizations. (1999). *Hospital accreditation standards.* Oakbrook Terrace, IL: Author.

Joint Commission on Accreditation of Healthcare Organizations. (2003). *Joint commission guide to patient and family education.* Oakbrook Terrace, IL: Author.

Knowles, M. (1970). *The modern practice of adult education: Andragogy versus pedagogy.* New York: Association Press.

Knowles, M., Swanson, R., & Holton, E. (1998). T*he adult learner: The definitive classic in adult education and human resource development.* Houston, TX: Gulf.

Lengetti, E., Ordelt, K., & Pyle, N. (2007, November). Patient teaching competency for staff. *Patient Education Management,* 123–124.

Lorig, K. (2001). *Patient education: A practical approach* (3rd ed.). Thousand Oaks, CA: Sage.

Mager, R. (1997). *Preparing instructional objectives* (3rd ed.). Atlanta, GA: Center for Effective Performance.

Majumdar, B., Browne, G., Roberts, J., & Carpio, B. (2004). Effects of cultural sensitivity training on health care provider attitudes and patient outcomes. *Journal of Nursing Scholarship, 36*(2), 161–166.

Masters, K. (2001). The effect of education that is modified to accommodate for age-related barriers to learning in older adult home health patients with congestive heart failure. Unpublished doctoral dissertation, Louisiana State University Health Sciences Center.

McLaughlin, G. H. (1969). SMOG grading—a new readability formula. *Journal of Reading, 12,* 639–646.

Merriam, S. B., & Caffarella, R. S. (1999). *Learning in adulthood: A comprehensive guide.* San Francisco, CA: Jossey-Bass.

Miller, C. A. (2004). *Nursing for wellness in older adults: Theory and practice* (4th ed.). Philadelphia: Lippincott.

National Center for Education Statistics. (2007). *Literacy in everyday life: Results from the 2003 National Assessment of Adult Literacy.* Retrieved December 14, 2007, from http://nces.ed.gov/naal

National Institute on Deafness and Other Communication Disorders. (1997). *Hearing impairment and deafness.* Retrieved July 13, 2004, from http://www.nih.gov/nidcd/hearing.htm

Nightingale, F. (1860/1969). *Notes on nursing: What it is and what it is not.* New York: Dover.

Office of Cancer Communications, National Cancer Institute. (1989). *Making health communications work.* Rockville, MD: Author.

Oldaker, S. M. (1992). Live and learn: Patient education for the elderly orthopaedic client. *Orthopaedic Nursing, 11*(3), 51–56.

Prohaska, T. R., & Lorig, K. (2001). What do we know about what works: The role of theory in patient education. In K. Lorig (Ed.), *Patient education: A practical approach* (3rd ed., pp. 163–182). Thousand Oaks, CA: Sage.

Rankin, S. H. (2005). *Patient education in health and illness.* Philadelphia: Lippincott.

Rankin, S. H., & Stallings, K. D. (2001). *Patient education: Principles & practice* (4th ed.). Philadelphia: Lippincott.

Redman, B. K. (2001). *The practice of patient education* (9th ed.). St. Louis, MO: Mosby.

Redman, B. K. (2003). Measurement tools in patient education (2nd ed.). New York: Springer Publishing Company.

Stephenson, P. L. (2007). Before teaching begins: Managing patient anxiety prior to providing education. *Clinical Journal of Oncology Nursing, 10*(2), 241–246.

US DHHS. (1993). *Check your weight and heart disease I.Q.* Publication No. 93-3034. Washington, DC: U.S. Government Printing Office.

Weinrich, S. P., Boyd, M., & Nussbaum, J. (1989). Continuing education: Adapting strategies to teach the elderly. *Journal of Gerontological Nursing, 15*(11), 17–21.

Weinrich, S. P., Weinrich, M. C., Boyd, M. D., Atwood, J., & Cervenka, B. (1994). Teaching older adults by adapting for aging changes. *Cancer Nursing, 17*(6), 494–500.

Weiss, B. D. (1999). *Twenty common problems in primary care.* New York: McGraw-Hill.

Williams, M. V., Baker, D. W., Honig, E. G., Lee, T. M., & Nowlan, A. (1998). Inadequate literacy is a barrier to asthma knowledge and self-care. *Chest, 114,* 1008–1015.

Informatics and Technology in Professional Nursing Practice

Kay Coltharp Cater

LEARNING OBJECTIVES

After completing this chapter, the student should be able to:

1. Define nursing informatics.
2. Discuss levels of nurse informatics competencies.
3. Discuss common electronic communication technologies.
4. Use electronic databases to obtain information.
5. Evaluate information found on the Internet.
6. Discuss principles that apply to Web site accessibility.
7. Describe components of a health information system.
8. Explain security and privacy issues for electronic health records.
9. Discuss the privacy regulations of the Health Insurance Portability and Accountability Act.
10. Envision future trends in healthcare technology.

Key Terms and Concepts

- Nursing informatics
- E-mail
- Listserv
- Asynchronous
- Search engine
- Boolean logic
- Database
- EBSCO
- CINAHL
- MEDLINE
- PsycINFO
- Health Source
- ERIC
- PDA
- Electronic health record
- HIPAA
- Telehealth

Healthcare delivery is largely dependent on information for effective decision making. Every nursing action is reliant on knowledge based on information. The nursing process begins with the acquisition of information in the initial and ongoing assessment. Nursing informatics (NI) is the management of

As we enter the era of the electronic health record (EHR), NI has become an indispensable element in the practice of nursing.

information relevant to nursing. As we enter the era of the electronic health record (EHR), NI has become an indispensable element in the practice of nursing. All nurses utilize informatics skills in their practice.

Nursing Informatics Defined

Nursing informatics (NI) is together a field of study and an area of specialization. In the mid-1900s NI was first identified as the use of information technology in nursing practice (Hannah, 1985). Graves and Corcoran (1989) defined nursing informatics as the synthesis of computer science, information science, and nursing science in the organization and comprehension of data that directs nursing practice. In 1992, the American Nurses Association (ANA) recognized NI as a nursing specialty. ANA's *Scope and Standards of Nursing Informatics Practice* published in 2001 defined NI as

> a specialty that integrates nursing science, computer science, and information science to manage and communicate data, information, and knowledge in nursing practice. Nursing informatics facilitates the integration of data, information, and knowledge to support patient, nurses, and other providers in their decision making in all roles and settings. This support is accomplished through the use of information structures, information processes, and information technology. (ANA, 2001, p. 17)

Informatics contributes to the discipline of nursing by connecting the art of nursing to the science of nursing (Saba, 2001). The specialty of NI is focused on developing and implementing solutions for the management and communication of health information pertinent to providing better quality patient/client care (Zykowski, 2003).

The definition of NI continues to evolve as technology is incorporated into health care. The roles of an informatics nurse may include project manager, consultant, educator, researcher, or developer. Topics addressed may include budget management, telenursing, distance learning, electronic health, and the computerized patient record. The informatics nurse contributes to selection, testing, and implementation of healthcare systems as well as maintenance and evaluation of the systems. NI provides the support for information management for all other nursing specialties. The American Nursing Informatics Association Web site (www.ania.org) and the Alliance for Nursing Informatics Web site (http://www.allianceni.org/) both offer information related to nursing in the digital world, including membership, conferences, and online resources.

Informatics Competencies

All nurses need informatics competencies. Defined levels of competencies vary from beginning nurse, experienced nurse, informatics specialist, and informatics innovator (Staggers, Gassert, & Curran, 2001). The beginning nurse entering practice is expected to have computer literacy and basic information management skills. Computer literacy skills include those of word processing, database and spreadsheet applications, presentation software, and e-mail. Information literacy skills enable a nurse to locate, access, and evaluate clinical data. Access includes the ability to perform bibliographic retrievals using the Internet and library-based resources (McNeil et al., 2003). A national survey identified the most critical technology skills of the entry-level nurse as those involved in knowing nursing-specific software, such as computerized documentation and medication dispensing (McCannon & O'Neal, 2003).

The experienced nurse should be skilled in information management and computer technology to sustain their specific area of practice. These skills include making judgments based on trends of data in addition to collaboration with informatics nurses in the development of nursing systems. An informatics nurse specialist has advanced informatics preparation and assists the practicing nurse in meeting his or her needs for information. The informatics innovator also has advanced informatics preparation and possesses skills for conducting informatics research along with theory development (Thede, 2003).

Certification for NI became available in 1995 through the American Nurses Credentialing Center. Eligibility for the exam requires an active registered nurse license within the United States or legally recognized equivalent from another country, 2 years of full-time experience as a registered nurse, a baccalaureate or higher degree in nursing or a related field, 30 hours completed of continuing education within the past 3 years, and a practice hour requirement of one of the following:

- A minimum of 2000 hours of experience in the field of NI in the past 3 years
- A minimum of 1000 hours of experience in the field of NI in the past 3 years and completed 12 hours of academic credits in informatics courses at the graduate level
- Completion of a graduate program in informatics with 200 hours of clinical practicum (American Nurses Credentialing Center, 2007).

Information on test content is available at www.nursecredentialing.org/cert/TCOx/BSN27_Info_TCO.html.

E-Mail

E-mail (electronic mail) is the most common use of the Internet (Nicoll, 2001). Today, e-mail can be sent to anyone in the world who has an e-mail address. This allows many healthcare providers to be able to communicate with patients. Messages can be sent in moments across time zones, allowing instant communication. For several reasons, attention must be taken relative to the content of messages sent by e-mail. It is possible for others to access a message while it is being sent over the Internet. Also, forwarding messages accidentally or purposefully can occur. These concerns make privacy a legal and ethical issue (Thede, 2003).

E-mail requires an individual address that consists of two main parts separated by an *at* (@) sign. The first part is called a login name or a user ID. The part after the @ is the name of the computer used to access the Internet. The characters after the last dot in an e-mail address indicate the domain or main subdivision of the Internet to which the computer belongs. The Internet uses standard domain suffixes at the end of the address to indicate the type of organization providing the e-mail service. For example, an e-mail address for someone located at a university may appear as first.last@university.edu. Additional common organizations' domains are:

- .com for commercial organizations
- .gov for governments
- .net for networking organizations
- .org for nonprofit organizations

Addresses are case sensitive and must be accurate for the message to be sent. Appropriateness of address must be considered when selecting your login name. Professionals should not use suggestive or insensitive wording for their login name.

E-mail is a special form of communication and carries its own form of etiquette. Pagana (2007) suggests the following guidelines for consideration when sending a business or professional message:

- Don't use all uppercase letters. Typing in all caps is deemed shouting.
- Include a specific subject line.
- Sign your messages including your e-mail address and contact information.
- Use the "reply to all" function appropriately, as not everyone is interested in receiving your comments.
- Avoid forwarding chain letters, and delete all unnecessary information.
- Do not send confidential information, and check for correct recipients before sending.
- Use the spell check and grammar function.
- Do not use e-mail for thank-you correspondence.

Listserv Groups or Mailing Lists

Mailing lists or **listservs** are a form of group e-mail that provides an opportunity for people with similar interests to share information. Subscribing to the list usually requires no fee. Once subscribed, you can send and receive messages from the list. The communication is **asynchronous**, or not occurring in real time. Someone posts a question or comment to the list, and other members reply. List groups are usually layperson oriented or professional oriented. Nursing has numerous groups that can be joined. To find a list, ask friends and colleagues or visit L-Soft, a searchable database that can be accessed at www.lsoft.com/catalist.html.

To join a mailing list, subscribe by sending an e-mail message to the computer that is hosting the list. Send the message "subscribe," followed by your first and last name. Most listservs provide specific instructions on subscribing when requested. Every listserv has two addresses. One address is used to join, and the second is used to send messages that will be read by the group. Listserv groups may be open to anyone, or you must have permission to join.

It is important to remember that by sending a message to the listserv your message will be read by everyone subscribed to that listserv. Posting a personal message to an individual on a listserv is generally not considered appropriate. Do not send attachments to the list. The list may have hundreds of members, and some will not have computers that support sophisticated graphics or large files. Additionally, viruses may be transmitted in attachments.

The ability to send and receive messages between multiple people in multiple places is having a direct impact on health care. Nurses can easily and efficiently facilitate a virtual support group through the use of e-mail for families and patients with chronic conditions or limitations to accessing health care. The lists connect the participants to individuals with similar health concerns where they may share experiences, receive advice on difficulties, and alleviate the feeling of isolation (Mendelson, 2003).

Internet Resources

Not since the invention of the printing press has the speed with which new information could be obtained changed as with the development of the Web. Search tools or **search engines** assist in finding specific topics on the Web by compiling a database of Internet sites. Popular search engines are AltaVista, InfoSeek, WebCrawler, Yahoo, Northernlight, and Hotbot. All have different search features and produce somewhat differing information. In addition to search engines, there are metasearch engines. A metasearch engine conducts a search of a variety of search engines. Metacrawler (www.metacrawler.com), Google (www.google.com), and Dogpile (www.dogpile.com) are examples of metasearch engines. Each search engine queries different databases with different search techniques (Bliss & DeYoung, 2002) and uses a range of engines for retrieval of information.

Searching on the Internet can be frustrating because of the vast amount of information that is available. Using keywords or phrases will produce several sites that contain information on a particular subject. Most search engines use **Boolean logic** to combine terms. The most frequently used Boolean operators are AND, OR, and NOT. These terms can be used in most electronic database systems as well as on the Internet. The use of AND requires both keywords and phrases to be present, resulting in narrowing of the search. OR requires either of the keywords to be included and enlarges the search. Another way to narrow the search is with the use of NOT, which excludes information about the keyword. Some search engines use plus (+) or minus (−) signs in place of AND or NOT (Mascara, Czar, & Hebda, 2001).

Electronic Databases

An increasing number of **databases** are available over the Internet and can be accessed through local libraries or by subscription from a vendor such as **EBSCO** Publishing, which provides access to online databases and e-journals. Most of the databases use keyword searches and are capable of limited or advanced searching as well as limiting to full text. Some of the most beneficial to nursing include the following:

- **CINAHL** is the authoritative resource for nursing and allied health professionals, students, educators, and researchers. This database provides indexing and abstracting for over 1700 current nursing and allied health journals and publications dating back to 1982, totaling over 880,000 records.
- **MEDLINE**, created by the National Library of Medicine, is the largest biomedical literature database that provides authoritative medical information on medicine, nursing, dentistry, veterinary medicine, the healthcare system, and preclinical sciences. MEDLINE has the capabilities to search abstracts from over 4600 current biomedical journals. Included are citations from *Index Medicus, International Nursing Index, Index to Dental Literature,* PREMEDLINE, AIDSLINE, BIOETHICSLINE, and HealthSTAR.
- **PsycINFO** contains nearly 2 million citations and summaries of journal articles, book chapters, books, dissertations, and technical reports, all in the field of psychology. It also includes information about the psychological aspects of related disciplines such as medicine, psychiatry, nursing, sociology, education, pharmacology, physiology, linguistics, anthropology, business, and law.
- **Health Source**, the Nursing/Academic Edition, provides more than 550 scholarly full-text journals, including more than 450 peer-reviewed journals focusing on many medical disciplines, including nursing and allied health.
- **ERIC**, the Educational Resource Information Center, is a national information system supported by the US Department of Education, the National Library of Education, and the Office of Educational Research and Improvement. It provides access to information from journals included in the *Current Index of Journals in Education* and *Resources in Education Index.* ERIC provides full text of more than 2200 digests along with references for additional information and citations and abstracts from over 1000 educational and education-related journals.

Web access to government organizations and nonprofit organizations is also available. The US National Library of Medicine (www.nlm.nih.gov/hinfo.html) offers a wealth of health information Web sites. PubMed and MedlinePlus permit search of multiple retrieval systems and provide excellent information. Guidelines for evaluations should be applied to all Internet sites before using it in patient teaching (Thede, 2003).

Web Site Evaluation

The Web has grown rapidly since the beginning, and information can be published easily and inexpensively. An Internet site can be created by anyone with the ability to create a Web page. Many sites can be for commercial purposes, and others can simply be the opinions of the Web site developer. Web sites are under no required guidelines or standards. Additionally, no official organization is responsible for site evaluation. As a result, a vast amount of information is available on the Web, but not all information is reliable. Thede (2003) recommended six guidelines for evaluating a resource on the Web:

- Accuracy—Is the information accurate, reliable, and free from error? Spelling and punctuation errors may indicate an untrustworthy site.
- Authority—Look for the credentials of the author or the reputation of the hosting organization. A good indication of authority is peer review.
- Objectivity—What are the goals and objectives of the site? What biases are present? Is the site trying to present a specific or neutral point of view?
- Currency or timeliness—Look for publication and updates dates. Dead links may indicate old information.
- Coverage—Is the subject matter presented on the site of appropriate quality for the intended audience?
- Usability—Is the site designed for easy navigation? Are there excessive graphics that require long download times?

Applying these guidelines will assist you in acquiring reliable information from the Web.

> **CRITICAL THINKING QUESTION**
>
> What is your role as a nurse in the evaluation of information on the Internet?

Health Information Online

The number of people accessing health information online continues to grow. The Harris Poll (2004) found that 69% of all adults in the United States are now online, and 15% of those who use the Internet are often obtaining information related to health or disease. These numbers demonstrate the critical importance of healthcare Web sites to provide reliable and credible information. Nurses are responsible for assisting the public in evaluating health information available on the Web. Additionally, nurses are in the ideal position to provide health promotion education to their patients and to the public at large. Whether nurses are developing online materials or using existing online information, it is important for them to understand what makes the information accessible to all people (Thede, 2003) and to be able to make informed recommendations about online Web sites to individuals with disabilities (Smeltzer, Simmerman, Frain, DeSiltes, & Duffin, 2003). Contents of the sites should be presented in a way that people with disabilities and with low-end technology are able to navigate and use. Web sites displaying the "Bobby Approved" icon (bobby.watchfire.com/bobby/html/en/about.js) have been screened for accessibility for individuals with disabilities, and the icon is an indication of the site's appropriateness for patient use.

Additional tools are available for health Web site evaluation. The Health on the Net Foundation (HON), founded in 1995, is a nonprofit organization dedicated to assisting people in obtaining reliable health information on the Web. The HON Code of Conduct (HONcode) is available at www.hon.ch/honcode/conduct.htm (Health on the Net Foundation, 1995). To obtain certification, a Web site applies for registration. The site is evaluated and, if approved, qualifies to display the HONcode seal. The site is randomly checked for compliance. From this Web site, the HON toolbar can be downloaded and added to your Web browser. The seal illuminates when a certified site is accessed.

As the use of the Internet continues to gain in popularity, more people are using the Web for health information. Web-knowledgeable nurses need to assist patients and their families in the evaluation of the quality of Web resources. An additional organization that is a resource of knowledge is the Hardin MD (Hardin Meta Directory) at www.lib.uiowa.edu/hardin/md. The site is maintained by Hardin Library for the Health Sciences at the University of Iowa and lists several directors for health and medicine. MedlinePlus (available at www.nlm.nih.gov/medlineplus) is a consumer-oriented site that combines information from the National Library of Medicine (NLM), the National Institutes of Health (NIH), and other government agencies and health-related organizations. The site is maintained by the National Library of Medicine.

PDAs

Personal digital assistants (**PDAs**) are handheld devices that have wireless connectivity and can synchronize data and information between the PDA and a computer. Use of the PDA is becoming widely popular in health care and nursing. The device can be used as a digital reference for obtaining drug information, dosage calculations, and diagnostic test results, as well as decision protocols for administration. It is a useful tool for data collection and management of patient outcomes. PDAs can be interfaced with the electronic medical record to obtain and update vital patient information. Immediate access to the Internet allows the healthcare provider to obtain valuable information through national and international resources. HIPAA guidelines should be strictly followed when using PDAs and other wireless technology (Thompson, 2005).

Electronic Health Records

In 2004 President Bush, as part of the National Health Information Infrastructure, established a technology agenda authorizing the development of an **electronic health record** for all Americans by 2014. This initiative is intended to benefit the consumer through increased quality in health care and benefit the public through early detection and prevention of disease. Information on this agenda can be found at the US Department of Health and Human Services Web site: www.hhs.gov/infocus/technoogy/economic_policy200404/chap3.htm.

"The goal of nursing informatics (NI) is to improve the health of populations, communities, families, and individuals by optimizing information management and communication" (ANA, 2001, p. 17). Information management is integral to providing high-quality health care with a cost-effective approach. To provide this level of care, it is important to have accurate clinical information. The health information system or electronic health record (EHR) represents multiple systems that are interfaced to share data and networked to support information management and communication within a healthcare organization. The EHR has numerous advantages compared with the traditional paper record. It can store large amounts of data that are accessible from remote sites by many people at the same time. Information can be accessed easier and quicker, allowing for more time for patient care. The EHR can provide clinical alerts and reminders, identify abnormal parameters of laboratory and assessment data, and prompt clinicians on important tasks and protocols (Young, 2000).

Thede (2003) identified the following types of information systems within healthcare organizations:

- Admission, discharge, and transfer—This system collects and tracks patient information, such as demographics, hospital number, relatives, and primary physician. All patient contacts are connected to the information in this system.
- Financial systems—This system is responsible for the fiscal operations of an organization.
- Order entry—A clinician places an order for a specific service from a computer screen. Through selection of one service, the system is capable of scheduling, reporting, and billing. The system may have the potential of programmed patient safety functions that identify and report potential errors.
- Ancillary systems—Ancillary applications permit sharing of information among multiple systems and specialty areas such as those of radiology, laboratory, physical therapy, or pharmacy.
- Clinical documentation—This system enables the chart to be accessed at any time.

As data are entered into the system, the application can prompt the clinician for additional information that might be missed. The same data can be used in a variety of reports, leading to decreasing the redundancy of charting. Data such as pulse rate or blood pressure can be collected directly from monitors attached to the client and fed into the system (Hunter, 2002). Clinical documentation systems have the advantage of collection of data to use in planning and research:

- Scheduling applications are used for staff, patients, supplies, and procedures.

- Acuity applications attempt to predict the resources necessary for patient care. They are integrated with other systems such as staffing to create adequate staffing.
- Specialty systems are found in specialized units within the healthcare setting. Examples include monitoring equipment in intensive care units that automatically measure and record physiologic data, generate trends, sound alarms for abnormalities, and interact with other information systems with the patient environment.
- Communication systems such as e-mail and Internet accessibility facilitate communication among various disciplines within the organization.
- Critical pathways, generated by information systems, identify specific patient outcomes and make documentation by different disciplines possible. This promotes cost-effective care through effective communication.

Electronic information systems contribute to more effective communication and collection of patient information, resulting in more effective patient care (Thede, 2003). The electronic information system can maximize the time nurses spend on direct patient care, improve the accuracy of documentation, decrease medication errors, and promote patient safety.

Confidentiality, Security, and Privacy of Healthcare Information

Protecting an individual's personal and private information from others has historically been a significant issue for nursing. Healthcare information is a collection of data relating to acutely personal aspects of an individual's life. Improper disclosure can cause devastating consequences. Many people depend on the understanding that information provided to a healthcare provider will not be disclosed. It is possible for patients not to disclose certain types of information essential to their care if they believe the information would not continue to be confidential. The introduction of electronic documentation and communication has increased the difficulty of maintaining privacy. Improved access to healthcare information can and does increase efficiency and improve patient care, but accompanying the increased access to information are greater difficulties in maintaining privacy and confidentiality. Preserving security of the system becomes critical. By gaining entrance to the computerized healthcare information system, it becomes easy to access many personal records.

Protection against unauthorized access to a system can be achieved with a login process that verifies that the person has permission to use the system. The majority of systems rely on a user ID and password for verification. Passwords are changed frequently for protection from breach of security. Users should never divulge or share passwords. Healthcare agencies have written policies regarding the penalties of misuse of the system. These policies are usually severe and may result in termination of the employee (Thede, 2003).

Health Insurance Portability and Accountability Act

In 1996, Congress passed the Health Insurance Portability and Accountability Act (**HIPAA**) to improve the efficiency and effectiveness of the healthcare system by encouraging the development of a health information system. Several areas are addressed by the act, including simplifying healthcare claims, developing standards for data transmission, and implementing privacy regulations. The privacy regulations protect clients by limiting the ways that health plans, pharmacies, hospitals, and other entities can use clients' personal medical information. The regulations protect medical records and other individually identifiable health information, whether it is communicated orally, on paper, or electronically. Accompanying the privacy regulations are specific security rules that protect health information in electronic form. To be in compliance, agencies must ensure the confidentiality and integrity of all electronic health information that is created, received, transmitted, or stored; protect against threats to security; protect against disclosures of information; and ensure compliance of its employees (Garner, 2003). HIPAA, when fully implemented, will contribute to a "fully integrated healthcare system" (Thede, 2003, p. 327).

> **CRITICAL THINKING QUESTION**
>
> What is your role as a nurse in protecting patient healthcare information?

Telehealth

Telehealth is defined as "using electronic communication for transmitting healthcare information such as health promotion, disease prevention, professional or lay education, diagnosis, or actual treatments to people located at different geographical locations" (Thede, 2003, p. 129). Electronic communication can use wireless technology in the form of radio signals to transmit data. Hardware and software such as personal digital assistants, pagers, cellular phones, laptop computers, and mobile hardware peripherals are being used by clinicians in increasing numbers. Healthcare providers can monitor and send messages to patients in their homes regarding changes in health status. Information and images can be communicated digitally for consultation with other healthcare providers. This form of healthcare promises to provide many solutions for patient care in the future (Newbold, 2003).

Future Trends

Clearly, computerized technology will be shaping the future of health care. Recognizing this fact, *Healthy People 2010* objectives (US Department of Health and Human Services, 2000) call for increasing the number of households with access to the Internet. Many healthcare organizations and public service agencies use the Internet as the main avenue for information delivery. Thus, having access to the Internet will be essential to acquiring health information and services. Changes in delivery of patient care are common in clinical facilities in many areas of the country. Nurses and healthcare providers have become accustomed to computerized order entry for medical directives and point-of-care technology for patient care, automated medication dispensing, physiologic monitoring systems, and "smart" infusion pump deliver systems (Sabb & McCormick, 2006).

Nelson (2003) proposed the following ideas for the future of health care. The traditional office visit will be replaced with the virtual appointment through the use of videophones and monitoring equipment. Shopping malls will have ambulatory surgery centers and health booths providing access to healthcare providers. Treatment information obtained by e-mail will be common practice for patients and caregivers. Online communities and support groups will assist patients in self-care and disease management. Patients will be able to download personal physiologic data from any site. Wearable technology will monitor, detect, and send data wirelessly to health facilities. It will be possible to predict disease as a result of technology installed in the home or worn on the person.

Advances in technology may make vaccines for cancer and medications to prevent vascular disease available someday. New organs and body parts that correct or improve function may be commonly accessible. It is conceivable that bloodless surgery will be performed and drugs without side effects will be developed. Computer programs and clinical simulators will be universally used for practice in health education. Robotics will perform nursing support services for patient care through providing medication administration and physiologic monitoring.

Informatics technologies will have roles in protection and response for bioterrorism and national security. These capabilities will include emergency response systems, health alert networks, automated access to governmental support networks, and enlistment of workforce solutions. Informatics nurses will be called upon to establish, implement, and evaluate these initiatives.

Conclusion

Nursing informatics provides the solution to many of the challenges that health care is facing—from easing the strain of the nursing shortage to improving patient safety. Nurses must embrace technology and integrate it into their nursing practice. Technology will not go away. It will continue to transform healthcare delivery systems. Because of technology, individuals and groups communicate in new ways, the method in which we teach and learn has changed, and the way health care is delivered and acquired has changed. Nursing must continue to take a leadership role in the incorporation of technology in health care. Nursing informatics will provide the tools and skills to assist health care to move ahead in the ever-changing world.

Nursing informatics provides the solution to many of the challenges that health care is facing—from easing the strain of the nursing shortage to improving patient safety.

References

American Nurses Association. (2001). *Scope and standards of nursing informatics practice.* Washington, DC: American Nurses Publishing.

American Nurses Credentialing Center. (2007). *Informatics nurse certification exam.* Retrieved November 30, 2007, from http://www.nursecredentialing.org/cert/TCOs/BSN27_Info_TCO.html

Bliss, J. B., & DeYoung, S. (2002). *Working the Web: A guide for nurses.* Upper Saddle River, NJ: Prentice Hall.

Bush, G. W. (2004). *Transforming health care: The president's health information technology plan.* Retrieved November 12, 2007, from http://www.whitehouse.gov/focus/technology/economic_policy200404/chap3.html#

Garner, J. C. (2003). Final HIPAA security regulations: A review. *Managed Care Quarterly, 3*(11), 15–27.

Graves, J. R., & Corcoran, S. (1989). The study of nursing informatics. *IMAGE: Journal of Nursing Scholarship, 21*(4), 227–231.

Hannah, K. (1985). Current trends in nursing informatics: Implications for curriculum planning. In K. Hannah, E. J. Builenmin, & D. N. Corkin (Eds.), *Nursing uses of computer and information science.* Amsterdam: North-Holland.

Harris Poll. (2004, January 21). *Online activity grows as more people use Internet for more purposes.* Retrieved February 20, 2004, from http://www.harrisinteractive.com/harris_poll

Health on the Net Foundation. (1995). *HON code of conduct.* Retrieved November 12, 2007, from http://www.hon.ch/index.html

Hunter, K. M. (2002). Electronic health records. In S. Englebardt & R. Nelson (Eds.), *Health care informatics: An interdisciplinary approach* (pp. 209–230). St. Louis, MO: Mosby.

Mascara, C., Czar, P., & Hebda, T. (2001). *Internet resource guide for nurses and healthcare professionals* (2nd ed.). Upper Saddle River, NJ: Prentice Hall.

McCannon, M., & O'Neal, P. V. (2003). Results of a national survey indication information technology skills needed by nurses at time of entry into the work force. *Journal of Nursing Education, 42*(8), 337–340.

McNeil, B. J., Elfrink, V. L., Bickford, C. J., Pierce, S. T., Beyca, S. C., Averill, C., & Klappenbach, C. (2003). Nursing information technology knowledge, skills, and preparation of student nurses, nursing faculty, and clinicians: A US survey. *Journal of Nursing Education, 42*(8), 341–349.

Mendelson, C. (2003). Gentle hugs: Internet listservs as source of support for women with lupus. *Advances in Nursing Science, 26*(4), 299–306.

Nelson, A. (2003). Using simulation to design and integrate technology for safer and more efficient practice environments. *Nursing Outlook, 51*(3), S27–S29.

Newbold, S. K. (2003). New uses for wireless technology. *Nursing Management, 34*(10) (Supplement: IT Solutions), 22–23, 32.

Nicoll, L. H. (2001). *Nurses' guide to the Internet* (3rd ed.). Philadelphia: Lippincott.

Pagana, K. D. (2007). E-mail etiquette *American Nurse Today, 2*(7), 45.

Saba, V. K. (2001). Nursing informatics: Yesterday, today and tomorrow. *International Nursing Review, 48,* 177–187.

Sabb, V. K., & McCormick, K. A. (2006). *Essentials of nursing informatics* (4th ed.). New York: McGraw-Hill.

Smeltzer, S., Simmerman, V., Frain, M., DeSiltes, L., & Duffin, J. (2003). Accessible online health promotion information for persons with disabilities. *Online Journal of Issues in Nursing.* Retrieved February 20, 2004, from http://www.nursingworld.org/ojin/topic/tpc16_5.htm

Staggers, N., Gassert, C. A., & Curran, C. (2001). Informatics competencies for nurses at four levels of practice. *Journal of Nursing Education, 40*(7), 303–316.

Thede, L. Q. (2003). *Informatics and nursing: Opportunities & challenges* (2nd ed.). Philadelphia: Lippincott Williams & Wilkins.

Thompson, B. W. (2005). HIPAA guideline for using PDAs. *Nursing, 99*(35), 24.

US Department of Health and Human Services. (2000, November). *Healthy People 2010* (2nd ed.). With understanding and improving health and objectives for improving health (2 vols.). Washington, DC: U.S. Government Printing Office.

Young, K. M. (2000). *Informatics for healthcare professionals.* Philadelphia: F. A. Davis Company.

Zykowski, M. E. (2003). Nursing informatics: The key to unlocking contemporary nursing practice. *AACN Clinical Issues, 14*(3), 271–281.

Future Directions in Professional Nursing Practice

Katherine Elizabeth Nugent

LEARNING OBJECTIVES

After completing this chapter, the student should be able to:

1. Identify present trends associated with the profession of nursing that affect the transition of professional nursing practice for the future.
2. Articulate the vision for the future of nursing practice.
3. Reflect on the appropriate response of nursing leadership concerning issues affecting the future of nursing practice.

Key Terms and Concepts

- Nursing shortage
- Nurse faculty shortage
- Cultural competence
- Clinical nurse leader (CNL)
- Doctor of Nursing Practice (DNP)
- Gap between education and practice

The hardest thing is not to get people to accept new ideas; it is to get them to forget old ones.

—John Maynard Keyes

Peter Drucker stated that the best way to predict the future is to create it. The practice of nursing is facing a compilation of challenges: nursing shortage, workforce issues, cost and access of care, the education–practice gap, and changes in population demographics. While it is true that each of these issues is not a new challenge to nursing practice, it is critical to now acknowledge the collective impact of all of these challenges culminating in a "perfect storm" scenario. Nursing is rich in its history, resilient in its journey to develop as a profession and a discipline, and adaptive in its practice to meet the healthcare needs of the patient. Throughout its history, nursing has had identifiable periods of time in which the practice and education of nurses responded to the evolving changes in health care and in society. Today, nursing is again at the crossroads of a major transition in its education and practice. An awareness of the merging of these issues creates an urgency when contemplating the role, practice, and education of nurses.

It is almost a cliché to state that nothing is the same—nor will ever be again. Due to the explosion of knowledge and extraordinary innovation in technology, change is occurring so rapidly that our sphere of contact is expanded through instant communication, boundaryless relationships, and globalization of economics and politics (Porter-O'Grady & Malloch, 2003). This phenomenon of fluidity is characterized by conflict, complexity, and chaos resulting in instability within organizations. The convergence of chaos and complexity signals a transition between the past, present, and the future. This phenomenon is true of healthcare institutions, educational institutions, and the practice of nursing. Evidence, as reflected in quality outcomes, exists daily signaling that the healthcare system and the practice of nursing are straining to adapt to the forces of change. It is critical for nursing to analyze existing evidence and control nursing's transition for future success. Porter-O'Grady and Malloch state, "Moving into a new age does not mean leaving everything behind. It does mean thinking about what needs to be left behind and reflecting on what does go with us as we move into an age with a different set of parameters" (2003, p. 10).

This chapter will explore the phenomenon of nursing shortage, workforce issues, cost and access to care, the education–practice gap, and changes in population demographics and their cumulative effect on the practice of nursing. Since the proposition of this chapter is that the culmination of each of the issues creates the urgency for transition, the discussion of these challenges will be explored as one model with each issue as a concept that relates to and confounds other issues.

Nurse Shortage

Data from the Health Resources and Service Administration, Bureau of Health Professions, National Center for Health Workforce Analysis ("the center") has documented that the projected demand for nurses has exceeded the projected supply (HRSA, 2002). This data reflected that the **nursing shortage** began in the year 2000 when there was an estimated supply of 1.89 million nurses and with a projected demand of 2 million or 6% more than what existed. This scenario of excess demand continues today and is predicted to worsen each year for the next 12 years. The center projected the anticipated demand for nurses should continue to exceed the supply until 2010 when the shortage would reach 12%. "At that point demand will begin to exceed supply at an accelerated rate and by 2015 the shortage, a relatively modest 6% in the year 2000, will have almost quadrupled to 20%. If not addressed, and if current trends continue, the shortage is projected to grow to 29% by 2020" (HRSA, 2002).

It is difficult to fully comprehend the seriousness of this shortage, especially if it is viewed from a historical perspective of the frequent cycles of nursing shortages and if it is viewed as a separate issue. What is different about this nursing shortage? The answer to this question is complex and reflective of the other challenges that face the practice of nursing. The data reflecting the current profile of practicing nurses provides us with some insight into the phenomenon.

The average age of the practicing nurse has climbed steadily in the past decade resulting in a significant proportion of nurses approaching retirement. Data collected in the *National Sample Survey of Registered Nurses* (HRSA, 2004) document that the average age of the RN population is 46.8 years of age. Also, only 26.3% of the RN population is under 40 and only 8% is under the age of 30. Twenty-five percent of the RNs are over the age of 50. The data reflect fewer young nurses entering the RN population and larger cohorts of the RN population moving into their 50s and 60s.

Several factors served as antecedents to this scenario. The first was a period of declining enrollment in nursing schools and a higher age of the students graduating from nursing programs. Even with the recent increased enrollment of students in nursing programs, the number of new graduates is not increasing fast enough to balance the supply-and-demand ratio. Another precipitating factor is that in 2007, a report was released by the Pricewaterhouse Cooper's Health Research Institute that found that the average nurse turnover rate in hospitals was 8.4% and that the turnover rate for nurses in their first year of employment was 27.1%. The third major reason for this projected nurse shortage for the future is the increased number of baby boomers who will be accessing the healthcare system and thus increasing the projected number of hospital admissions.

Nursing Practice Setting

It is understandable how the shortage of nurses affects the practicing nurse and influences nurse turnover rate. However, there are other issues associated with the nurse practice setting that result in problematic quality outcomes. It is evident that health care and healthcare delivery has changed significantly in the past two decades. Most of these changes have been associated with response to the increasing cost of care, the decreasing cost of reimbursement to healthcare providers, increase in the use of technology in practice, and the knowledge explosion concerning disease management. A full discussion of each of these issues is beyond the scope of this chapter. However, it is important to note that most of the changes have resulted because of a focus on reducing the cost of health care. The move over the past decade to a system of managed care is the best example of this movement. The focus on cost containment has resulted in strategies aimed at determining the setting of the delivery of care, the length of stay in the hospital, the cost reimbursed to providers of care, and the designation of the appropriate provider of care. To date, it is fair to say that the changes in health care have resulted in chaos and complexity for both the provider and the recipient of care. Evidence has indicated that this environment of chaos and complexity has also created an environment that promotes a concern about access to care, quality of care, and patient safety (Adams & Corrigan, 2003; Institute of Medicine, 2000, 2004). The implementation of these various strategies has also resulted in nurse dissatisfaction.

"Although the percentage of nurses (68.1%) working in hospitals has decreased steadily since 1984: hospitals remain the major employer of nurses" (HRSA, 2004). The nursing staff provides continuous care for acute patients in a complex environment with highly technical equipment and involving multidisciplinary providers (Lin & Liang, 2007). The issues associated with the hospital work environment have been shown to dominate problems and outcomes associated with nursing practice. It is because of this environment that the practice of nursing has been challenged to evaluate its practice and outcomes. In fact, 75% of nurses completing a survey stated that they perceived that the unsafe working environment interfered with their ability to provide quality patient care (ANA, 2001a).

Nurses in the hospital are providing care for patients that are sicker, older, and have more complex physical, psychosocial, and economic needs (Brown, 2004; Clark, 2004). The combination of older patients with higher acuity, the sophisticated technology, and shorter hospital stays creates a chaotic environment and demands that nurses assume greater responsibility (Grando, 2006). This chaos also increases not only the risk of errors in patient care but the risk of health concerns of the nurse. Health concerns include the threat of infection, risks from needle sticks, and ever increasing sensitivity to latex, back injuries, and stress-related health problems. In addition to these health risks, nurses are susceptible to workplace violence (e.g., physical violence, horizontal violence) and sexual harassment (Smith-Pittman & McKoy, 1999; Valente & Bullough, 2004; Longo & Sherman, 2006; Ray & Ream, 2007).

The Institute of Medicine (2004) in exploring issues associated with errors in patient care, reported that as the primary work of the nurse is the "surveillance" of the patient and the coordination of the care, the work environment for nurses needs to be substantially transformed to support the nurses' practice and better protect patients. It further stated that the current healthcare environment is leading to patient harm and nurse burnout.

Other surveys of practicing nurses have documented that job dissatisfaction, patient safety concerns, decrease in quality care, inadequate staffing, patient care delays, and mandated overtime are issues negatively affecting their practice (Institute of Medicine, 1996; American Nurses Association, 2001b; Aiken et al., 2002; Cooper, 2004). Nurses have also reported being concerned about health and safety issues; with job stress being the most frequent health problem reported. Other health problems reported include back injuries, HIV, and hepatitis (ANA, 2001a).

Despite, the effort to address the issues of the chaotic and potentially harmful work environment, strategies to address these issues have fallen short of the target, and the dissatisfaction of hospital nurses has persisted. In a recent study, 41% of nurses currently working reported being dissatisfied with their jobs; 43% scored high in a range of burnout measures; and 22% were planning to leave their jobs in the next year. Of the latter group, 33% were under the age of 30 (JACHO, 2002). These factors help to create a scenario that further fuels the shortage of nurses.

Confounding the chaos is the shortage of healthcare workers, the supervision of unlicensed personnel, and the appropriate delegation of care, mandatory overtime, and staffing ratios. The debate over the use of unlicensed personnel and the use of other licensed personnel in providing patient care has been well documented in the literature (American Nurses Association, 1992, 1997, 1999; Barter & Furmidge, 1994; Manuel & Alster, 1994; Zimmerman, 2006). Research studies indicate that a decrease in RN staff increased patient care errors, infection rates, readmission, and morbidity (Aiken, Smith, & Lake, 1994; Aiken et al., 2002; Needleman et al., 2002; Stanton & Rutherford, 2004; Sofer, 2005).

If research indicates that a decrease in RN staff or use of unlicensed personnel and other licensed personnel influence quality patient outcomes, then what is a rationale for this practice? One answer that is quickly provided is the financial costs of a higher RN–patient ratio. The employment of nurses represents about 23% or higher of the hospital workforce. It is also known that the salary of the licensed RN is higher compared to other nonphysician healthcare providers. Thus, the basic assumption is that to employ more unlicensed personnel or other licensed personnel (LVN) would reduce the cost of care. This assumption is not necessarily true. One must consider costs other than salary, such as hiring, benefits, training, and staff turnover, and responsibilities that must be assumed by a licensed care provider. Aiken et al. (2002) found that nurses in hospitals with low nurse–patient ratios are more than twice as likely to experience job-related burnout and dissatisfaction with their jobs when compared to nurses in hospitals with the highest nurse–patient ratios. Cooper (2004) has noted that lower nursing staff ratios also indicate higher costs in a plethora of areas that reflect the actual reality of nursing practice. McCue, Mark, and Harless (2003) found that a 1% increase in nonnurse personnel increased the operating costs by 0.18% and diminished profits by 0.021%. One would question if these data are significant in the overall budget and considering the rising costs of health care. Zimmerman (2006) stated, "Futurescan: Health Trends and Implications, 2005–2010 (American College of Healthcare Executives, 2005) indicates the concept of healthcare organizations competing on value, which includes cost and quality dimensions, has become a reality. In the end, the question that may drive the debate concerning the use of the non-RN is what should the spending priorities of a hospital be?" (p. 325).

CRITICAL THINKING QUESTION

As a nursing student preparing to enter the profession of nursing, what do you think about the statistics presented in relation to the practice setting?

Nurse Faculty Shortage

In previous cycles of nursing shortage, the primary solution was to increase the enrollment in nursing programs. However, there is ample evidence that supports the conclusion that a national **nursing faculty shortage** also exists. In a survey conducted by AACN in June 2004, a total of 614 faculty vacancies were identified at 300 nursing schools across the nation. An interesting aspect of this survey was that the response rate for this survey was only 52.7%, and the population surveyed were baccalaureate and higher degree institutions only, leading to speculation that the vacancy rate is even higher (AACN, 2004). This shortage is limiting student capacity in nursing programs across the nation (AACN, 2004; SREB, 2002).

The number of nurses employed in nursing education has changed little since 1980. When the number of nurse educators is compared to the increase in number of RNs, the result is actually a decline (2.4%) in the percentage of nurses working in education (HRSA, 2004). Even though the American Association of Colleges of Nursing (AACN) has reported 7 consecutive years of enrollment growth in baccalaureate programs, the rate of growth has not been enough to meet the projected supply demand. In 2007, AACN reported that "Though enrollment increased by almost 5% in baccalaureate nursing programs, more than 30,000 qualified applicants were turned away from schools nationwide in 2007" (AACN, 2007).

An additional concern in the statistics of the nurse faculty shortage is that the average age of nurse faculty is 51.6 years of age, with the average age of PhD faculty being 58.6 (professor rank), 55.8 (associate professor rank), and 50.1 (assistant professor rank) (Fange, Wilsey Wisniewski, & Bednash, 2007). The age of the doctoral-prepared faculty is concerning, considering that 59.8% of the faculty vacancies reported in the 2003 AACN survey were positions requiring a doctoral degree. Berlin (2002) wrote that the average age at retirement of nurse faculty was 62.5 years. The author further projected that between the years of 2003 and 2012, 200–300 doctoral faculty will retire. An additional 220–280 master's-prepared faculty will be eligible for retirement between 2012 and 2018.

Changing Demographics

Despite national trends of increasing diversity with ethnic and racial minorities reaching almost one third of the US population, minorities are overall underrepresented in the healthcare profession. The 2004 US census reported that 67.4% of the population is white and non-Hispanic and 32.6% are nonwhite or Hispanic. In contrast, the registered nurse population remains predominantly female (94.2%) and 81.8% white, non-Hispanic (HRSA, 2004). The Sullivan Commission (2004) highlighted the diversity gap in its hallmark report *Missing Persons: Minorities in the Health Professions.* Together, African Americans, Hispanic Americans, and American Indians make up more than 25% of the US population but only 9% of the nation's nurses, 6% of its physicians, and 5% of dentists. Similar disparities show up in the faculties of health professional schools. For example, minorities make up less than 10% of baccalaureate nursing faculties, 8.6% of dental school faculties, and only 4.2% of medical school faculties. If the trends continue, the health workforce of the future will resemble the population even less than it does today. If these data are viewed in the context of the prediction that no racial or ethnic group will compose a majority by the year 2050, such a decline in a diverse workforce could be catastrophic.

In 2003, the Institute of Medicine (IOM) warned of the "unequal treatment" minorities face when encountering the health system. Cultural differences, a lack of access to health care, combined with high rates of poverty and unemployment, contribute to the substantial ethnic and racial disparities in health status and health outcomes (Institute of Medicine, 2003b). Health services research has shown that minority health professionals are more likely to serve minority and medically underserved populations. Increasing the number of underrepresented minorities in the health professions as well as improving the cultural competency of providers present key strategies of reducing health disparities (Betancourt, Green, Carrillo, & Ananeh-Firempong, 2003; Institute of Medicine, 2003b).

Cultural competence in multicultural societies continues as a major initiative for health care and nursing, specifically.

> The mass media, healthcare policy makers, the Office of Minority Health, and other governmental organizations, professional organizations, the workplace, and health insurance payers are addressing the need for individuals to understand and become culturally competent as one strategy to improve quality and eliminate racial, ethnic, and gender disparities in health care. (Purnell & Paulanka, 2008)

Culturally competent healthcare providers will reduce patient care error and increase access to and satisfaction with health care. The beginning of cultural competence is self-awareness. Culture has a powerful unconscious impact on health professionals and the care they provide. Purnell and Paulanka believe that self-knowledge and understanding promote strong professional perceptions that free healthcare providers from prejudice and facilitate culturally competent care.

Nursing has a long history of incorporating culture into nursing practice (DeSantis & Lipson, 2007). Yet, some maintain, no matter how culturally competent the nurse may be, the patient's experience remains structured in the nurse's culture (Dean, 2005). Despite nurses' best efforts to understand the culture of the patient, nurses often fail to understand that the patient may be experiencing health care for the first time, not in his or her own culture, but in the nurse's culture of healthcare delivery. The understanding of this concept associated with cultural competence increases the reality of the urgency in increasing the diversity in the nursing workforce.

Nursing Education

As the gap between nursing education and expected performance in practice appears to widen, questions are being raised about the knowledge, skill, and education needed in nursing to ensure issues of quality and safety.

The changes in health care, the chaos and complexity of the hospital practice environment, the advances in technology, the change in population demographics, and the nursing shortage, including the nurse faculty shortage, have prompted a need for nursing education reform. As the gap between nursing education and expected performance in practice appears to widen, questions are being raised about the knowledge, skill, and education needed in nursing to ensure issues of quality and safety. The issues around nursing education extend into the practice setting. Whether a nurse graduates from a 2-year, 3-year, or 4-year nursing program, the transition into practice is quick, with little time for mentoring or on-the-job training (JACHO, 2002).

Throughout the years, nursing education has made an effort to transition its curriculum and programs to accommodate the knowledge explosion and the advanced technology associated with health care. However, the transition within the programs of nursing has assumed a patchwork approach instead of significant reform. This is due in part to the tradition associated with the history of nursing education, the inability to resolve the differences in prelicensure programs, and faculty propensity to be reluctant to "leave behind" what is no longer successful in a changing practice arena.

In 2003, the Institute of Medicine issued a report titled *Health Professions Education: A Bridge to Quality* (Institute of Medicine, 2003a). This report, which focused on knowledge that healthcare professionals needed to provide quality care, stated that students in the health professions are not prepared to address the shifts in the country's demographics nor or they educated to work in interdisciplinary teams. They further stated that students were not able to access evidence for use in practice, determine the reasons for or prevent patient care errors, or access technology to acquire the latest information. Specifically, the report expressed concern with the adequacy of nursing education at all levels, yet focused intensely on education at the prelicensure level. The report identified five core competencies that all clinicians should possess: (1) provide patient-centered care; (2) work in interdisciplinary teams; (3) use evidence-based practice; (4) apply quality improvement and identify errors and hazards in care; and (5) utilize informatics (IOM, 2003).

In response to the IOM (2003a) and the JACHO (2002) reports, the American Association of Colleges of Nursing proposed two new educational programs for nursing. The first is the **clinical nurse leader (CNL)**, an advanced generalist role prepared at the master's level of education. The CNL oversees the coordination of care for a group of patients, assesses cohort risk, provides direct patient care in complex situations, and functions as a part of an interdisciplinary team (AACN, 2007). The lateral integration of care has been what is missing in the delivery of care to patients with complex needs. There has been no single person who oversees patient care laterally and over time and who is able to intervene, facilitate, or coordinate care for the entire patient experience. The CNL will be instrumental in helping all disciplines see the interdependencies that exist between and among them (Begun et al., 2006).

What makes the CNL movement different from past efforts within nursing? There has been thoughtful and broad engagement in looking at both the educational and competency needs of nursing to function in an environment that has changed dramatically and become extremely complex. This change requires advanced knowledge, new skills, and interdependent relationships. The uniqueness of the inception and implementation of the CNL is the approach that is: (1) being advanced as a partnership with education and practice, (2) occurring at a broad national level of activity, (3) being structured with milestones for the partnerships to attain, and (4) being facilitated by nurses and administrators at the highest levels within healthcare organizations (Begun et al., 2006).

Another new program within nursing is the **Doctor of Nursing Practice (DNP)**. The need for this terminal practice degree was based upon the series of reports from the Institute of Medicine (IOM) that address quality of health care, patient safety, and educational reform, as well as following the movement of other healthcare professions to the practice doctorate. In 2002, the American Association of Colleges of Nursing (AACN) established a task force to examine the current status of existing advanced practice programs, current existing practice doctorates, and future need for such a program. AACN in collaboration with the National Organization of Nurse Practitioner Faculties met with other constituencies and held regional meetings to discuss the nature of this terminal degree and the need for a terminal degree in practice. After much national discussion and debate, it was determined that a practice doctorate was needed that encompassed any form of nursing intervention that influences healthcare outcomes for individual patients, management of care for individuals and populations, administration of nursing and health organization, and the development and implementation of health policy (AACN, 2004). It was clearly stated that this practice degree was not the same as the research doctoral degree and that graduates would be prepared to blend clinical, economic, organizational, and leadership skills and to use science in improving the direct care of patients, care of patient populations, and practice that supports patient care (Champagne, 2006).

At the AACN 2004 annual meeting, the recommendations of the task force were endorsed by the membership, supporting the need for a DNP degree. The recommendations also stated that the educational preparation of advanced practice nurses, broadly defined, would be transitioned from the master's level to the practice doctorate level (DNP) by 2015 (AACN, 2004). Two years later, *The Essentials for Doctoral Education for Advanced Practice Education* was endorsed by the membership (AACN, 2006). Even though the implementation of the DNP has raised much concern and many questions, 59 programs exist and another 140 additional institutions are planning to establish the degree (AACN, 2008).

The development of the DNP and the CNL programs of study represents a bold effort by the profession of nursing to address the issues of educational reform needed to prepare graduates to meet the healthcare needs of the future. Although, many questions and concerns surround the implementation of these two new programs, and the evaluation of the implementation of these programs is yet to be determined, one must applaud the spirit of evidence-based educational innovation.

Conclusion

The challenges of the nursing shortage, workforce issues, cost and access to care, the education–practice gap, and changes in population demographics have merged together to create a crisis point for the profession of nursing.

This chapter supports the concept that the challenges of the nursing shortage, workforce issues, cost and access to care, the education–practice gap, and changes in population demographics have merged together to create a crisis point for the profession of nursing. Individually, each identified challenge in itself would create a need for some degree of change in the practice of nursing, and considered individually, nursing would have continued to patch together a response. Together, the compounding consequences of these challenges signal the need for major transformation in nursing. The culminating results of these issues have been connected to a decline in quality care, dissatisfaction in the achieved outcomes of practice, and a wider gap between education preparation and performance in the practice setting.

The issue of the employment of non-RN personnel for patient care is not one that will disappear in the future, given the predicted increase in patient population and the nurse shortage. Currently, 97% of hospitals employ UAP (Zimmerman, 2006). The issue may indeed be how will nursing practice transition? Will the move continue to be from the hospital to other healthcare settings? Will nurses redefine who they are and what constitutes their practice?

The **gap between education and practice** looms larger as the healthcare setting continually changes as a result of advanced technology, knowledge explosion, shorter hospital stays, and rapid changes in disease management. Emphasis is now placed on evidence-based medicine and evidence-based practice. In general, curriculums in nursing programs have not evolved to keep pace with changes in the practice setting. The reasons are varied and include limited funding sources, confinement of higher education boundaries and standards, past success in educational outcomes, inability to differentiate between levels of nursing practice, multiple entry into practice and licensure, and pedagogical methods that emphasize receiving content rather than discovery of evidence. The current emphasis on integrating clinical simulation as a teaching and evaluation strategy and the development of the clinical nurse leader (MSN generalist) and doctor of nursing practice are steps in the right direction.

Evidence supports that a better educated nurse is needed in practice. The initial educational preparation for the largest proportion of RNs is the associate degree. In 2004, the initial educational level of registered nurses indicated that 733,000 (25.2%) were diploma, 1,227,000 (42.2%) were associate degree, and 903,000 (31%) were baccalaureate (HRSA, 2004). In 2004, 33.7% of nurses (981,238) reported the associate degree as their highest level of nursing education, 34.2% (994,276) reported the baccalaureate degree as their highest level, and 13% (376,901) reported a master's or doctoral degree as their highest level of education. Leaders in nursing education must identify a way to move younger students to the desired graduate level of education more expediently.

> **CRITICAL THINKING QUESTIONS**
>
> Can you think of some incentives or strategies to move younger nurses into graduate-level education? Do you have plans to pursue graduate-level education soon after you complete your undergraduate nursing education? What do you think will be the impact on professional nursing if we are able to accomplish the goal of increasing the educational level of nurses in practice?

Clearer roles in practice must be developed, answering the question what do nurses do. The answer will probably be different than the traditional role of nursing practiced by those who are nearing retirement. As the future evolves, an increase in the movement of nurses from the hospitals into other settings of care will be realized. Entrepreneurial opportunities will be available for nurses, and nurses will be able to implement their theory-based practice in providing quality health care to the population.

The theme of promoting cultural competence in health care will be explored from two perspectives: creating practice environments that support culturally competent care and developing educational programs that foster cultural awareness and sensitivity among students in the healthcare professions. As the population continues to become more diverse, culturally competent care will be the basis for quality care, access to care, and alleviation of health disparities, thus promoting healthier population outcomes.

The nursing profession must be able to navigate the high-speed, convoluted pace of the current healthcare delivery system. Nurses must be competent to meet the demands of the current patient population, the complex technology, more responsibility, and cost-contained care. In reality, the changes in advanced technology, the updates in pharmacological interventions, the knowledge explosion, and the advancements in gene therapy will significantly change not only the practice of the nurse but that of all healthcare providers. The innovation in technology, the culture of violence, terrorism, and the increase in natural disasters resulting from global warming will change the practice of nursing. It is imperative that professional nurses control their future and redefine their roles in practice. Noel Tichy (1997) stated, "In the future, the real core competence of organizations will be the ability to continuously and creatively destroy and remake themselves." The same might be applied to the profession of nursing. Are you ready to be a part of transforming professional nursing practice as we transition our profession into the future?

CLASSROOM ACTIVITY

Divide into five groups. Each group should have markers and large pieces of paper such as newsprint. Each group should consider the information and data presented in one section of the chapter: (1) nurse shortage, (2) nurse practice setting, (3) nurse faculty shortage, (4) changing demographics, or (5) nursing education. In your group develop a plan to address the issues identified. What are the obstacles to implementing your plan? What would be the benefits of implementing your plan? Would your plan have any impact on the issues presented in the other sections of the chapter? If so, what impact? Each group should briefly present its plans to the class. Finally, as a class discuss how the individual group plans might be integrated into a comprehensive plan to create the future of professional nursing practice.

References

Adams, K., & Corrigan, J. (Eds.) (2003). *Priority areas for national action: Transforming health care quality.* Quality Chasm Series. Washington, DC: National Academies Press.

Aiken, L., Clarke, S., Sloane, D., Sochalski, J., & Silber, J. (2002). Hospital nurse staffing and patient mortality, nurse burnout, and job dissatisfaction. *Journal of the American Medical Association, 288*(16), 1987–1993.

Aiken, L., Smith, H., & Lake, E. (1994). Lower Medicare mortality among a set of hospitals known for good nursing care. *Medical Care, 32,* 771–787.

American Association of Colleges of Nursing. (2002). *Nursing faculty shortage fact sheet.* Washington, DC: Author.

American Association of Colleges of Nursing. (2003). *Special survey on vacant faculty positions.* Washington, DC: Author.

American Association of Colleges of Nursing. (2004). *AACN position statement on the practice doctorate in nursing.* Press Release. Retrieved February 20, 2008, from http://www.aacn.nche.edu/DNP/index.htm

American Association of Colleges of Nursing. (2006). *Essentials of doctoral education for advanced nursing practice.* Retrieved February 10, 2008, from http://www.aacn.nche.edu/DNP/index.htm

American Association of Colleges of Nursing. (2007, February). *White paper on the education and role of the clinical nurse leader.* Washington, DC: Author.

American Association of Colleges of Nursing. (2008). *List of programs offering the DNP.* Retrieved February 10, 2008, from http://www.aacn.nche.edu/DNP/index.htm

American Nurses Association. (1992). *Position statement on registered nurse utilization of unlicensed assistive personnel.* Washington, DC: Author.

American Nurses Association. (1997). *Implementing nursing's report card: Study of RN staffing, length of stay, and patient outcomes.* Washington, DC: Author.

American Nurses Association. (1999). *Principles for nurse staffing.* Washington, DC: Author.

American Nurses Association. (2001a). *Nursing world health and safety survey.* Retrieved February 4, 2008, from http://www.nursingworld.org/surveys/hssurvey.pdf

American Nurses Association. (2001b). *Analysis of American Nurses Association: Staffing survey.* Retrieved February 4, 2008, from http://www.nursingworld.org/staffing/ana_pdf.pdf

Barter, M., & Furmidge, M. (1994). Unlicensed assistive personnel: Issues related to delegation and supervision. *Journal of Nursing Administration, 24*(4), 36–40.

Begun, J., Hamilton, J., Tornabeni, J., & White. K. (2006). Opportunities for improving patient care through lateral integration: The clinical nurse leader. *Journal of Healthcare Management, 51*(1), 19–25.

Berlin, L. (2002). The shortage of doctorally prepared nursing faculty: A dire situation. *Nursing Outlook, 50*(2), 50–56.

Betancourt, J. R., Green, A. R., Carrillo, J. E., & Ananeh-Firempong, O. (2003). Defining cultural competence: A practical framework for addressing racial/ethnic disparities in health and health care. *Public Health Report, 118*(4), 293–302.

Brown, B. (2004). From the editor: Restoring caring back into nursing. *Nursing Administration Quarterly, 28*, 237–238.

Champagne, M. (2006). The future of nursing education: Educational models for future care. In P. Cowen and S. Moorhead (Eds.), *Current issues in nursing* (7th ed.). St. Louis, MO: Mosby/Elsevier

Clark, J. (2004). An aging population with chronic disease compels new delivery systems focused on new structures and practice. *Nursing Administration Quarterly, 28*, 105–115.

Cooper, P. (2004). Nurse-patient ratios revisited. (Editorial). *Nursing Forum, 39*(2), 3–4.

Dean, P. (2005). Transforming ethnocentricity in nursing: A culturally relevant experience of reciprocal visits between Malta and the Midwest. *Journal of Continuing Education in Nursing, 36*(4), 163, 167.

DeSantis, L., & Lipson, J.(2007). Brief history of inclusion of content on culture in nursing education. *Journal of Transcultural Nursing, 18*(7), 7s–9s.

Drucker, P. *A personal quote.* Retrieved February 10, 2008, at http://www.famous-quotes.com/topic.php?tid=502

Fange, D., Wilsey Wisniewski, S., & Bednash, G. (2007). *2006–2007 salaries of instructional and administrative nursing faculty in baccalaureate and graduate programs in nursing.* Washington, DC: American Association of Colleges of Nursing.

Grando, V. (2006). Staff nurses working in hospitals: Who they are, what they do, and what are their challenges? In P. Cowen and S. Moorhead (Eds.), *Current issues in nursing* (7th ed.). St. Louis, MO: Mosby/Elsevier.

HRSA. (2002). *Projected supply, demand, and shortages of registered nurses: 2000–2020.* Washington, DC: Health Resources and Services Administration, Bureau of Health Professions National Center for Health Workforce Analysis.

HRSA. (2004). *The registered nurse population: Finding from the March 2004 National Sample Survey of Registered Nurses.* Washington, DC: Health Resources and Services Administration, Bureau of Health Professions.

Institute of Medicine. (1996). *Nursing staff in hospitals and nursing homes: Is it adequate?* Washington, DC: National Academy Press.

Institute of Medicine. (2000). *To err is human: Building a safer health system.* Washington, DC: National Academy Press.

Institute of Medicine. (2003a). *Health professions education: A bridge to quality.* Washington, DC: National Academy Press.

Institute of Medicine. (2003b). *Unequal treatment: Confronting racial and ethnic disparities in health care.* Washington, DC: National Academy Press.

Institute of Medicine. (2004). *Keeping patients safe: Transforming the work environment of nurses.* Washington, DC: National Academies Press.

JACHO. (2002). *Healthcare at the crossroads: Strategies for addressing the evolving nurse crisis* (2002). Joint Commission on Accreditation of Healthcare Organizations. Retrieved February 9, 2008, from http://www.jointcommission.org/NR/rdonlyres/5C138711-ED76-4D6F-909F-B06E0309F36D/0/health_care_at_the_crossroads.pdf

Lin, L., & Liang, B. (2007). Addressing the nursing work environment to promote patient safety. *Nursing Forum, 42*(1), 22–29.

Longo, J., & Sherman, R. (2006). Leveling horizontal violence. *Nursing Management, 38*(3), 34–37, 50–51.

Manuel, P., & Alster, L. (1994). Unlicensed personnel no cure for an ailing health care system. *Nursing & Health Care, 15*(1), 18–21.

McCue, M., Mark, B., & Harless, D. (2003). Nurse staffing, quality, and financial performance. *Journal of Healthcare Finance, 29*(4), 54–76.

Needleman, J., Buerhaus, P., Mattke, S., Stewart, M., & Zelevinsky, K. (2002). Nurse staffing levels and the quality of care in hospitals. *New England Journal of Medicine, 346,* 1715–1722.

Porter-O'Grady, T., & Malloch, K. (2003). *Quantum leadership: A textbook of new leadership* (p. 1). Sudbury, MA: Jones and Bartlett.

Pricewaterhouse Cooper's Health Research Institute. (2007, July). *What works: Healing the healthcare staffing shortage.* Retrieved February 4, 2008, from http://www.pwc.com/ext web/pwcpublications.nsf/docid/674D1E79A678A0428525730D006B74A9

Purnell, L., & Paulanka, B. *Transcultural health care: A culturally competent approach* (3rd ed.). Philadelphia: F. A. Davis.

Ray, M., & Ream, K. (2007). The dark side of the job: Violence in the emergency department. *Journal of Emergency Nursing 2007, 33*(3), 257–261.

Smith-Pittman, M., & McKoy, Y. (1999). Workplace violence in healthcare environments. *Nursing Forum, 34*(3), 5–13.

Sofer, D. (2005). You get what you pay for: News flash: Higher nurse-patient ratios still saves lives. *American Journal of Nursing, 105*(11), 20.

SREB (Southern Regional Education Board), Council on Collegiate Education for Nursing. (2002). *SREB study indicates serious shortage of nursing faculty.* Atlanta, GA: Author.

Stanton, M., & Rutherford, M. (2004). How many nurses are enough? Hospital staff nursing and quality care research. *Accidents and Emergency Nursing, 15*(1), 1–2.

Sullivan Commission. (2004). *Missing persons: Minorities in the health professions. A report of the Sullivan Commission on diversity in the health care workforce.* Retrieved February 9, 2008, from http://www.sullivancommission.org

Tichy, N. (1997). *The leadership engine: How winning companies create leaders at all levels.* New York: HarperCollins.

Valente, S., & Bullough, V. (2004). Sexual harassment of nurses in the workplace. *Journal of Nursing Care Quality, 19*(3), 234–241.

Zimmerman, P. (2006). Who should provide nursing care? In P. Cowen and S. Moorhead (Eds.), *Current issues in nursing* (7th ed., pp. 324–331). St. Louis, MO: Mosby Elsevier.

American Nurses Association *Standards of Nursing Practice*

Standards of Care (Use of the Nursing Process)

Standard I   Assessment: The nurse collects client health data.

Standard II   Diagnosis: The nurse analyzes assessment data in determining diagnoses.

Standard III   Outcome identification: The nurse identifies expected outcomes individualized to the client.

Standard IV   Planning: The nurse develops a plan of care that prescribes interventions to attain expected outcomes.

Standard V   Implementation: The nurse implements the interventions identified in the plan of care.

Standard VI   Evaluation: The nurse evaluates the client's progress toward attainment of outcomes.

Standards of Professional Performance (Professional Behavior)

Standard I   Quality of care: The nurse systematically evaluates the quality and effectiveness of nursing practice.

Standard II   Performance appraisal: The nurse evaluates his or her own nursing practice in relation to professional practice standards and relevant statutes and regulations.

Standard III   Education: The nurse acquires and maintains current knowledge in nursing practice.

Standard IV   Collegiality: The nurse contributes to the professional development of peers, colleagues, and others.

Standard V   Ethics: The nurse's decisions and actions on behalf of clients are determined in an ethical manner.

Standard VI   Collaboration: The nurse collaborates with the client, significant others, and healthcare providers in providing client care.

Standard VII   Research: The nurse uses research findings in practice.

Standard VIII   Resource use: The nurse considers factors related to safety, effectiveness, and cost in planning and delivering client care.

Source: American Nurses Association. (1991). *Standards of clinical nursing practice.* Washington, DC: Author.

American Nurses Association *Code of Ethics*

Provision 1 The nurse, in all professional relationships, practices with compassion and respect for the inherent dignity, worth, and uniqueness of every individual, unrestricted by conditions of social or economic status, personal attributes, or the nature of health problems.

Provision 2 The nurse's primary commitment is to the patient, whether an individual, family, group, or community.

Provision 3 The nurse promotes, advocates for, and strives to protect the health, safety, and rights of the patient.

Provision 4 The nurse is accountable and responsible for individual nursing practice and determines the appropriate delegation of tasks consistent with the nurse's obligation to provide optimum patient care.

Provision 5 The nurse owes the same duties to self as to others, including the responsibility to preserve integrity and safety, to maintain competence, and to continue personal and professional growth.

Provision 6 The nurse participates in establishing, maintaining, and improving healthcare environments and conditions of employment conducive to the provision of quality healthcare and consistent with the values of the profession through individual and collective action.

Provision 7 The nurse participates in the advancement of the profession through contributions to practice, education, administration, and knowledge development.

Provision 8 The nurse collaborates with other health professionals and the public in promoting community, national, and international efforts to meet health needs.

Provision 9 The profession of nursing, as represented by associations and their members, is responsible for articulating nursing values, for maintaining the integrity of the profession and its practice, and for shaping social policy.

The *ANA Code of Ethics with Interpretive Statements* is available in its entirety in print from the American Nurses Association and is also available in its entirety at http://nursingworld.org/ethics/code/ethicscode150.htm.

Source: American Nurses Association. (2001). *Code of ethics with interpretive statements.* Washington, DC: Author.

Glossary

5-year plan: A plan that has clear objectives and follows specific steps to meet those objectives while allowing for flexibility in adjusting to changing life circumstances.

Academic Center for Evidence-Based Nursing (ACE) Star Model of Knowledge Transformation: This model involves five steps: discovery, summary, translation, implementation, and evaluation.

Access to care: Living in rural areas has unique concerns regarding access to care. As finances influence the closing of many rural hospitals, more communities find themselves struggling to find primary care providers who will work in those areas.

Active euthanasia: Active euthanasia occurs when a person takes an action to end a life (including one's own life). Active euthanasia may include a lethal dose of medication, such as in physician-assisted suicide.

Administrative or regulatory law: The regulatory process is itself governed by statutory law called administrative procedure acts at both federal and state levels. These acts provide that before regulations can be adopted a published notice of the proposed rules and where they are available must occur. The published notice and availability of the proposed rules provide concerned persons with the opportunity to comment on and suggest changes to the rules before final adoption. When rules are adopted they become administrative law within a set period of time. Thus, the process has three steps: (1) proposal of regulations, (2) consideration of proposed regulations, and (3) adoption of regulations with or without changes.

Advance directive: A written expression of a person's wishes about medical care, especially care during a terminal or critical illness.

Advanced beginner: Benner's stage 2, the advanced beginner, the student is able to formulate principles that dictate action. For example, the advanced beginner would grasp the rationale behind why different medications require different injection techniques.

Advocate: The nurse speaks for the patient or maintains the patient's rights in the face of the healthcare system. As the nurse–client relationship develops, the nurse needs professional knowledge to assist the clients in their decision making. The nurse fills the role of advocate in the delivery of health care, intervening in crises of AIDS, homelessness, drug and alcohol abuse, teenage pregnancy, child and spouse abuse, and increasing healthcare costs. A client advocate is a person who pleads the cause for clients' rights.

Age-related changes: Changes in cognition, vision, and hearing that occur as one ages. Research has demonstrated that teaching is not as effective if it does not accommodate for age-related cognitive and sensory changes.

AGREE instrument: A framework for determining the quality of guidelines for diagnoses, health promotion, treatments, or clinical interventions.

Alternative program: Alternative programs for nurses with drug and alcohol addictions exist. Nurses must qualify for the program.

American Journal of Nursing: Mary Adelaide Nutting, Lavinia L. Dock, Sophia Palmer, and Mary E. Davis were instrumental in developing the first nursing journal, the *American Journal of Nursing* (AJN) in October of 1900. Through the

ANA and the AJN, nurses then had a professional organization and a national journal with which to communicate with each other.

American Nurses Association: The American Nurses Association (ANA) is the only full-service professional organization representing the nation's 2.9 million registered nurses (RNs) through its 54 constituent member associations. The ANA advances the nursing profession by fostering high standards of nursing practice, promoting the rights of nurses in the workplace, projecting a positive and realistic view of nursing, and by lobbying the Congress and regulatory agencies on healthcare issues affecting nurses and the public.

Andragogy: Initially defined as "the art and science of helping adults learn," andragogy has taken on a broader meaning over the past 35 years and is currently used to refer to learner-focused education for people of all ages.

Assumptions: Assumptions describe concepts or connect two concepts and represent values, beliefs, or goals. When assumptions are challenged, they become propositions.

Asynchronous: Not occurring in real time.

Autonomy: Autonomy involves one's ability to self-rule and to generate personal decisions independently.

Barton, Clara: In 1882 Barton was able to convince Congress to ratify the Treaty of Geneva, thus becoming the founder of the American Red Cross.

Basic dignity: Basic dignity is intrinsic, or inherent, and dwells within all humans, with all humans being ascribed this moral worth.

Beliefs: Beliefs indicate what we value and often have a faith component. Rokeach (1973) identified three categories of beliefs: existential, evaluative, and prescriptive/proscriptive beliefs.

Beneficence: Beneficence in nursing implies that nurses take actions to benefit patients and to facilitate their well-being.

Best interest standard: Based on the goal of the surrogate's doing what is best for the patient or what is in the best interest of the patient.

Bioethics: A specific domain of ethics that is focused on moral issues in the field of health care.

Black Death: During the Middle Ages, a series of horrible epidemics, including the Black Death or bubonic plague, ravaged the civilized world. In the 1300s, Europe, Asia, and Africa saw nearly half their populations lost to the bubonic plague.

Bolton, Frances Payne: This congressional representative from Ohio is credited with the founding of the Cadet Nurse Corps through the Bolton Act of 1945. By the end of WWII, over 180,000 nursing students had been trained through this act, while advanced practice graduate nurses in psychiatry and public health nursing had received graduate education to increase the numbers of nurse educators.

Boolean logic: The use of Boolean operators AND, OR, and NOT to enhance searching efforts on the Web.

Boundaries: In nursing, boundaries can be thought of in terms of appropriate professional behavior that serves to maintain trust between patients and nurses and to maintain nurses' good standing within their profession.

Breckenridge, Mary: Founder of the Frontier Nursing Service.

Brewster, Mary: A colleague of Lillian Wald, Brewster established the Henry Street Settlement in the same neighborhood in 1893. She quit medical school and devoted the remainder of her life to "visions of a better world" for the public's health.

Brown Report: *Nursing for the Future* or the Brown Report, authored by Esther Lucille Brown in 1948 and sponsored by the Russell Sage Foundation, was critical of the quality and structure of nursing schools in the United States. The Brown Report became the catalyst for the implementation of educational nursing program accreditation through the National League for Nursing.

Burnout: Burnout occurs when nurses can no longer cope with the stresses and strains of professional nursing and choose to leave the profession to seek employment elsewhere.

Cadet Nurse Corps: WWII and the resulting severe shortage of nurses on the home front resulted in the development of the Cadet Nurse Corps.

Capitalistic society: Profit motivated. Even though we live in a capitalistic society, nursing in the United States has been protected against the details of healthcare finance.

Career management: A planned logical progression of one's professional life that includes clearly defined goals and objectives and a plan for achievement.

Caregiver: The role as a dependent person to the physician who only provided personal care has evolved to that of the educated nurse who is an autonomous and informed professional. As a caregiver, the nurse practices nursing as a science.

Case law: Case law is established from court decisions, which may explain or interpret the other sources of law.

Case management: A current nursing model of nursing care delivery is case management, which relies on clinical pathways to evaluate care. The critical pathway refers to expected outcomes and interventions that the collaborative practice team establishes. The professional nurse is responsible for initiating and updating the plan of care, care map, or clinical pathway used to consistently guide and evaluate client care.

Case manager: Organizes patient care by major diagnoses or DRGs and focuses on specific time frames to achieve predetermined patient outcomes and contain costs. The case manager makes referrals to other healthcare providers and manages the quality of care.

Chadwick Report: Edwin Chadwick became a major figure in the development of the field of public health in Great Britain by drawing attention to the cost of the unsanitary conditions that shortened the life span of the laboring class and the threats to the wealth of Britain. One consequence of the report was the establishment of the first board of health, the General Board of Health for England, in 1848.

CINAHL: The authoritative resource for nursing and allied health professionals, students, educators, and researchers.

Civil law: The law of civil or private rights, as opposed to criminal law.

Clinical judgment skills: Use of the clinician's experience and knowledge in assessment, diagnosis, planning, intervention, and evaluation.

Clinical nurse leader (CNL): An advanced generalist role prepared at the master's level of education.

Clinical practice guidelines: Developed to guide clinical practice and represent an effort to put a large body of evidence into a manageable form.

Cochrane Library: The Cochrane Library is a collection of databases that contain high-quality, independent evidence to inform healthcare decision making.

Collaboration: To work jointly with others.

Collaborative critical path: Refers to expected outcomes and interventions that the collaborative practice team establishes emphasizing the interdisciplinary collaboration of the critical pathway.

Collaborative practice: The purpose of collaboration is to achieve high-quality client care and client satisfaction. A collaborative framework with an interdisciplinary team can also limit costs as well as improve quality of care.

Comanagement: Comanagement and referral represent the highest level of collaboration, in which providers are responsible and accountable for their own aspects of care, and then patients are directed to other providers when the problem is beyond their expertise.

Competent: Benner's stage 3, competent, is characterized by the ability to analyze problems and prioritize. The nurse has a solid grasp of the rules and principles. The nurse at this stage has had experience in a variety of clinical situations and is able to draw on prior knowledge and experience.

Complementary and alternative medicine: Complementary medicine refers to an approach that *combines* conventional medicine with less conventional options, whereas alternative medicine is an approach used *instead of* conventional medicine.

Concept: A concept is a term or label that describes a phenomenon. The phenomenon described by a concept may be either empirical or it may be abstract.

Conceptual model: A conceptual model is defined as a set of concepts and statements that integrate the concepts into a meaningful configuration.

Confidentiality: To fulfill their social contract to provide nursing care, nurses must often gather sensitive information from patients. Thus, the nurse, along with other caregivers, has the obligation to keep healthcare information confidential. Privacy is the right of the patient. Confidentiality is the obligation of all healthcare providers.

Consultation: Obtaining the opinion of a specialist or other caregiver.

Consumerism: The concept of consumers having more control of their healthcare experiences.

Continuity of care: The primary nurse provides for continuity of care with the initiation of appropriate interventions and assessment for collaboration, changing the current plan of care with continuous evaluation of outcomes.

Core values: Those values that are most important to us; the values that define who we are as human beings. In 1998 the American Association of Colleges of Nursing (AACN, 1998) developed five core values to facilitate the development of professional nursing values. The core values embraced by the AACN are human dignity, integrity, autonomy, altruism, and social justice.

Critical pathway: Refers to expected outcomes and interventions that the collaborative practice team establishes.

Critical thinking: Critical thinking is the ability to think in a systematic and logical manner, solve problems, make decisions, and establish priorities in the clinical setting. Critical thinking is the competent use of thinking skills and abilities to make sound clinical judgments and safe decision making.

Cultural competence: The ability to interact effectively with people of different cultures. Cultural competence comprises of awareness of one's own worldviews, attitude toward cultural differences, knowledge of different cultural practices, and cross-cultural skills.

Database: A collection of electronic data into individual records that are systematically organized, indexed, and cross-referenced. A database allows for the rapid collection, organization, manipulation, and analysis of data.

Deaconesses: Nursing was most influenced by Christianity with the beginning of deaconesses, or female servants, doing the work of God by ministering to the needs of others. This role of the deaconess in the church was considered a forward step in the development of nursing, and in the 1800s would strongly influence the young Florence Nightingale.

Delano, Jane A.: Director of Nursing in the American Red Cross, she initiated a national publicity campaign to recruit young women to enter nurses' training.

Delegation: The process by which responsibility and authority for performing a certain task are transferred to another individual.

Deontology: Refers to actions that are duty based, not based on their rewards, happiness, or consequences. One of the most influential philosophers for the deontologic way of thinking was Immanuel Kant, a German philosopher from the 1700s.

Dignity: In general terms, a person has dignity if he or she is in a situation where his or her capabilities can be effectively applied.

Disaster preparedness: Plans designating response during an emergency and often coordinated by local, state, and federal groups. Firefighters, police officers, and healthcare professionals are part of response teams.

Dix, Dorothea: A Boston schoolteacher, Dix became aware of the horrendous conditions in prisons and mental institutions. For the rest of her life, Dorothea Dix stood out as a tireless zealot for the humane treatment of the insane and imprisoned. She had exceptional savvy in dealing with legislators.

Dock, Lavinia Lloyd: Became a militant suffragist linking women's roles as nurses to the emerging women's movement in the United States.

Doctor of Nursing Practice (DNP): This practice degree encompasses any form of nursing intervention that influences healthcare outcomes for individual patients, management of care for individuals and populations, administration of nursing and health organization, and the development and implementation of health policy. This practice degree is not the same as the research doctoral degree, and graduates are prepared to blend clinical, economic, organizational, and leadership skills and to use science in improving the direct care of patients, care of patient populations, and practice that supports patient care.

Durable power of attorney: The legal document with the most strength, this is a written directive in which a designated person is allowed to make either general or healthcare decisions for a patient.

EBSCO: An electronic journals service available to both academic and corporate subscribers. It aggregates access to electronic journals from various publishers.

Electronic health record: Represents multiple systems that are interfaced to share data and networked to support information management and communication within a healthcare organization.

Electronic mail (e-mail): A method of composing, sending, receiving, and storing messages over electronic communication systems; the most common use of the Internet.

Environment: One of the four concepts of the metaparadigm of nursing; the environment within which the person exists.

ERIC: The Educational Resource Information Center is a national information system supported by the US Department of Education, the National Library of Education, and the Office of Educational Research and Improvement. It provides access to information from journals included in the *Current Index of Journals in Education* and *Resources in Education Index*.

Ethic of care: Personal relationships and relationship responsibilities are emphasized in this ethic. Important concepts in this approach are compassion, empathy, sympathy, concern for others, and caring for others.

Ethical dilemma: An ethical dilemma is a situation in which an individual is compelled to make a choice between two actions that will affect the well-being of a sentient being and both actions can be reasonably justified as being good, neither action is readily justifiable as good, or the goodness of the actions is uncertain. One action must be chosen, thereby generating a quandary for the person or group who must make the choice.

Ethical principlism: A popular approach to ethics in health care, involves using a set of ethical principles that are drawn from the common or widely shared conception of morality. The four principles that are most commonly used in bioethics are autonomy, beneficence, nonmaleficence, and justice.

Ethics: The study of ideal human behavior and ideal ways of being. The approaches to ethics and the meanings of ethically related concepts have varied over time among philosophers and ethicists. As a philosophical discipline of study, ethics is a systematic approach to understanding, analyzing, and distinguishing matters of right and wrong, good and bad, and admirable and deplorable as they exist along a continuum and as they relate to the well-being of and the relationships among sentient beings.

Evidence-based practice: Allows nurses to provide high-quality patient care based upon research evidence and knowledge rather than tradition, myths, hunches, advice from peers, outdated textbooks, or even what the nurse learned in school 5, 10, or 15 years ago.

Expert: Benner's final stage, expert, has moved beyond a fixed set of rules. There is an internalized understanding grounded in a wealth of experience as well as depth of knowledge. The expert is always learning and always questioning using subjective and objective knowing.

Expert witness: Someone who has complex knowledge beyond the general knowledge of most people in the court or on the jury.

Feedback: Information that we receive from others about the impact of our behavior on them; it allows us to view ourselves from another's perspective.

Frontier Nursing Service: The first organized midwifery service in the United States was the Frontier Nursing Service. It served isolated Appalachian communities on horseback until WWII.

Functional nursing: In the functional nursing system, client needs are divided into tasks, and each task is assigned to RNs, LPNs, or UAPs. This system is advantageous because each assigned caregiver becomes highly efficient in performing the assigned tasks.

Futile care: When a treatment has no physiologic benefit for a terminally ill person.

Gap between education and practice: Looms larger as the healthcare setting continually changes as a result of advanced technology, knowledge explosion, shorter hospital stays, and rapid changes in disease management.

Global aging: In the post-WWII era, fertility rates have increased as death rates decreased in both developed and developing countries, leading to the aging of the global population at an unprecedented rate.

Goldmark Report: A significant report, known simply as *The Goldmark Report, Nursing and Nursing Education in the United States,* was released in 1922 and advocated the establishment of university schools of nursing to train nursing leaders.

Goodrich, Annie: First dean of the Army School of Nursing.

Greek era: The periods of Greek history in classical antiquity, lasting ca. 750 BC (the archaic period) to 146 BC (the Roman conquest). It is generally considered to be the seminal culture that provided the foundation of Western civilization. Time of Hippocrates, father of medicine. In Greek society, health was considered to result from a balance between mind and body.

Group discussions: Group discussions can assist nursing students in connecting clinical events or decisions with information obtained in the classroom. This form of cooperative learning occurs when groups work together to maximize their own and each other's learning.

Health: One of the four concepts of the metaparadigm of nursing; the health–illness continuum within which the person falls at the time of the interaction with the nurse.

Health Belief Model: This model was originally developed to predict the likelihood of a person following a recommended action and to understand the person's motivation and decision making regarding seeking health services.

Health literacy: The ability to read, understand, and act on health information.

Health Source: The Nursing/Academic Edition provides more than 550 scholarly full-text journals, including more than 450 peer-reviewed journals focusing on many medical disciplines, including nursing and allied health.

Healthcare delivery system: The healthcare delivery system has changed profoundly over the past several decades for several reasons. Population shifts (demographic changes), cultural diversity, the patterns of diseases, advances in technology, and economic changes have all impacted the delivery of health care.

Henry Street Settlement: The Henry Street Settlement was an independent nursing service where Wald lived and worked. This later became the Visiting Nurse Association of New York City, which laid the foundation for the establishment of public health nursing in the United States.

HIPAA: The Health Insurance Portability and Accountability Act (HIPAA) was enacted by the U.S. Congress in 1996. It was intended to improve the efficiency and effectiveness of the healthcare system by encouraging the development of a health information system. Several areas are addressed by the act, including simplifying healthcare claims, developing standards for data transmission, and implementing privacy regulations.

Holistic care: Holistic care is a philosophical approach that emphasizes the uniqueness of the individual, in which interacting wholes are more important than the sum of each part. That is, the whole person is greater than merely each component part of the client: their biophysical, psychological, social, and spiritual parts.

Idealism: Idealism contains these assumptions: The world is evolving. There is more than meets the eye. The social world is created. Reality is a conception perceived in the mind. Thinking is dynamic and constructive.

Informed consent: Mandates to the physician or independent healthcare practitioner the separate legal duty to disclose needed material facts in terms that patients can reasonably understand so that they can make an informed choice. Meaningful information must be disclosed even if the clinician does not believe that the information will be beneficial.

Integrity: Maintaining integrity involves acting consistently with personal values and the values of the profession. In a healthcare system often burdened with constraints and self-serving groups and organizations, threats to integrity can be a serious pitfall for nurses.

Interdisciplinary healthcare team: The interdisciplinary healthcare team can be especially effective in outpatient services. Here, the physician or nurse practitioner sees the client, and consultations are put into practice as needed. The teams deal with client-related problems and help the patients progress through the clinic and hospital efficiently.

Iowa Model of Evidence-Based Practice: Resembles a decision-making tree that identifies either problem-focused or knowledge-focused triggers that initiate the process in the organization.

Jenner, Edward: In Britain, Edward Jenner discovered an effective method of vaccination against the dreaded smallpox virus in 1798.

Journaling: The process by which one sits down quietly on a daily or regular basis to think and record one's thoughts and ideas in writing. Keeping a journal of clinical experiences that were meaningful or troubling to you is a recommended way to help enhance and develop reasoning skills.

Justice: The fair distribution of benefits and burdens. In regard to principlism, justice most often refers to the distribution of scarce healthcare resources.

Klebs, Edwin: Edwin Klebs (1834–1913) proved the germ theory, that is, that germs are the causes of infectious diseases. This discovery of the bacterial origin of diseases may be considered the greatest achievement of the 1800s.

Koch, Robert: Robert Koch (1843–1910), a physician known for his research in anthrax, is regarded as the father of microbiology. By identifying the organism that caused cholera, *Vibrio cholerae*, he also demonstrated its transmission by water, food, and clothing.

Learning domains: Identification of the learning domain reflects the type of learning desired as a result of the patient education process. Learning occurs in three domains: the cognitive, the psychomotor, and the affective.

Licensure: The granting of permission to perform professional actions that may not be legally performed by persons who do not have this permission.

Life management: Entails determining what is truly important to you and making positive choices about how, where, and with whom you spend your precious hours.

Lifelong learning: A professional and personal approach that embraces opportunities to increase one's understanding and skills throughout one's career and life.

Lister, Joseph: Joseph Lister (1827–1912) was a physician who set out to decrease the mortality resulting from infection after surgery. He used Pasteur's research to eventually arrive at a chemical antiseptic solution of carbolic acid for use in surgery. Widely regarded as the father of modern surgery, he practiced his antiseptic surgery with great results, and the Listerian principles of asepsis changed the way physicians and nurses practice to this day.

Listserv: A form of group e-mail that provides an opportunity for people with similar interests to share information.

Living will: A formal legal document that provides written directions concerning medical care that is to be provided in specific circumstances.

Lobbyist: Lobbyists develop expertise on proposed legislation and learn to present to legislators that information clearly and concisely.

Malpractice: The failure of a professional to use such care as a reasonably prudent member of the profession would use under similar circumstances, which leads to harm.

Managed care: Managed care is a market approach based on managed competition as a major strategy to contain healthcare costs and is still the dominant approach today.

Manager: All nurses are managers. They direct the work of professionals and nonprofessionals in order to achieve expected outcomes of care.

Medical directive: A medical directive is not a formal legal document but provides specific written instructions concerning the type of care and treatments that individuals want to receive if they become incapacitated.

MEDLINE: The largest biomedical literature database that provides authoritative medical information on medicine, nursing, dentistry, veterinary medicine, the healthcare system, and preclinical sciences.

Mental health: A level of cognitive or emotional well-being. The definition of mental health is affected by cultural differences, subjective assessments, and competing professional theories. As professional nurses experience the stresses that come with today's healthcare environment, they are obliged to assess their own mental health needs.

Mentoring: A developmental, empowering, and nurturing relationship that extends over time and in which mutual sharing, learning, and growth occur in an atmosphere of respect, collegiality, and affirmation.

Metaparadigm: A metaparadigm is the most global perspective of a discipline and acts as an encapsulating unit, or framework, within which the more restricted structures develop.

Mind mapping: The technique of arranging ideas and their interconnections visually; a popular brainstorming technique. It is used to generate, visualize, structure, and classify ideas and is used as an aid in organization, problem solving, and decision making.

Mission statement: A clear, concise statement of who you are and what you are about in life. It can be a powerful tool for helping you find meaning and give direction to your life.

Models of patient care: Nurses are leaders and managers within various models of patient care delivery. The methods might differ significantly from one organization to another. The purpose of a nursing care delivery system is to provide a framework for nurses to deliver care to a specific group of patients.

Moral reasoning: Pertains to making decisions about how humans ought to be and act.

Moral right: The right to perform certain activities (a) because they conform to the accepted standards or ideas of a community (or of a law, or of God, or of conscience); or (b) because they will not harm, coerce, restrain, or infringe on the interests of others; or (c) because there are good rational arguments in support of the value of such activities.

Moral suffering: Moral suffering can be experienced when nurses attempt to sort out their emotions when they find themselves in situations that are morally unsatisfactory or when forces beyond their control prevent them from influencing or changing these perceived unsatisfactory moral situations. Suffering may occur because nurses believe that situations must be changed in order to bring well-being to themselves and others or to alleviate the suffering of themselves and others.

Morals: Specific beliefs, behaviors, and ways of being based on personal judgments derived from one's ethics. One's morals are judged to be good or bad through systematic ethical analysis.

Multiculturalism: There is diversity among the members of the nursing profession in race, age, and socioeconomic backgrounds. However, the presence of this multiculturalism force can lead to people feeling threatened, especially if the culture within the profession does not encourage mutual respect and acceptance.

National Guideline Clearinghouse: Includes structured summaries containing information about each guideline, including comparisons of guidelines covering similar topics that show areas of similarity and differences; full text or links to full text; ordering details for full guidelines; annotated bibliographies on guideline development, evaluation, implementation, and structure; weekly e-mail updates; and guideline archives.

Negligence: Negligence is defined as the failure to act as a reasonably prudent person would have acted in a specific situation.

Networking: The process by which you get to know people within your organization and within your profession.

Nightingale, Florence: Nightingale was identified as a true "angel of mercy," having reformed military health care in the Crimean War and having used her political savvy to forever change the way society views the health of the vulnerable, the poor, and the forgotten. She is perhaps one of the most written about women in history.

Nonmaleficence: The injunction to "do no harm" is often paired with beneficence, but a difference exists between the two principles. Beneficence requires taking action to benefit others, whereas nonmaleficence involves refraining from action that might harm others.

Nonvoluntary euthanasia: Occurs when persons are not able to express their decision about death.

Novice: Benner's model identifies the stages of novice, advanced beginner, competent, proficient, and expert that are based on the nurse's experience in practice. The first stage, novice, is characterized by a lack of knowledge and experience. In this stage, the facts, rules, and guidelines for practice are the focus. Rules for practice are context free, and the student task is to acquire the knowledge and skills.

Nurse-managed centers: Also called nursing clinics and nurse practice arrangements, these healthcare delivery options are meeting needs in communities across the country. Based on the philosophy of primary care and education, nurses are offering vital services at a lower cost.

Nursing: (1) Attention to the full range of human experiences and responses to health and illness without restriction to a problem-focused orientation; (2) integration of objective data with an understanding of the subjective experience of the patient; (3) application of scientific knowledge to the processes of diagnosis and treatment; (4) provision of a caring relationship that facilitates health and healing; and (5) one of the four concepts of the metaparadigm of nursing; the nursing actions themselves.

Nursing ethics: Nursing ethics is sometimes viewed as a subcategory of the broader domain of bioethics, just as medical ethics is a subcategory of bioethics. However, controversy continues about whether nursing has unique moral problems in professional practice.

Nursing faculty shortage: This shortage is limiting student capacity in nursing programs across the nation.

Nursing informatics: The synthesis of computer science, information science, and nursing science in the organization and comprehension of data that directs nursing practice.

Nursing process: The nursing process is the tool by which all nurses can become equally proficient at critical thinking. The nursing process contains the following criteria: (1) assessment, (2) diagnosis, (3) planning, (4) implementation, and (5) evaluation.

Nursing shortage: Due to the growing complexity of health care, limited educational opportunities for nursing students, the aging of the population, and the overall growth of the population, a shortage of registered nurses has occurred and will continue to worsen. The current nursing shortage began in the year 2000 when there was an estimated supply of 1.89 million nurses and with a projected demand of 2 million, or 6%.

Nursing's Agenda for Health Care Reform: A demand for healthcare reform in the late 1980s. The nursing profession heralded the way in healthcare reform with an unprecedented collaboration of more than 75 nursing associations, led by the American Nurses Association and the National League for Nursing, in the publication of *Nursing's Agenda for Health Care Reform.*

Objectives: Specific measures that you will take to achieve your goal. Objectives should be specific and measurable, serving as milestones that mark your progress.

Osborne, Mary D.: Supervisor of public health nursing for the state of Mississippi from 1921 to 1946, Osborne had a vision for a collaboration with community nurses and granny midwives, who delivered 80% of the African-American babies in Mississippi.

Palliative care: Providing comfort rather than curative measures for terminally ill patients.

Paradigm: A paradigm is the lens through which you see the world. Paradigms are also philosophical foundations that support our approaches to research.

Passive euthanasia: Passive euthanasia means that a person allows another person to die by not acting to stop death or prolong life. An example of this type of euthanasia may include withholding treatment that is necessary to prevent death at a point in time.

Pasteur, Louis: A French chemist, Pasteur first became interested in pathogenic organisms through his studies of the diseases of wine. He discovered if wine was heated to a temperature of 55°C to 60°C, the process killed the microorganisms that spoiled wine. This discovery was critical to the wine industry's success in France. This process of pasteurization led Pasteur to investigate many fields and save many lives from contaminated milk and food.

Paternalism: Nurses may decide to act in ways that they believe are for a patient's "own good" rather than allowing patients to exercise their autonomy. The deliberate overriding of a patient's autonomy in this way is called paternalism.

Patient education: Any set of planned, educational activities designed to improve patients' health behaviors, health status, or both.

Patient Self-Determination Act: Legislation designed to facilitate the knowledge and use of advance directives.

Patient teaching: Activities aimed at improving knowledge are known as patient teaching.

PDA: Personal digital assistants (PDAs) are handheld devices that have wireless connectivity and can synchronize data and information between the PDA and a computer. Use of the PDA is becoming widely popular in health care and nursing.

Performance improvement: Collaboration and evidence-based practice are key elements of successful quality programs, or performance improvement programs.

Person: One of the four concepts of the metaparadigm of nursing; the person receiving the nursing.

Personal dignity: Often mistakenly equated with autonomy; judging others and describing behaviors as dignified or undignified are of an evaluative nature.

Philosophy: Philosophy is the discipline concerned with questions of how one should live; what sorts of things exist and what are their essential natures; what counts as genuine knowledge; and what are the correct principles of reasoning. Philosophies set forth the general meaning of nursing and nursing phenomena through reasoning and the logical presentation of ideas. Philosophies are broad and address general ideas about nursing. Because of its breadth, nursing philosophy contributes to the discipline by providing direction, clarifying values, and forming a foundation for theory development.

Physician-assisted suicide: According to Oregon's Death with Dignity Act, "lethal medications, expressly prescribed by a physician for that purpose."

PICO: PICO is an acronym that assists in the formatting of clinical questions: P = Patient, Population, or Problem; I =Intervention or Exposure or Topic of Interest; C = Comparison or Alternate Intervention (if appropriate); O = Outcome. Using this format helps the nurse to ask pertinent clinical questions, focus on asking the right questions, and choose relevant guidelines.

Primary nursing care: The primary nursing care model of delivery was developed in the 1960s after team nursing first became popular and was designed to put the nurse back at the bedside. Primary nursing allows the nurse to provide care to a small number of clients for their entire stay. The nurse provides and is accountable for care, communicates with clients and their families and other healthcare providers, and performs discharge planning. The actual care is given by the primary RN or associate nurses (other RNs).

Privacy: The right of a person to be free from unwanted intrusion into the person's personal affairs.

Professional values: Professional values are beliefs or ideals that guide interactions with patients, colleagues, other professionals, and the public.

Proficient: Benner's stage 4 refers to the professional who is able to grasp the situation contextually and as a whole. Such nurses have a solid grasp of the norms as well as solid experiences that shed light on the variations from the norm. Incorporated into practice is the ability to test knowledge against situations that might not fit and to solve problems with alternative approaches.

Propositions: Propositions are statements that describe relationships between events, situations, or actions.

PsycINFO: Contains nearly 2 million citations and summaries of journal articles, book chapters, books, dissertations, and technical reports, all in the field of psychology.

Public speaking: By being a spokesperson for the organization a nurse can increase his or her visibility dramatically. This a daunting task for many nurses who are otherwise fearless in their other professional activities.

Pure autonomy standard: Decisions made on behalf of an incompetent person based on decisions that the formerly competent person made.

Quality improvement: Quality improvement focuses on systems, processes, satisfaction, and cost outcomes, usually within a specific organization.

Rathbone, William: William Rathbone, a wealthy ship owner and philanthropist, is credited with the establishment of the first visiting nurse service, which eventually evolved into district nursing in the community. He was so impressed with the private duty nursing care that his sick wife had received at home that he set out to develop a "district nursing service" in Liverpool, England.

Rational suicide: Rational suicide is a self-slaying and is categorized as voluntary active euthanasia.

Readiness to learn: Patient's readiness or evidence of motivation to receive information at that particular time.

Realism: Realism contains these assumptions: The world is static. Seeing is believing. The social world is a given. Reality is physical and independent. Logical thinking is superior.

Referral: The practice of sending a patient to another practitioner for consultation or service.

Reformation: Religious changes during the Renaissance were to influence nursing perhaps more than any other aspect of society. During the Reformation, the monasteries were abolished. The effects on nursing were drastic: monastic-affiliated institutions, including hospitals and schools, were closed, and orders of nuns, including nurses, were dissolved.

Research utilization: Research utilization involves critical analysis and evaluation of research findings and then determining how these findings fit into clinical practice.

Respondeat superior: The doctrine that indicates the employer may also be responsible if the nurse was functioning in the employee role at the time of the incident.

Robb, Isabel Hampton: In 1896 she founded the Nurses' Associated Alumnae, which in 1911 officially became known as the American Nurses Association (ANA).

Role of the professional nurse: The role of the professional nurse has expanded in response to changing populations and the philosophical shift toward health promotion rather than illness cure. The list could be exhaustive, but roles of nurses include caregiver, advocate, educator, leader, manager, and researcher.

Roman era: The periods of Roman history in classical antiquity, lasting ca. 146 BC (the Roman conquest of Greece) or 31 BC (defeat of Mark Antony by Augustus at the Battle of Actium) to ca. AD 476 (fall of the Roman Empire). Roman civilization is often grouped into classical antiquity with ancient Greece, a civilization that inspired much of the culture of ancient Rome. The development of policy, law, and protection of the public's health was an important precursor to our modern public health systems.

Rule of double effect: Usually defined narrowly in health care as the use of high doses of pain medication to lessen the chronic and intractable pain of terminally ill patients even if doing so hastens death.

Saint Vincent de Paul: In 1633, Saint Vincent de Paul founded the Sisters of Charity in France, an order of nuns who traveled from home to home visiting the sick.

Sanger, Margaret: Margaret Sanger worked as a nurse on the Lower East Side of New York City in 1912 with immigrant families. She was astonished to find widespread ignorance among these families about conception, pregnancy, and childbirth. After a horrifying experience with the death of a woman from a failed self-induced abortion, Sanger devoted her life to teaching women about birth control. A staunch activist in the early family planning movement, Sanger is credited with founding Planned Parenthood of America.

Scales, Jessie Sleet: Scales is considered the first African-American public health nurse. Scales provided district nursing care to New York City's African-American families and is credited with paving the way for African-American nurses in the practice of community health.

Search engine: Search engines assist in finding specific topics on the Web by compiling a database of Internet sites.

Self-care: Acknowledging and meeting your own physical, psychological, social, and spiritual needs. It means caring for yourself *before* you care for others, not after you have tended to everyone else.

Self-efficacy: A person believes that he or she is capable of performing a behavior.

Shattuck Report: Lemuel Shattuck, a Boston bookseller and publisher who had an interest in public health, organized the American Statistical Society in 1839 and issued a census of Boston in 1845. Shattuck's census revealed high infant mortality rates and high overall population mortality rates. In his *Report of the Massachusetts Sanitary Commission in 1850*, Shattuck not only outlined his findings on the unsanitary conditions but made recommendations for public health reform. He also called for services for well-child care, school-age children's health, immunizations, mental health, health education for all, and health planning. The report was revolutionary in its scope and vision for public health.

Snow, John: John Snow, a prominent physician, is credited with being the first epidemiologist by demonstrating in 1854 that cholera rates were linked with water pump use in London.

Social justice: A virtue that guides us in creating those organized human interactions we call institutions. In turn, social institutions, when justly organized, provide us with access to what is good for the person, both individually and in our associations with others. Social justice also imposes on each of us a personal responsibility to work with others to design and continually perfect our institutions as tools for personal and social development.

Social learning theory: If a person believes that he or she is capable of performing a behavior (self-efficacy) and also believes that the behavior will lead to a desirable outcome, the person will be more likely to perform the behavior.

Socialization: Professional socialization involves a process by which a person acquires the knowledge, skills, and sense of identity that are characteristic of a profession.

Statutory law: Consists of ever-changing rules and regulations created by the United States Congress, state legislators, local governments, and constitutional law. The statutes are the rights, privileges, or immunities secured and protected for each citizen by the US Constitution.

Stereotypes: A standardized mental picture that is held in common by members of a group and that represents an oversimplified opinion, prejudiced attitude, or uncritical judgment. For example, Nightingale defined nursing as "female work." Nurses need to face the stereotypes present in our society and erase the lines that define us.

Substituted judgment standard: Used to guide medical decisions that involve formerly competent patients who no longer have any decision-making capacity.

Success: Success in life can be defined as doing what you want, where you want, and with the people you want to do it with. This implies balance within the various arenas of your life: professional, personal, social, and spiritual.

Team nursing: The team nursing model of care is used in the United States most frequently in hospitals and in long-term and extended-care facilities. This arrangement evolved after the functional nursing of the 1940s. With this approach, the nursing staff is divided into teams, and total patient care is provided to a group of patients.

Telehealth: Using electronic communication for transmitting healthcare information such as health promotion, disease prevention, professional or lay education, diagnosis, or actual treatments to people located at a different geographical location.

Terminal sedation: When a suffering patient is sedated to unconsciousness, usually through the ongoing administration of barbiturates or benzodiazepines. The patient then dies of dehydration, starvation, or some other intervening complication, as all other life-sustaining interventions are withheld.

Theory: A theory is an organized, coherent, and systematic articulation of a set of statements related to significant questions in a discipline that are communicated in a meaningful whole.

Tort: Refers to acts that result in harm to another.

Total patient care: As early as the 1920s, the first model of patient care delivery was total patient care. In this model, the RN has the responsibility for all aspects of care of the patient(s). The RN works directly with the client, other nursing staff, and physician in implementing a plan of care. The objective of total patient care is to have one nurse provide all care to the same patient(s) for the entire shift. Currently this model is practiced in areas such as critical care units or postanesthesia recovery units, where a high level of expertise is required.

Tyler, Elizabeth: Lillian Wald hired African-American nurse Elizabeth Tyler in 1906 as evidence of her commitment to cultural diversity. Although unable to visit white clients, Tyler made her own way by "finding" African-American families who needed her service.

Unavoidable trust: Zaner's contention that patients, in most cases, have no option but to trust nurses and other healthcare professionals when the patient is at the point of needing care.

Utilitarianism: Contrasted with deontology, the ethical approach of utilitarianism is to promote the greatest good that is possible in situations (i.e., the greatest good for the greatest number).

Values: Refer to a group's or individual's evaluative judgments about what is good or what makes something desirable. Values refer to what the normative standard should be, not necessarily to how things actually are. Values are the principles and ideals that give meaning and direction to our social, personal, and professional life. Professional values are integral to moral reasoning. Values in nursing encompass appreciating what is important for both the profession and nurses personally, as well as what is important for patients.

Values clarification: The process of values clarification can occur in a group or individually and helps us understand who we are and what is most important to us. The outcome of values clarification is positive because the outcome is growth.

Violence: The exertion of physical force so as to injure or abuse. Objectives toward the prevention of violence and abuse are included in *Healthy People 2010*.

Virtues: *Arête* in Greek; refer to excellences of intellect or character.

Voluntary euthanasia: Voluntary euthanasia occurs when persons with a sound mind authorize another person to take their life or to assist them in achieving death. Also, this type may include the taking of one's own life.

Wald, Lillian: A wealthy young woman with a great social conscience, Wald graduated from the New York Hospital School of Nursing in 1891 and is credited with creating the title "public health nurse."

Wholeness of character: Pertains to knowing the values of the nursing profession and one's own authentic moral values, integrating these two belief systems, and expressing them appropriately. Integrity is an important feature of wholeness of character.

Index